GERIATRIC
CARE PLANS

DIANE KASCHAK NEWMAN, RN, MSN, CRNP
DIANE A. JAKOVAC SMITH, RN, MSN, CRNP

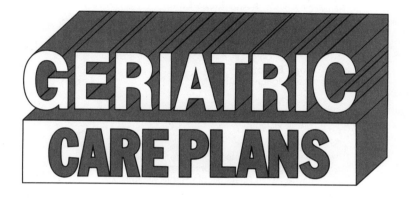

DIANE KASCHAK NEWMAN, RN, MSN, CRNP
DIANE A. JAKOVAC SMITH, RN, MSN, CRNP

Springhouse Corporation
Springhouse, Pennsylvania

Staff

Executive Director, Editorial
Stanley Loeb

Director of Trade and Textbooks
Minnie B. Rose, RN, BSN, MEd

Art Director
John Hubbard

Associate Acquisitions Editor
Bernadette M. Glenn

Editors
Diane Labus, David Moreau, Gale Sloan

Copy Editor
Mary Hohenhaus Hardy

Designers
Stephanie Peters (associate art director),
StellarVisions

Typography
David Kosten (director), Diane Paluba
(manager), Elizabeth Bergman,
Joyce Rossi Biletz, Robin Rantz, Valerie
Rosenberger

Manufacturing
Deborah Meiris (manager), T.A. Landis,
Jennifer Suter

Production Coordination
Aline S. Miller (manager), Laurie Sander

Library of Congress Cataloging-in-Publication Data

Newman, Diane Kaschak.
  Geriatric care plans/Diane Kaschak Newman,
Diane A. Smith.
    p.   cm.
  Includes bibliographical references.
  Includes index.
  1. Geriatric nursing. 2. Nursing care plans. I. Title.
  [DNLM: 1. Geriatric Nursing. 2. Nursing
Assessment. 3. Patient Care Planning. WY 152
N552g]
RC954.N39 1991
610.73′65—dc20
DNLM/DLC   90-9856
ISBN 0-87434-263-5   CIP

Contents

Acknowledgments

The authors would like to thank their company, Golden Horizons, Inc., for providing the opportunity and time to complete this book.

Special thanks to Mary Frances Szpila for her secretarial expertise and time.

DEDICATION

In memory of our parents, Amelia Dzurinko and Amelia and Jacob Jakovac, who were never given the chance to grow old

To Michael, for his never-ending love and support; Carolyn Beth and Michelle Amelia, for all those missed hours; and my father, John Dzurinko, who has shown me the intricacies of aging

DKN

To David, with whom I will grow old, and Jacklyn and Rebecca, my inspirations for the future

DAJS

Consultants and Contributors

Consultants

Ann L. Cupp Curley, RN, MSN
Department of Education and Practice
New Jersey State Nurses Association
Trenton, N.J.

Mary Snyder Knapp, MSN, CRNP, NHA
Vice-President
John Whitman & Associates
Geriatric Healthcare Consultants
Philadelphia

Deanna Gray Miceli, RN,C, MSN
Geriatric Nurse Practitioner
University of Medicine and Dentistry of
    New Jersey
School of Osteopathic Medicine
Stratford, N.J.

Rosemary Carol Polomano, RN, MSN, CS
Oncology and Pain Clinical Specialist
Hospital of the University of Pennsylvania
Philadelphia

Contributors

Diane Kaschak Newman, RN, MSN, CRNP
Nurse Practitioner and Vice-President
Golden Horizons, Inc.
Newtown Square, Pa.
Director of Clinical Services
Continence Management Specialists, Inc.
Hightstown, N.J.
(Assessment; Clinical Care Plans; General Care Plans)

Diane A. Jakovac Smith, RN, MSN, CRNP
Nurse Practitioner and President
Golden Horizons, Inc.
Newtown Square, Pa.
Director of Research
Continence Management Specialists, Inc.
Hightstown, N.J.
(Assessment; Clinical Care Plans; General Care Plans)

Barbara L. Brush, RN,C, MSN
Clinical Lecturer and Nurse Practitioner
University of Pennsylvania School of
    Nursing
Philadelphia
(Benign Prostatic Hypertrophy and
    Prostate Cancer)

Regina L. Burdette, MS, CCC-SLP
Speech-Language Pathologist
Rehabilitation Institute of Sarasota
Sarasota, Fla.
(Dysphagia)

Linda G. Canonica, RN, MSN, GNP
Former Coordinator of Long-Term Care
University of Medicine and Dentistry of
    New Jersey
School of Osteopathic Medicine
Stratford, N.J.
(Angina Pectoris; Transient Ischemic
    Attack)

Elizabeth Capezuti, RN,C, MSN
Project Director
Restraint Reduction Project
University of Pennsylvania School of
    Nursing
Philadelphia
Program Director
Elder Mistreatment Program
University of Dentistry and Medicine of
    New Jersey
Stratford, N.J.
(Elder Abuse)

Elizabeth B. Chapman, RN, MSN, CRNP
Program Manager
Incontinence Treatment Center
Presbyterian Medical Center
Philadelphia
(History Taking in the Older Client;
    Delirium)

Valerie Telford Cotter, RN, MSN
Geriatric Nurse Practitioner in Joint Appointment with University of Pennsylvania School of Nursing and University of Medicine and Dentistry of New Jersey
Stratford, N.J.
(Pneumonia; Chronic Obstructive Pulmonary Disease; Influenza)

Ann L. Cupp Curley, RN, MSN
Department of Education and Practice
New Jersey State Nurses Association
Trenton, N.J .
(Skin Cancer; Pruritus and Xerosis; Bunions, Calluses, and Corns; Psoriasis)

Bonnie Doren, PhD
Professional Writing Consultant
In-Home Geriatric Case Management, Inc.
Eugene, Ore.
(Chronic Pain)

Cynthia Lee Dzurinko, RN
Emergency Nurse
Homewood Hospital Center South
Johns Hopkins Health Care System
Baltimore
(Congestive Heart Failure)

William F. Edwards, MSN, CRNP
Gerontologic Nurse Practitioner and Director of the Department of Geriatrics
The Good Samaritan Hospital
Pottsville, Pa.
(Parkinson's Disease)

Carol Lyn Gerhard, RN, MSN, CRNP
Faculty
Department of Nursing
Community College of Philadelphia
(Hypothermia)

Gail L. Goetz, RN,C, MSN, CRRN
Nurse Practitioner
McGee Rehabilitation Hospital
Philadelphia
(Aphasia)

Margaret T. Goldberg, RN, BSN, CETN
Enterostomal Therapist
Crozer-Chester Medical Center
Chester, Pa.
(Pressure Sores)

Janice M. Haddad, RN, CS, MSN, CDE
Diabetes Program Coordinator
Diabetes Center of New Jersey
Muhlenberg Regional Medical Center
Muhlenburg, N.J.
(Diabetes Mellitus)

Wendy A. Halbert, RN, MSN
Family and Gerontologic Nurse Practitioner and Clinic Coordinator
UroClinic
Sarasota, Fla.
(Hiatal Hernia; Dysphagia)

Mary Snyder Knapp, MSN, CRNP, NHA
Vice-President
John Whitman & Associates
Geriatric Healthcare Consultants
Philadelphia
(Sexual Dysfunction; Falls; Osteoarthritis and Rheumatoid Arthritis; Gout; Cerebrovascular Accident; Sensory Deprivation; Disruptive Behavior; Insomnia and Sleep Anea)

Rebecca Sload McCarron, RN, MSN
Homecare Coordinator
Skilled Nursing Homecare, Inc.
Liaison
University of Pennsylvania Homecare Hospice Program
Philadephia

Deanna Gray Miceli, RN,C, MSN
Geriatric Nurse Practitioner
University of Medicine and Dentistry of New Jersey
School of Osteopathic Medicine
Stratford, N.J.
(Physical Examination of the Older Client; History Taking in the Older Client; Diabetes Mellitus)

Shirley Morgan, RN, MSN, CS, CNOR
Operating Room Staff Development Instructor
Fox Chase Cancer Center
Philadelphia
(Surgical Care)

Rosemary Carol Polomano, RN, MSN, CS
Oncology and Pain Clinical Specialist
Hospital of the University of Pennsylvania
Philadelphia
(Chronic Pain; Cancer)

Molly A. Rose, RN, PhD, CRNP
Assistant Professor
LaSalle University
Philadelphia
(Malnutrition; Dehydration)

Elizabeth von Wellsheim, MSN, MA, GNP
President
In-Home Geriatric Case Management, Inc.
Eugene, Ore.
(Chronic Pain)

Christine K. Wanich, RN,C, MSN
Geriatric Nurse Practitioner
Director of Continence Program
The Ralston-Penn Center
Philadelphia
(Tuberculosis)

Meta M. Wisinger, RN,C, MSN
Clinical Nurse Specialist
Veterans Administration Medical Center
Lake City, Fla.
(Dehydration)

Preface

The number of Americans over age 65 has increased dramatically over the last 50 years, now totaling about 26 million, or 12% of the U.S. population; by 2030, demographers expect this figure to double. Consequently, older adults, particularly those over age 85, are now the fastest growing population segment in the United States.

Corresponding with the increased number of older adults is the growing number of elderly clients seeking health care treatment. Because of the various physiologic and psychosocial changes that accompany aging, these clients typically require highly specialized care. Despite this need, many nurses and other health care professionals know little about geriatric care and have difficulty coping with the complex problems and needs of this age-group.

Geriatric Care Plans, written for practicing nurses, nursing students, and nurse educators, will be especially useful for those who care for elderly clients in acute care hospitals, outpatient clinics, extended care facilities, and home care settings. It contains numerous nursing care plans that focus on the most common diseases, disorders, and problems affecting the geriatric population and includes specific sections on assessment, clinical care plans, and general care plans.

Section I, Assessment, provides a thorough review of the steps involved in obtaining a detailed health history and performing a comprehensive physical examination. Accurate health information and an assessment of the client's functional abilities enable the nurse to determine the client's current health status and need for supportive services. Section I stresses the importance of considering age-related changes when performing an assessment or conducting a physical examination.

Section II, Clinical Care Plans, contains a series of nursing care plans on the most common diseases, disorders, and problems of elderly clients. Categorized according to body system, these plans provide concise, accurate information on the medical and nursing aspects of the presenting problem. Each plan includes a definition of the disease or disorder, etiologic and precipitating factors, health history findings, physical findings, pertinent diagnostic studies, potential complications, relevant nursing diagnoses, and appropriate nursing actions.

Each of the nursing diagnoses, approved by the North American Nursing Diagnosis Association (NANDA), contains specific nursing goals; a list of related signs and symptoms; detailed dependent and interdependent interventions with corresponding rationales; and client outcome criteria.

Section III, General Care Plans, contains a series of care plans on age-related problems common to elderly clients. Although unrelated to specific body systems, these care plans follow the format established in Section II and include specific information on such problems as cancer, surgical care, chronic pain, and elder abuse.

As the number of elderly clients entering the health care system continues to increase, so will the need for current, reliable nursing resources to help in planning and administering care. *Geriatric Care Plans,* which can be used by nurses in any health care setting, provides this kind of practical information. Nurses will find it an invaluable reference and indispensable care plan tool.

Diane Kaschak Newman
Diane A. Jakovac Smith

Introduction

According to recent demographic findings, the American population will be overwhelmingly over age 65 within a few decades. Currently, those over age 65 constitute approximately 12% of the U.S. population and their number is increasing at a dramatic rate, growing twice as fast as that of the younger population.

Americans are beginning to understand the serious social, economic, political, and personal implications of an enlarging older population. We have been living in a cultural milieu that has usually celebrated youth over age, cure over care, acute intervention over long-term rehabilitation, and highly specialized technology over nurturing and support. Not surprisingly in such a milieu, the elderly population has been overlooked and neglected in many ways.

U.S. Census Bureau statistics reveal that about one of every seven elderly Americans lives in poverty. Elderly women, the fastest growing segment of our population, are almost twice as likely as elderly men to be poor, and half of all elderly widowed black women live in a state of chronic poverty. Although the general health of Americans is remarkably good, most of those over age 65 have at least one chronic health problem, and three of every four can expect to die of heart disease, cancer, or cerebrovascular accident.

Although the number of hospitalized older adults has remained fairly constant, the rate of nursing home use has almost doubled since the introduction of Medicare and Medicaid in 1965. About one in every four older adults can expect to be placed in a nursing home at some future date, and the chances increase with age.

As the number of elderly adults increases, so do the incidence of chronic illness and the need for health care services. The greatest need for service will continue to be in maintaining elderly clients' functional abilities and independence. The greatest barriers to the delivery of those services, however, will be escalating health care costs, reduced access to care (especially long-term care) in an increasingly fragmented system, and a short supply of nurses who are prepared to practice geriatric nursing.

Of great concern to health practitioners and society at large is nurses' general lack of interest in becoming involved in the care of elderly clients. Currently, only 8% of all active registered nurses work in nursing homes, and only 5% of recent graduates intend to join them. Contributing to the problem are stereotypical images of aging, inadequate salaries, and difficult working conditions.

Efforts are being made, however, to try to attract more nurses to the geriatric field. A small but growing number of innovative educational programs at the undergraduate and graduate level, demonstration projects like the Robert Wood Johnson Foundation Teaching Nursing Home Program, and significant strides in nursing research aimed at clinical problems of older adults may draw more nurses to geriatrics as a career.

One of the most significant and growing areas in geriatric nursing involves the long-term care of elderly clients. As older adults live longer and are more productive, nurses are increasingly needed to help promote and maintain health. Health promotion, which aims to facilitate healthful living and reinforce healthful practices, focuses on ensuring adequate nutrition, weight control, and physical activity and on eliminating physical and psychological stresses. Health maintenance, which aims at the early detection and treatment of diseases and disorders, concentrates on problems commonly encountered by older adults, such as arthritis, sensory deficits, cardiovascular disease, genitourinary conditions, dehydration, inappropriate drug use, and changes in cognitive awareness and mobility.

Because geriatric nursing is growing less rapidly than the elderly population, nurses entering the field can look forward to diverse job opportunities and increasingly responsible and independent roles in care management. For those already involved in geriatric nursing, this is a time of great excitement. Advances in nursing research, knowledge, and practice are fostering an atmosphere of creativity and challenge. Such advances, and the sophisticated decision making required to implement them, should help dispel any notions of geriatric nursing as simplistic, commonplace, or unchallenging. *Geriatric Care Plans,* in keeping with the American Nurses' Association's recently revised "Scope and Standards of Gerontological Nursing Practice," will add considerably to nurses' understanding of the pathophysiologic and psychosocial changes of aging. This reliable and comprehensive book will help nurses distinguish between normal and abnormal clinical findings, evaluate functional status, and devise appropriate interventions for each client's changing health needs.

Geriatric nursing will continue to play a major role in assuring that the elderly client is well cared for in the decades ahead. Although meeting this challenge will not be easy, nurses can do so if they remain informed, knowledgeable, and, above all, caring. *Geriatric Care Plans* provides essential, authoritative information to guide nurses toward that end.

Neville E. Strumpf, RN,C, PhD, FAAN
Associate Professor and Director
Gerontological Nurse Clinician Program
University of Pennsylvania
Philadelphia

SECTION I

ASSESSMENT

History Taking in the Older Client

Collecting an accurate history is an essential part of nursing care. When performed correctly, it allows for early diagnosis of the problem and prompt intervention and enables the client to maintain or return to his previous state of health. At the same time, it provides the client and interviewer with an opportunity to develop a trusting relationship. In the older client, history taking requires special skills and preparation.

PREPARING FOR THE INTERVIEW
Before collecting a history from the older client, the nurse must be aware of how age-related changes can affect vision and hearing and how these changes can interfere with effective communication during history taking.

For example, older clients who squint or exhibit poor eye contact may be experiencing reduced visual acuity or environmentally induced blindness from bright lights, shiny floors, or direct sunlight. Before the history taking session, the nurse should reduce the effects of sun glare by closing the blinds, shielding bright light sources from view. During the interview, she should face the client closely at eye level.

Hearing impairments can be detected during the initial conversation with a client. The older client may have difficulty discriminating fast-paced speech. The nurse may notice that the client seems distracted, unable to follow the conversation, or puzzled by the questions posed.

To compensate for these age-related changes, the nurse should speak slowly and periodically repeat facts during the interview. Ascertaining which is the client's better ear and speaking toward it will help to ensure that the client hears the information being delivered. Speaking in a low voice will help reduce the effects of presbycusis. Background noise can be reduced by closing the door and turning off any radio or television in the room.

GREETING THE CLIENT
Initial contact with the older client should focus on ensuring that the client knows the purpose of the interview and how he can be of assistance during history taking and in establishing a trusting relationship.

An older client should always be addressed as Miss, Mrs., or Mr. and the surname unless he or she requests otherwise. The use of touch is also recommended—for example, shaking the client's hand when saying hello and then holding it briefly—to convey concern.

OBTAINING THE HEALTH HISTORY
Depending on the length of the interview, conducting the health appraisal on two separate occasions may prevent tiring the client. The older client should always

be informed of the time frame for the interview and physical examination and the methods of data collection. Data usually can be gathered directly from the client, from a family member or significant other, through direct observation, or through a combination of these techniques.

A comprehensive nursing assessment of the older client must focus on current health status (including a review of systems [ROS]), past medical history, and ability to function in the environment. This information establishes the client's baseline health status, allowing the nurse to evaluate any progress or decline in his condition over time and to determine the need for support services. Because the client may forget important health information, the nurse must be patient and gather information from significant others, such as family members or friends.

Following the Client Health History form (see pages 6 to 9), the nurse should begin by asking the client his full name, address, age, date of birth, birthplace, and contact persons in case of an emergency.

Although mental status is usually assessed toward the end of the ROS or physical examination, the nurse can assess certain aspects of mental status in a nonthreatening way during general conversation. Typical questions posed in a dementia profile include ability to recall birth date and place and ability to calculate. Asking the client to state his date of birth and then to calculate his age tests for the higher cognitive function of calculation as well as for remote (recall of birth date), recent (recall of current year), and immediate memory (recall of instructions). To avoid a false assessment of the client's ability to calculate, the nurse must first ascertain the client's educational level.

Medical status
The medical record should begin with the reason for admission, or chief complaint, as explained by the client. Each complaint should be evaluated in terms of onset, location, duration, timing, intensity, aggravating or alleviating factors, treatment measures, and impact on the client's life-style. The client's address should be included in this section.

List current medications (including prescription and over-the-counter drugs) and treatments next, including the name of the medication and the dosage. (Elderly clients' use of multiple drugs increases the risk for interactions among drugs and adverse drug reactions.) Examples of treatments to list in this section are pulmonary treatments, wound care and irrigation, catheter management, and pain control.

Next, list any devices that the client uses, such as mobility assistance devices; adaptive aids, such as reacher tongs and special eating utensils; corrective lenses; hearing aids or assistive listening devices; and dentures. Also ask if the patient has any home-safety devices, such as grab rails in the shower or tub and near the toilet, smoke alarms, adequate lighting, and nonskid floor surfaces, and whether carpeting is in good repair.

Begin the psychosocial assessment by asking about the client's use of alcohol and tobacco. Research indicates that the stresses of aging—including bereavement, loneliness, depression, marital stress, and physical illness—lead to or exacerbate drinking problems for 2% to 10% of elderly people. Note the quantity and type of alcoholic beverages consumed—for example, 1 oz of sherry at bedtime or one-fifth of whiskey per week. Document tobacco use in terms of "pack years"—the number of packs smoked per day multiplied by the number of years the client has been smoking. (For example, a person smoking two packs per day for the last 40 years has an 80-pack-year history.) Also list cigar and chewing tobacco use if appropriate. Finally, note whether the client uses barbiturates (sedatives or tranquilizers), a class of drugs commonly used by the older population, and add to the medication list.

Other aspects of the psychosocial history include the client's support systems, participation and satisfaction in community activities, and employment status. Try to determine the answers to the following questions:
• Does the client rely on assistance from family or friends to perform activities of daily living (ADLs)?
• Is a primary caregiver available when required?
• Is the caregiver stressed?
• How often does the client have social contacts?
• What is the client's employment status?
• What are his hobbies?

Also discuss the client's income, listing each income source (such as social security, pension funds, and revenues from stocks and bonds) in dollar amounts per month. Ask the client if his income meets his monthly expenditures for food, rent, household items, clothing, and other bills. A client whose income falls below his monthly expenditures should be referred to social services for possible assistance.

Finally, note the use of community support services (such as nutritional support; free transportation for seniors; adult day care; and home health care services), and ask about current living arrangements. (Does the client live alone or with a spouse, friend, or family member? Does he own a home, rent, or live in a retirement, boarding, or nursing home?)

Medical history

The medical history includes:
• an overview of the client's general state of health
• a history of adult illnesses
• a record of past hospitalization for medical, surgical, or psychiatric purposes
• frequency of physician visits
• current medications and treatments
• reason for current admission (chief complaint).

Before asking specific questions about the medical history, the nurse should ask the client an open-ended question, such as "How would you describe your health over the years?" This can provide specific information about the health history and reveal how the client perceives his health status. The nurse should also try to determine the client's reaction to previous hospitalizations. A client who has had a bad experience may fear readmission to the hospital and, thus, withhold important information.

Ask the client whether he has a history of heart disease or heart attacks; angina; hypertension; transient ischemic attacks or cerebrovascular accident (CVA); arthritis; diabetes; pulmonary disorders, such as emphysema, bronchitis, or asthma; pneumonia or influenza; tuberculosis; asbestos exposure; cancer; ulcers; thyroid disorder or treatment with a thyroid preparation; seizure disorder; prostate problems; renal disease; urinary or fecal incontinence; and falls, trauma, or fracture.

Try to obtain a chronological listing of medical events—for example, "1968 (age 50) developed hypertension; 1975 (age 57) admitted to Memorial Hospital under Dr. Smith's care for myocardial infarction." Because the older client usually has been treated by many physicians, eliciting their names, reasons for treatment, and dates of visits can yield significant information.

REVIEW OF SYSTEMS

Begin with a general overview of the client's health. Ask if he has recently experienced anorexia, unusual fatigue, frequent falls, night sweats, chills or fever, confusion, immobility, forgetfulness, decreased food or fluid intake, or agitation. Frequent falls are a sign of serious illness in elderly persons, often accompanying silent myocardial infarction, cholelithiasis, and generalized infection. Falling is also observed in clients with diabetes, transient ischemic attacks (TIAs), seizure disorders, and osteoarthritis of the hips. (See "Falls," pages 165 to 171.)

Keep in mind that older clients often have an atypical disease presentation—for example, subtle changes in appetite and mental status may be their only symptoms.

After the general overview, begin reviewing specific body areas and systems, using either the head-to-toe method or the major-body-systems method used in this book. Because both methods provide a systematic and organized framework to help you collect assessment data, either method is appropriate, and you can choose the method most comfortable for you.

Integumentary

Ask the client if he has an unhealed sore or mole or an irregularly shaped lesion. Ask him to describe whether his skin feels dry, oily, or normal. Does he experience pruritus, easy bruising, rashes, calluses, or bunions? Rashes may occur more commonly among older clients as side effects of certain medications or secondary to contact allergens. Calluses and bunions can affect ambulation and other ADLs.

Eyes

Ask the client if he is experiencing eye swelling or infection, pain, double vision, blurring, difficulty reading, or loss of vision. Clients with foreign bodies in the eyes will complain of inflammation, discharge, or eye pain. Symptoms of closed-angle glaucoma include eye pain, redness, and sudden vision loss. Eye disorders common among the aged, such as cataracts, macular degeneration, and diabetic retinopathy, present with vision loss. Also ask the client if he uses corrective lenses and when he last had an eye examination.

Ears

Question the client about ear pain, tinnitus, cerumen, ear discharge, and hearing problems. Older clients often have difficulty hearing high-pitched sounds, such as those produced by smoke detectors. The client should be free of any ear pain (otalgia) or discharge (otorrhea). Tinnitus (ringing in the ears) has been observed in older clients without hearing impairment; when no other clinical symptoms are present, this disorder is considered benign. Conductive hearing loss can be attributed to cerumen plugs; unilateral hearing loss should be investigated to rule out acoustic neuroma. In general, older clients are expected to have diminished hearing. Noting which ear is affected helps improve communication and plan for the use of a hearing aid.

Mouth

Note the language the client speaks, and ascertain if he has slurred speech or appears to have difficulty expressing himself or understanding. A client who complains of a change in his speech or an inability to express himself or understand a conversation should be evaluated for possible TIA or CVA.

Ask the client if he is experiencing dry mouth, halitosis, periodontal disease, mouth sores, bleeding, excessive thirst, or a coated tongue, and determine the date of his last dental checkup. A client with diabetes mellitus may present with oral infections and polydipsia (excessive thirst). Any persistent ulcer or lesion must be evaluated (oral carcinoma commonly occurs in older men who smoke). Leukoplakia, a precancerous lesion, appears on the mucous membranes of the mouth, tongue, or lips and can present as a coated tongue. A client who has difficulty chewing should be referred to the dentist and undergo a thorough examination of the teeth. Ill-fitting dentures, caries, or jagged teeth can make eating difficult.

Respiratory

Ask the client if he experiences dyspnea on exertion or when supine. Older clients commonly experience dyspnea on exertion and lung infections, such as bronchitis or pneumonia. To monitor the client's tolerance level, note the distances travelled or the type of exertion that normally produces dyspnea (for example, the client may experience dyspnea after ascending 10 stairs or when carrying two packages of groceries on an incline).

If the client has a cough, ask whether it is productive or nonproductive, and note the color of the sputum (especially if it is bloody). Document complaints of wheezing or pain on breathing. A chronic cough is often observed in clients with heart disease. A persistent productive cough with clear sputum may be observed in smokers; however, yellow or green sputum is abnormal and indicates infection. Hemoptysis is observed in bronchitis, tuberculosis, bronchiectasis, lung abscesses, and lung cancer. Wheezing, an often overlooked symptom in elderly clients, may indicate asthma. Finally, note if chest X-rays are available and whether the cleint has received a pneumococcal or influenza immunization or a purified protein derivative (PPD) test.

Cardiovascular

Ask the client if he has been experiencing any chest pain, pressure, tightness, or heaviness; shortness of breath; light-headedness; palpitations; or numbness in an extremity. Because of the high incidence of cardiovascular disease in elderly persons, always ask about the use of sublingual nitrates. A client complaining of palpitations may be experiencing cardiac dysrhythmias. Light-headedness on sitting or standing may indicate orthostatic hypotension.

Intermittent claudication (pain in the legs induced by exercise and relieved with rest) may indicate an arterial disease of the legs. Claudication must be differentiated from spinal stenosis, a common condition in elderly people that presents with low back pain and radiating leg pains to the calves with forward flexion of the spine. Clients with low back pain that radiates beyond the knees must receive a neurological examination.

Ask about edema, a symptom that is especially important in a client with a history of congestive heart failure. Edema typically occurs bilaterally in the legs or in the most dependent area. Determine whether the client experiences edema all the time or only at the end of the day after prolonged sitting or standing. In the latter instance, edema may indicate chronic venous disease or leg varicosities. Ask the client how his clothing fits around his waist. Abdominal fluid retention may result from worsening congestive heart failure or hepatic failure.

Gastrointestinal

Ask the client if he is experiencing indigestion, nausea, vomiting, or diarrhea. Weight loss, change in bowel habits, rectal bleeding, and melena are key signs of possible GI cancer. Common causes of rectal bleeding in the elderly (in order of least clinical significance) include hemorrhoids, polyps, angiodysplasia, and carcinoma.

Abdominal pain may stem from constipation, diverticulitis, gallstones, or peptic or duodenal ulcer disease.

Diseases of the abdominal cavity present atypically in older clients—for example, diffuse abdominal pain may signify severe fecal impaction. Constipation is a frequent complaint and must be addressed (see "Constipation and Fecal Incontinence," pages 97 to 104). Fecal incontinence is abnormal at any age; in older clients, it is commonly seen with laxative abuse, advanced dementia, CVA, or spinal cord disease. Note the presence of an ostomy or an enteral feeding tube.

Genitourinary

Older men tend to develop prostatic obstruction, which may be manifested by frequent urinary infections, urinary incontinence, dribbling after urination, and a decrease in the size and force of the urine stream.

Urinary tract infection usually presents with complaints of dysuria, increased frequency, incontinence, urgency, burning, or hematuria. Urinary infection can also present atypically as acute confusion. Many cases of infection occur secondary to the use of instrumentation, such as urinary catheters. Urinary incontinence, the most underreported health problem in the United States, should be documented in terms of duration, onset, and frequency. Most older people believe that urinary incontinence results from aging. When questioning a client about incontinence, ask if he uses incontinence pads or experiences enuresis. Common causes of urinary incontinence include fecal impaction, prostatic obstruction, atrophic vaginitis, infection, and certain medications. (See "Urinary Incontinence," pages 128 to 137.)

Ask the older female client if she is experiencing vaginal pruritus, discharge, or pain. Postmenopausal bleeding or breast masses are abnormal and require prompt evaluation. Ask the client if she performs monthly breast self-examinations and, if so, whether she has detected any abnormalities.

Ask all clients about sexual activity, and encourage them to express any concerns or questions they may have about sexual dysfunction. Sexual activity continues through old age despite some myths to the contrary. Complaints of impotence should be evaluated for physiological or psychological etiology.

Musculoskeletal

Ask the client if he is experiencing any joint pain, low back pain, or weakness or stiffness in an extremity. Is he afraid of falling? If so, why? Does he have a deformity or wear a prosthesis? Osteoarthritis commonly accounts for older people's complaints of pain, stiffness, or limitation in the weight-bearing joints. Focal pain may occur in individuals who have other rheumatoid diseases, such as rheumatoid or gouty arthritis or carpal tunnel syndrome. Unsteady gait may explain an older individual's fear of falling, especially if he has a past history of falls, hip pain, foot pain, cerebellar disorder, or neurologic disease.

Neurologic

An older client doesn't usually complain of focal upper extremity weakness unless he has experienced a CVA. Lower extremity weakness, on the other hand, which presents bilaterally, often occurs secondary to osteoarthritis of the weight-bearing joints. Pain along an extremity and paresthesia commonly occur in nerve root entrapment or secondary to a CVA involving the thalamic region.

Dizziness and vertigo must be differentiated from one another: vertigo is the sensation that the room is rotating around the person or that the person himself is rotating, whereas dizziness is a sensation of unsteadiness and movement within the head or of light-headedness. Vertigo in the elderly may be attributed to inner ear disorders, such as labyrinthitis, Ménière's disease, or benign positional vertigo, and to posterior circulatory diseases, such as vertebrobasilar insufficiency or CVA.

Syncope (loss of consciousness) may represent a cardiac, neurologic, or metabolic event. Common complaints are a feeling of "blacking out" or complete amnesia of events during a specific time period. Ask the client about events leading up to the syncope as well as the initial events remembered once he regained consciousness.

Ask the client to identify any sensory loss that he has experienced. A patient with sensory loss may withdraw, creating further sensory deprivation.

Psychological

Ask the client if he is experiencing any difficulty sleeping, unresolved problems, sadness, depression, or loss of interest in his usual activities. A client with a major depressive disorder commonly has changes in appetite and difficulty sleeping. Ask any older client, regardless of mood, about sleep habits:
• When does he go to bed, and when does he wake up?
• Does he use sleeping aids, such as alcohol or sedatives?
• Does he take naps during the day?
• Has his activity level decreased?

A client who frequently forgets recent events (amnesia), names of objects or family members (anomia), or how to perform tasks previously learned (apraxia), or one who wanders, should be evaluated for dementia. Complaints of visual or auditory hallucinations or excessive fear or anxiety are unusual.

ASSESSING FUNCTION

Functional assessment determines an individual's ability to maintain himself within his environment given his physical, mental, and social health. According to a recent survey by the National Center for Health Statistics, 45% of persons age 65 and older and 60% of those age 85 and older require assistance in performing ADLs or instrumental activities of daily living (IADLs). ADLs include personal care activities, such as bathing, dressing, grooming, toileting, eating, and am-

(Text continued on page 12.)

CLIENT HEALTH HISTORY

Name: _____ Date: _____ Time: _____ Room: _____

Address: _____ Phone: _____ Sex: _____

Religion: _____ Date of birth: _____ Age: _____ Birth place: _____

Responsible person: _____ Address: _____ Phone: _____

Source of information: _____ Reliability: _____

Admitted from: ☐ Home ☐ Hospital ☐ Long-term care ☐ Other _____

Family physician: _____ Address: _____ Phone: _____

Reason for admission: _____

_____

Present illness: _____

_____

General health (describe past health, dates and frequency of visits to physician): _____

_____

MEDICAL HISTORY (check whichever is reported as a positive finding)

☐ Heart disease or angina   ☐ Cerebrovascular accident   ☐ Kidney or prostate disorder   ☐ Thyroid disorder   ☐ Myocardial infarction

☐ Diabetes mellitus   ☐ Tuberculosis   ☐ Asthma   ☐ Hypertension   ☐ Pulmonary disease

☐ Cancer   ☐ Seizures   ☐ Transient ischemic attack   ☐ Pneumonia   ☐ Fall or fracture

☐ Ulcers   ☐ Rheumatoid arthritis or osteoarthritis

Comments: _____

PAST HOSPITALIZATION

Illness: _____ Location: _____ Date: _____

_____ _____ _____

Operations: _____ Location: _____ Date: _____

_____ _____ _____

CURRENT MEDICATIONS (list all prescribed and over-the-counter drugs)

Name	Dosage (including frequency)	Prescribed
1. _____	_____	☐ Yes ☐ No
2. _____	_____	☐ Yes ☐ No
3. _____	_____	☐ Yes ☐ No
4. _____	_____	☐ Yes ☐ No

CURRENT TREATMENTS _____

ALLERGIES   ☐ Drug   ☐ Food   ☐ Contact   ☐ Seasonal

EQUIPMENT AND PROSTHESES

☐ Cane   ☐ Upper dentures   ☐ Walker   ☐ Adaptive devices   ☐ Corrective lenses

☐ Hearing aid   ☐ Lower dentures   ☐ Wheelchair   ☐ Other _____

SOCIAL HISTORY

Alcohol use (amount and type): _____

Tobacco use (amount and number of years): _____

Support systems (family, friends): _____

Description of relationship, frequency and type of contact: _____

_____

Participation and satisfaction in activities (leisure time, hobbies, work, adult education, travel): _____

_____

Income sources: _____ Income per month: _____ Income adequate to meet needs: ☐ Yes ☐ No

SERVICES CURRENTLY USED BY CLIENT

☐ Nutritional support ☐ Medical or social day care ☐ Social services ☐ Hospice

☐ Home health aide ☐ Senior transportation ☐ Visiting nurse ☐ Respite

☐ Other _____

CURRENT LIVING ARRANGEMENTS

☐ Alone ☐ Spouse ☐ Friend ☐ Family ☐ Long-term care

☐ Renter ☐ Homeowner ☐ Other _____

FUNCTIONAL ASSESSMENT (ask the client or caregiver to rate the client in the following categories)

Functional ability	Independent	Supervised	Assisted (mechanical, human)	Comment
Activities of daily living				
Bathing				
Dressing				
Grooming				
Eating				
Toileting				
Ambulation				
Instrumental activities of daily living				
Shopping				
Cooking				
Meal preparation				
Housekeeping				
Laundry				
Telephone				
Finances				
Medication				

REVIEW OF SYSTEMS (check any positive finding; note those not listed under *Comments*)

GENERAL

☐ Anorexia   ☐ Decreased fluids or food   ☐ Falls   ☐ Unusual fatigue   ☐ Fever

☐ Night sweats   ☐ Chills   ☐ Agitation   ☐ Immobility   ☐ Acute or worsening confusion

Comments: _____

INTEGUMENTARY

☐ No difficulty   ☐ Dry   ☐ Oily   ☐ Normal   ☐ Rash

☐ Sores or ulcers   ☐ Discoloration (location): _____

☐ Unhealed sores or moles   ☐ Calluses or bunions   ☐ Pruritus   ☐ Frequent infection   ☐ Bruises

Comments: _____

EYES

☐ No difficulty   ☐ Swelling   ☐ Infection   ☐ Pain   ☐ Diplopia

☐ Blurring   ☐ Difficulty reading   ☐ Discharge   ☐ Loss of vision   L   R

☐ Corrective lenses   Date of last eye examination: _____

Comments: _____

EARS

☐ No difficulty   ☐ Pain   ☐ Tinnitus   ☐ Discharge   ☐ Wax

☐ Deafness   L   R   ☐ Hearing loss   L   R

☐ Hearing aid   ☐ Improvement with aid

Comments: _____

MOUTH

Language spoken: _____   ☐ No difficulty   ☐ Slurred speech

☐ Difficulty expressing   ☐ Difficulty understanding

Comments: _____

☐ Dry mouth   ☐ Lesion   ☐ Coated tongue   ☐ Halitosis   ☐ Difficulty chewing

☐ Periodontal disease   ☐ Bleeding sore   ☐ Excessive thirst   Date of last dental check-up: _____

Comments: _____

RESPIRATORY

☐ No difficulty   ☐ Pain on exertion   ☐ Dyspnea   ☐ Dyspnea when supine   ☐ Persistent cough

☐ Wheezing   ☐ Sputum (color): _____   ☐ Hemoptysis   ☐ Frequent colds

Last chest X-ray: _____   Last PPD test: _____   Last influenza vaccine: _____   Last pneumovax vaccine: _____

Comments: _____

CARDIOVASCULAR

☐ No difficulty   ☐ Use of sublingual nitrates   ☐ Chest pain   ☐ Palpitations   ☐ Cyanosis

☐ Radiating jaw or arm pain   ☐ Light-headedness on sitting or standing   ☐ Calf pain with activity   ☐ Ankle swelling

☐ Varicosities   ☐ Numbness   ☐ Abdominal swelling

Comments: _____

GASTROINTESTINAL

☐ No difficulty   ☐ Indigestion   ☐ Dysphagia   ☐ Nausea   ☐ Vomiting   ☐ Diarrhea

Diet: _____   Appetite: ☐ good   ☐ fair   ☐ poor

Food likes and dislikes: _____   Weight loss or gain (amount): _____

☐ Abdominal pain   Bowel pattern: _____   ☐ Recent change in bowel habits

☐ Melena   ☐ Constipation   ☐ Fecal incontinence   ☐ Hemorrhoids

☐ Enteral feeding   ☐ Ostomy   ☐ Laxative use

Comments: _____

GENITOURINARY

☐ No difficulty   Incontinence: ☐ recent onset ☐ long or chronic duration   _____ incidents per week

☐ Leakage of urine   ☐ Dribbling   ☐ Nocturia   ☐ Urgency

☐ Painful urination   ☐ Hematuria   ☐ Frequency   ☐ Infection

☐ Hesitancy   ☐ Abnormal size or force   ☐ Catheter use   ☐ Wears perineal   Reason: _____
of urine stream   pads or diapers

☐ Impotence   ☐ Penile sores or lesions   ☐ Sexually active

Menses cessation: _____   ☐ Postmenopausal bleeding   ☐ Vaginal pruritus

☐ Frequent infections   ☐ Genital pain   ☐ Perineal itching   ☐ Lesion

☐ Breast mass   ☐ Monthly breast   ☐ Last pelvic examination: _____
self-examination

Comments: _____

MUSCULOSKELETAL

☐ No difficulty   ☐ Focal or diffuse joint pain   ☐ Low-back pain   ☐ Deformity

☐ Adequate calcium intake   ☐ Fear of falling   ☐ Focal or diffuse   ☐ Stiffness
(supplements): _____   weakness

☐ Unsteady gait   ☐ Contracture (location): _____

Comments: _____

NEUROLOGIC

☐ No difficulty   ☐ Dizziness   ☐ Vertigo   ☐ Headache   ☐ Paresthesia

☐ Upper extremity weakness: L   R   ☐ Lower extremity weakness: L   R   ☐ Paralysis

☐ Transitory focal   ☐ Loss of consciousness (duration): _____   ☐ Sensory loss: _____
symptoms

Comments: _____

PSYCHOLOGICAL

☐ No difficulty   ☐ Somatic concerns   ☐ Unresolved problems   ☐ Hallucinations

☐ Forgetful   ☐ Recent memory loss   Forgets: ☐ names of objects ☐ places ☐ family

☐ Loses way   ☐ Excessive fearfulness   ☐ Emotional lability   ☐ Sadness   ☐ Loss of interest

☐ Suicidal ideation   ☐ Anxiety   ☐ Difficulty sleeping

Retires at: _____   ☐ Arises at: _____   Usual number of hours of sleep: _____

Napping patterns: _____   Use of sleeping aids: _____

Comments: _____

ENVIRONMENTAL ASSESSMENT TOOL

Please examine each area and check the correct response.

Item	Satisfactory	Unsatisfactory	Not applicable	Comments
Lighting				
Hallways				
Stairwells				
Bathroom				
Bedroom				
Kitchen				
Living room				
Dining room				
Entrances and exits				
Sensory stimulation				
Pictures and mirrors present				
Wall hangings securely hung				
Radio, television present and used				
Plants, pets present				
Individual able to care for plants, pets				
Blankets and pillows present				
Color				
Use of easily seen colors, such as red, yellow, orange				
Objects well defined				
Noise Reduction				
Use of auditory stimulation, such as soft music				
Carpeting, window treatments used				
Temperature				
Heating, air conditioning				
Circulation, ventilation				
Floor covering				
Throw rugs tacked down				
Low pile carpeting				
Furniture				
Amount				
Sturdiness				
Table lamps firmly in place				
Arm chairs				
Firm seat cushions				
Furniture with smooth edges				
Tables and chairs at appropriate height				

Item	Satisfactory	Unsatisfactory	Not applicable	Comments
Furniture (continued)				
Reclining chair				
Furniture easily cleaned				
Bathroom				
Floors clear from clothes, rugs, debris				
Nightlight present				
Handrails and grab bars at toilet and bathtub				
Faucets with easy-to-turn knobs				
"Hot" and "Cold" labeled on faucets				
Electric appliances not present				
Raised toilet seat				
Nonskid mat in bathtub				
Bedroom				
Firm mattress				
Bed at appropriate height				
Telephone				
Alarm bell				
Side rails				
Dining room				
Tables set for groups				
Homelike atmosphere				
Kitchen				
Exhaust system				
Flammable items away from stove				
Safety				
Neighbor to check in				
Windows and doors with locks				
Smoke detectors				
Electrical wiring in good condition				
Electrical outlets covered				
Pipes covered				
Telephones on each floor				
Sturdy railing in stairwells				
Cabinets and light switches within reach				
Orientation devices (clocks, calendars) in place				
Doorways accessible to wheelchairs, walkers				
Ramps in place				
Fire sources away from blankets, towels, papers				
Other				
Personal items				
Areas for privacy				

bulation. IADLs include the ability to shop, do laundry, prepare meals, take public transportation, use the telephone, administer medication, keep house, travel, and handle personal finances. Functionally impaired clients may have more difficulty with IADLs than with ADLs because they require more skill to perform.

Regular functional assessments enable the nurse to note any positive or negative changes in the client's abilities and help her determine what kinds of services he needs. They should be performed by a professional, using an assessment tool such as the chart on page 7. An assessment tool reminds the interviewer which aspects of the client's functioning to check and keeps the information organized. It can also be used to communicate with other health professionals.

ASSESSING THE ENVIRONMENT

An environmental assessment can help the nurse determine whether any changes need to be made in the client's residence to accommodate physical changes he may have experienced. For example, ask the client if his home has adequate lighting, heating, and air conditioning, tacked-down carpeting, handrails in the bathroom, smoke detectors, enough telephones, and safe electrical wiring. An environmental assessment tool like the one on pages 10 and 11 will help you obtain a complete assessment and can be used for either the home or an extended care setting.

Perform an environmental assessment periodically to determine further necessary changes.

SELECTED REFERENCES

Bates, B. *A Guide To Physical Examination.* Philadelphia: J.B. Lippincott Co., 1987.

Brown, M.D. "Functional Assessment of the Elderly," *Journal of Gerontological Nursing,* 14(5):13-17, May 1988.

Burnside, I.M. *Nursing And The Aged.* New York: McGraw-Hill Book Co., 1988.

Carnevali, D.L., and Patrick, M. *Nursing Management for the Elderly.* Philadelphia: J.B. Lippincott Co., 1986.

Esberger, K.K., and Hughes, S.T. *Nursing Care of the Aged.* Norwalk, Conn.: Appleton & Lange, 1989.

Matteson, M.A., and McConnell, E.S. *Gerontological Nursing.* Philadelphia: W.B. Saunders Co., 1988.

ASSESSMENT
Physical Examination of the Older Client

The physical condition of a client does not typically change abruptly at age 65. However, normal changes from aging do occur in every organ system (See *Normal Physiologic Age-Related Changes*, pages 21 to 24), and can be detected during the physical examination.

Before beginning the physical examination, escort the older client to a private, well-lit examination area that has minimal background noise. Whenever possible, observe the client's posture, gait, and balance on the way to the examination area, paying particular attention to his ability to rise from the chair, ambulate, and use assistive devices.

Begin the physical examination with a check of vital signs and measurement of weight and height; then proceed to specific body areas and systems, using either the head-to-toe method or the major-body-systems method used here.

VITAL SIGNS
Encourage the client to rest for 10 to 15 minutes before obtaining vital signs, which include temperature, respiratory status, pulse rate, and blood pressure. If these measurements, especially the pulse and respiratory rates, are taken immediately after physical exertion, false readings are likely to occur.

Temperature
The aging process alters temperature regulation, making temperature an unreliable sign of infection—an older client may be afebrile even with a clinical infection. Normal body temperature in the elderly can range from 96° to 98.6° F (35.6° to 37° C). If the client is dyspneic or a "mouth breather," use rectal or axillary measurement instead of oral temperature readings. The older client is at a high risk for infection because of age-related changes in immunity and increased incidence of hospitalization, which can lead to nosocomial infections. Hypothermia, a core body temperature less than 96° F, is a medical emergency and must be evaluated immediately. (See "Hypothermia," pages 322 to 325).

Respiratory status
Respiratory status includes the rate, depth, rhythm, and quality of respirations. In the older client, respiratory rate, rhythm, and quality remain constant during rest, but periods of apnea followed by deep breaths may occur during sleep. With exercise, the respiratory rate will increase and take longer to return to the pre-exercise level.

The respiratory rate may be a reliable sign of infection and congestive heart failure in the elderly client, especially if the resting respiratory rate is tachypneic.

Pulse rate
The resting pulse rate remains fairly constant through old age, ranging from 60 to 100 beats/minute. The maximum obtainable heart rate during exercise, however, has been shown to decrease substantially with age, and the heart rate may also take longer to return to the baseline state after exercise. To obtain the most accurate pulse rate, count the apical pulse for 1 minute. All pulses should be measured in terms of rate, rhythm, strength, and equality. The incidence of dysrhythmias, such as premature ventricular contractions and atrial fibrillation, increases with age. Irregular rhythms should be reported to the physician for further evaluation.

Blood pressure
Changes in blood pressure reflect several physiologic age-related changes:
• a gradual increase in both systolic and diastolic values
• a widening of pulse pressure (the difference between the systolic and diastolic readings) influenced by an increase in arterial rigidity and a decrease in blood vessel resiliency
• a tendency to develop orthostatic hypotension, a drop in systolic blood pressure of 20 mm Hg or more or a drop in diastolic blood pressure of 10 mm Hg or more upon standing.

To assess for postural blood pressure changes in clients at risk for falls, measure blood pressure in each arm with the client lying, sitting, and standing. Note any differences and the arm with the higher pressure on the client's record, and use that arm consistently for routine blood pressure checks. Wait 3 to 5 minutes between readings because of the decrease in baroreceptor responsiveness.

WEIGHT AND HEIGHT
Obtain the client's weight, taking care to consistently weigh the client either with or without his shoes and at the same time of day. Sudden or profound changes in weight pattern are not a normal consequence of aging, but a gradual weight gain may occur over the years if the client continues to consume the same number of calories as he becomes more sedentary. Certain diseases, such as congestive heart failure and depression, may present with weight gain. Weight loss of more than 10% of the client's typical weight in a short time span (six months or less) requires medical evaluation.

Height usually decreases about 2″ to 3″ (5 to 7.6 cm) with age. The best way to determine an older client's height is to measure with a tape measure from the crown to the rump and then from the rump to the heels. This technique will account for changes in the curvature of the spine, such as senile kyphosis or widow's hump.

SKIN

Inspect the skin of the scalp, head, neck, trunk, and limbs, noting color, skin tears and lacerations, scars, lesions, ulcerations, edema, temperature, texture, tone, turgor, thickness, and moisture. Because the amount of subcutaneous tissue is reduced in older clients, skin turgor may be an unreliable sign of hydration. Checking skin turgor involves pinching the subcutaneous tissue at the forehead or over the xiphoid process and watching for a quick return of the tissue to the baseline state.

As the distances between the outer layer of the skin surface and the underlying bone of the bony prominences (elbow, heel, hip) become smaller, the "fat padding" and protective effects of the subcutaneous tissue diminish, increasing the likelihood of pressure sore formation. The first sign of a pressure sore is reactive hyperemia (local redness over the pressure site). Another type of sore commonly seen in the elderly population is stasis ulceration of the legs secondary to long-standing venous insufficiency.

Aging skin also becomes translucent, friable, and more susceptible to breakage with trauma—hence, the appearance of skin tears and senile purpura (red, dark purple, or brownish yellow skin discoloration secondary to hemorrhage into the subcutaneous tissue). The gradual decrease in total body water and sebum production with age leads to skin dryness, particularly of the legs.

Skin temperature is described as cool, cold, warm, or hot. Use the ball of the hand to get an accurate assessment and to feel for symmetrical changes in temperature. Unilateral changes in temperature along with other clinical findings suggest an aberration.

Certain diseases may change skin color. Typical discolorations include redness, pallor, jaundice, ashen gray color, cyanosis, and bronze or brawny color. Brawny discoloration of the legs typically signifies chronic venous disease in older people. Changes in the distribution of pigment also occur, such as hyperpigmentation in the solar regions (hands, face and neck). Ecchymoses and petechiae can occur from vitamin C deficiency.

Benign skin lesions that commonly accompany aging must be differentiated from precancerous or malignant lesions. Note the following lesion characteristics: size (more or less than 1 cm), pattern of distribution, shape (oval, round), color, consistency (soft, boggy, firm), borders (regular, irregular), and appearance (scaling, greasy). (See "Skin Cancer," pages 32 to 34.)

Skin typically becomes thicker with age. Corns (overgrowths of the horny layer of the epidermis) are round, hard, or soft and usually occur on the dorsal portion of the small toes. Skin texture may be described as smooth or rough.

HAIR AND NAILS

Inspect and palpate the hair noting its color, quantity, distribution, and texture (fine, silky, or coarse). Hair thinning and sparseness are readily observed around the axilla and pubis symphysis. Certain diseases prevalent among the aged, such as hypothyroidism and hyperthyroidism, produce changes in both hair texture and distribution.

Inspect the fingernails and toenails, noting color, shape, thickness, presence of lesions, and capillary refill. Hypertrophy of the nails (onychogryphosis) is a common clinical condition causing nail thickness and a hooked, clawlike deformity. A fungal infection of the nails (onychomycosis) commonly produces thickened, friable nails and a yellow discoloration. Ingrown nails (onychocryptosis) often cause infection and mobility problems for the older client. Changes in the shape or angle of the nails may indicate a pathologic etiology. Any client with a foot deformity or a nail aberration should be referred to the podiatrist promptly. Likewise, lesions of the nail beds such as splinter hemorrhages (linear streaks in the nail beds) must be referred to the podiatrist or physician for further evaluation.

Abnormal nail bed color can signal certain conditions. The normal color of the nail beds is pink; however, clients with anemia often exhibit pallid nail beds with poor capillary refill. Infection at the bed of the nail (paronychia) presents with redness and possibly heat, drainage, and (if severe) bulging at the nail base. Clients who experience respiratory distress or heart disease may have cyanotic nail beds and clubbing (increase in the angle of the nail beds).

HEAD

Inspect the head, noting its size, contour, and symmetry. The size and shape of the skull should not change as a function of age. Soft-tissue swelling or bulging of the cranium may indicate recent head trauma.

Palpate the skull, noting tenderness, masses, or lesions. Point tenderness or localized enlargement of the cranium should be evaluated by a physician.

Observe the older client's facial expression, noting the presence of masklike facies or the blank stare that often accompanies Parkinson's disease and certain psychiatric disorders.

EYES

A comprehensive eye examination requires the assessment of visual acuity, visual fields, extraocular eye movement, and external and internal eye structures. It will require the use of an ophthalmoscope, reading materials, and a Snellen eye chart. An older client should have his acuity assessed with and without corrective lenses and using monocular and binocular vision. (See *Assessing cranial nerve function.*)

An older person suffering from a transient ischemic attack (TIA), a cerebrovascular accident (CVA), or glaucoma may present with changes in the visual fields. A

ASSESSING CRANIAL NERVE FUNCTION

Cranial nerve I: Olfactory (Sense of smell)
To assess for a decreased sense of smell, occlude one of the client's nostrils, and ask him to close his eyes. Pass various aromas, such as lemon or alcohol, past the nonoccluded nostril.

Cranial nerve II: Optic (Vision)
Assessment of the optic nerve involves checking the client's visual acuity and visual fields. To check visual acuity, use the Snellen eye chart. Ask the client to stand about 20′ (6 m) away from the chart and to read the last (smallest) line from left to right. If the client cannot read more than half of the letters in the row, progress to the next largest row, and so on.

Visual acuity is expressed as a fraction with the numerator indicating the distance in feet from the Snellen chart (for example, 20′) and the denominator representing the standardized number for the smallest row read correctly. This fraction should be expressed for each eye. Thus, if the client can read the last line correctly with the right eye while standing 20′ away, the finding would be written as O.D. 20/20. Legal blindness is defined as 20/200.

Another method of assessing acuity is to ask the client to read the fine print in a book or newspaper. A client with profound visual impairment who may be unable to read even large printed materials should be assessed for perception of light and objects.

To assess visual fields, face the client closely at eye level, then cover one of the client's eyes and your opposite eye. Check the eight fields of vision by moving an object such as a pen, or by alternating fingers, from a distance into the client's field of vision. Large objects, such as a penlight, may be preferable to a pen or pencil because of the decreased visual acuity seen among older clients. Ask the client to signal or comment when he sees the object. This assessment will also identify decreased peripheral vision.

Other methods of assessing visual field losses include covering the client's eyes separately and asking him to look at your face or asking the client to draw the face of a clock with all 12 numbers. Visual field deficits may be identified if the client tells you he cannot see your whole face or if certain numbers are omitted from the drawing of a clock.

Cranial nerve III: Oculomotor (Pupillary constriction, elevation of upper eyelid, most extraocular eye movements [EOMs])
Assess for reaction to light accommodation by shining a bright light directly onto the pupil and observing for constriction (direct response). Assess for constriction in the opposite eye when the light is shined (consensual response).

Assess for EOMs by having the client face you, with his head still, and follow your finger or pen with both eyes. Move your finger or pen through the cardinal gazes, observing for parallel movements of the eye (conjugate gaze) and any abnormal movements or oscillations. Observe for convergence of the eyes by asking the client to follow your finger as you move it toward his nose.

Cranial nerve IV: Trochlear (Downward, inward movement of the eye)
Assess this nerve by having the client gaze upward and downward. The eyes should move together and no jerking movement should occur.

Cranial nerve V: Trigeminal (Corneal sensation)
Assess for corneal response by grazing a piece of cotton lightly over the cornea. Repeated stimulation may be necessary to elicit a normal response—closure of the eyelids—in an elderly client.

Cranial nerve VI: Abducens (Lateral deviation of the eye)
Assess the client's ability to perform lateral eye movements. Ask the client to follow your finger as you move it vertically and horizontally.

Cranial nerve VII: Facial (Taste on tip of tongue)
Assess for taste perception on the anterior part of the tongue by asking the client, with his eyes closed, to identify concentrated salty or sweet tastes on the tip of the tongue.

Cranial nerve VIII: Acoustic (Hearing)
Assess for hearing loss by performing the whisper test. Occlude one of the client's ears, then stand on the opposite side and whisper a series of words or numbers at a distance of 1′ to 2′ (0.3 to 0.6 m) toward the nonoccluded ear. Or, in a quiet environment, ask the client to detect the ticking of a watch.

Cranial nerve IX: Glossopharyngeal (Innervation of stylopharyngeus muscle, used in swallowing; taste at back of tongue)
Ask the client to lift his tongue, and inspect for abnormalities. An older client should be able to move the tongue unassisted. Repeat this manuever to examine the lateral sides of the tongue.

Assess for taste perception on the posterior part of the tongue by asking the client, with his eyes closed, to taste concentrated salty and sweet tastes on the back part of the tongue.

Cranial nerve X: Vagus (Control of swallowing, phonation, and movement of uvula and soft palate; sensation of mucosa of pharynx, soft palate, and tonsils)
Ask the client to say "ah," and observe the rise of the palate and uvula. Assess for the gag reflex by gently pressing a tongue blade against the back of the tongue toward the pharynx. Retract the tongue blade when the client exhibits the gag reflex.

Cranial nerve XI: Spinal (Movement of sternocleidomastoid muscles and upper portion of trapezius muscles)
Place your hands on the client's shoulders, and have him lift his shoulders against the force of your hands.

Cranial nerve XII: Hypoglossal (Tongue movements)
Ask the client to stick out his tongue; it should protrude along the midline. Then, hold a tongue blade against one side of his tongue, and ask him to push his tongue against the tongue blade, to test tongue strength. Repeat on the opposite side. Finally, ask him to move his tongue rapidly in and out and from side to side.

---

client with central or peripheral vision loss should be referred to an ophthalmologist.

In examining the external eye structures, observe the eyebrows and eyelids, lacrimal apparatus, conjunctiva, sclera, pupils, and iris. Inspect the eyebrows, noting symmetry and distribution of hair. Observe the eyelids, noting color, presence of lesions or edema, and direction of the eyelashes. Note whether the upper eyelid partially or completely covers the pupil, which indicates ptosis, an abnormal finding. Common findings affecting the eyelids in older clients include entropion (inversion of the margin of the eyelid) and ectropion (eversion of the margin of the eyelid). Compare eyelid color to the client's facial skin color; the lid should be free of any color changes, such as redness.

The lacrimal apparatus includes the lacrimal gland, which secretes tears, the lacrimal sac, and the nasolacrimal duct, which empties into the lacrimal cavity. The lacrimal duct opening can be readily observed at the nasal corner where the upper and lower eyelids meet (puncta lacrimale). Note any discharge, redness, edema, excessive tearing, and tenderness. Also assess the client for dry, lusterless eyes.

To examine the conjunctiva of the lower eyelid, ask the client to look upward while you retract the lower lid with the thumb pressed against the bony orbit. Note the color and the presence of lesions, edema, or discharge. The conjunctiva of older clients is often light pink color or slightly pale. To examine the conjunctiva of the upper lid, ask the client to look downward while you gently grasp the lid, pulling it first down and then forward. Next, place a cotton-tipped applicator above the lid margin and gently roll the lid inside out. Again, note the color and the presence of lesions or edema.

The sclera usually appears creamy white in color. Because of the presence of fat, however, the sclera and the conjunctiva may appear yellow. One common observation in the elderly is pinguecula, yellowish thickenings of the bulbar conjunctiva that are triangular in shape and that occur on the inner and outer margins of the cornea.

The pupil and iris must be inspected using a light, preferably a penlight. Note the pupils' size (including equality of size), shape, and reaction to light. In older clients, the pupils may be smaller than usual (senile miosis) and irregularly shaped. Cataracts (clouding of the crystalline lens) are readily observed. They appear as opacifications in the pupil and may obscure the transmission of light to the macula. Inspect the iris, noting any margin aberrations.

Ophthalmoscopic examination is necessary to inspect the retina and retinal blood vessels, optic disk, macula, and fovea centralis. These structures may be difficult to visualize in clients with senile miosis; to improve visualization, use a bright light and a dimly lit environment. During the examination, observe for the larger dark red veins, small light red arteries, yellowish oval optic disk, and avascular macula. Background eye changes characteristic of diseases common in the elderly client (such as diabetes, macular degeneration, hypertension, and arteriosclerosis) can be seen.

EARS

Inspect the auricle, noting color and any temperature change, discharge, or lesions. Palpate the auricle gently, pulling it upward and then downward to assess for tenderness. To inspect the ear internally, gently pull the auricle up and back and insert the otoscope. Examine the external canals and the tympanic membrane, and observe for the light reflex. Note any lesions, bulging of the tympanic membrane, or cerumen accumulation. Older men may develop hair in the ears.

NOSE AND SINUSES

Examination of the nose and sinuses involves inspection, using a nasal speculum and penlight, and palpation. First, observe the external portion of the nose, noting asymmetry or any abnormality, such as a structural deformity. Then ask the client to tilt his head backwards. Gently insert the speculum into the nasal cavity and observe the mucosa, noting color, discharge, swelling, bleeding, or lesions. Inspect the septum (the partition separating the two nasal cavities), noting any deviations or lesions.

Inspect the turbinates for discoloration, enlargement, inflammation, and lesions. An enlarged, boggy, often pale turbinate or mucosa may indicate allergic rhinitis.

Palpate the frontal and maxillary sinuses with the thumbs to check for tenderness. The frontal sinuses are located on either side of the midline, just above the brow; the maxillary sinuses are located directly over the maxillary bone (cheek bone).

MOUTH AND PHARYNX

An older client's mouth and oral structures can reveal important information about his state of health, including hydration status, ability to chew food, and the presence of numerous diseases, such as oral carcinoma, vitamin deficiencies, and anemia. Examine the client in a well-lit environment with his mouth open wide.

Inspect the oral cavity, beginning with the lips. Note color, symmetry, lesions or ulcerations, and hydration status. Clients suffering from dehydration may exhibit dry, parched lips. Clients with poorly fitting dentures may exhibit cheilosis (fissures or cracks at the corners of the mouth); those with vitamin B complex deficiencies exhibit cheilosis with reddened lips. Inspect the oral cavity with the client's dentures or bridges intact and then removed. Palpate any oral lesions or nodules with the index finger of a gloved hand, noting tenderness, pain, bleeding, and mobility. When the dentures are worn, observe for fit and the presence of sores or abscesses secondary to friction; poorly fitting dentures may need to be relined. Using a penlight, inspect the mucosa, noting color, texture, hydration status, lesions, or exudate. A white exudate coating the mucosa or tongue may be observed in older clients with poor oral hygiene. Gently remove this coating to prevent the growth of bacteria; if the exudate persists or bleeds easily, leukoplakia (a precancerous lesion) must be ruled out.

Inspect the gums for color, inflammation, lesions, and bleeding. They should appear pink and moist. Periodontal gum disease usually presents with inflamed gums that bleed easily. If the older client has his natural teeth, note their number and condition (caries, jagged or loose teeth).

Observe the tongue, noting its color, size, texture, and coating. The tongue normally is red, smooth, and free of involuntary movements. However, extrapyramidal side effects from psychotropic drugs can result in involuntary movements, such as lip smacking, tongue protrusion, and slow, rhythmic movements of the tongue, lips, or jaws. An enlarged tongue (macroglossia) may be observed in clients with hypothyroid disease. Assess the tongue's position. Deviation to the right or left in an older client suggests a neurologic disorder, such as TIA or CVA. Iron deficiency anemia, a common condition in the older population, may manifest with sublingual varicosities.

Observe the pharynx using a penlight and a tongue depressor. Place the tongue depressor over the back of the tongue, gently push the tongue down, and shine the light on the posterior pharynx. Observe for inflammation, discoloration, exudate, and lesions.

NECK

Examination of the neck involves palpation of the trachea, thyroid gland, and lymph nodes.

First, help the client to a comfortable sitting position and ask him to relax the neck. Inspect the neck, noting scars, masses, and asymmetry. If masses are evident, gently palpate them in a rotary motion with the fingertips, noting consistency (hard, firm, soft), size (length, width, depth), shape (oval, oblong), mobility (fixed, mobile), and tenderness. Then repeat this procedure for the lymph nodes. With the fingertips, palpate the submental, submaxillary, preauricular, occipital, supraclavicular, deep cervical chain, superficial cervical, and posterior cervical nodes. Note if nodes are found unilaterally or bilaterally.

Check the trachea for alignment by gently palpating both sides with the thumb and index finger at the level of the suprasternal notch. The trachea is normally located midline at the suprasternal notch. Note displacement and the presence of masses. Standing directly in front of the client, inspect his thyroid gland while he swallows a sip of water; note any masses or bulging. Next, standing behind the client, palpate the lower trachea with your fingertips. Displace the thyroid lobe with one hand, and palpate the opposite lobe while the client swallows a sip of water. Normally, the thyroid gland should not be palpable. Palpate the thyroid for masses and nodules as well as enlargement.

CHEST AND LUNGS

Examination of the chest and lungs requires inspection, palpation, percussion, and auscultation.

Inspection

The client should be in a sitting position and draped from the waist down. Inspect the chest's shape and symmetry both anteriorly and posteriorly. Note the anteroposterior (AP) to lateral diameter. The older person's thorax should be symmetrical despite the change in AP to lateral diameter. Symmetry can be judged by observing certain landmarks—for example, both tips of the scapulae should be aligned near the 7th thoracic vertebrae. Also, observe the chest for scars.

Observe for rib retraction along the intracostal spaces as the client inhales deeply; observe for bulging of the intracostal spaces as he exhales. An older client with asthma or emphysema secondary to chronic obstructive pulmonary disease (COPD) will typically present with intracostal retraction or bulging. During respirations, listen for inspiratory or expiratory wheezes (indicating airway turbulence), which may be audible from the oral airways.

Inspect the breasts, noting any mass, nodule, dimpling, or nipple retraction. Observe for breast symmetry and for a rash beneath the breast folds. Intertrigo (a local erythematous dermatitis) often occurs in the moist environment created by skin folds, as do fungal infections.

Finally, ask the client to stand, and note the position and curvature of the spine.

Palpation

Using the fingertips, palpate the anterior and posterior chest for tenderness, masses, or lumps. Localized tenderness over the costochondral junctions suggests costochondritis, a frequent cause of chest pain among elderly clients. To assess chest excursion anteriorly, stand in front of the client and place your hands on the lateral rib cage around the 11th rib along the costal margins, with thumbs separated about 2" (5 cm). Ask the client to inhale and assess the symmetry of chest excursion by observing thumb separation. To assess chest excursion posteriorly, stand behind the client and repeat the above procedure. In the older client, chest excursion should be symmetrical; however, lung expansion may be reduced secondary to decreased elasticity of the rib cage.

Using the ball of the hand, palpate the anterior and posterior chest symmetrically for tactile fremitus (vibratory tremors felt through the chest wall). Fremitus is usually most evident near the tracheal bifurcation.

The client should be in the supine position for breast palpation. Have her extend her right arm overhead when you palpate her right breast and her left arm overhead when you palpate her left breast. This position will help displace the breast tissue so that abnormalities can be detected more readily. Using the pads of the fingertips, palpate in a rotary and concentric fashion around the outer margins of the breasts toward the areola. Instruct the client in breast self-examination during this demonstration. Note any nodules or masses; if present, include their size, shape, consistency, mobility, and tenderness. The upper outer quadrant of the breast or the axillary tail is a common location of breast cancer. Next, gently squeeze the nipple between the thumb and index finger to check for discharge or tenderness.

Percussion

With the client sitting, percuss the lung fields anteriorly and posteriorly from bases to apices. Make certain to percuss in a symmetrical fashion for comparison. Normal lung fields will sound resonant on percussion; bony prominences, organs, or consolidated tissue will yield dullness.

Auscultation

In auscultating an older client, especially one who is obese or has COPD, an amplified stethoscope may be useful. Using the diaphragm of the stethoscope, auscultate from bases to apices, anteriorly and posteriorly, and in a symmetrical fashion for comparison. While auscultating, ask the client to take some deep breaths in and out through an open mouth. If he becomes dizzy, tell him to stop and rest.

In the absence of disease, rales at the bases can be attributed to reduced mobility. If rales are evident, ask the client to cough. Rales secondary to congestive heart failure will not clear with coughing; rales caused by physical immobility may clear. Older clients with pulmonary fibrosis or interstitial lung disease often present with "Velcro-type" rales. Rhonchi or wheezes signify bronchospasm and require further evaluation.

Clients showing evidence of adventitious lung sounds (rales, rhonchi) with dullness on percussion should be checked for consolidation. Assessing for egophony will help confirm consolidation. Ask the client to say "E-E-E" while you auscultate over the suspicious area. "A-A-A" sounds are positive findings.

CARDIOVASCULAR SYSTEM

Help the older client to a supine position, and carry out the cardiovascular assessment from the client's right side. First, inspect and palpate the point of maximal impulse (PMI). In young persons, the PMI is palpated around the fifth or sixth left intercostal space at the midclavicular line. In elderly persons however, the PMI may be displaced downward to the left.

Using the ball of the hand, palpate over the following landmarks, listing the presence of thrills, heaves, or vibrations: aortic area, located at the second right intercostal space at the sternum (base of the heart); pulmonic area, located at the second left intercostal space at the sternum (base of the heart); tricuspid area, located at the fifth left intercostal space at the sternum (apex of the heart); and the mitral area, located at fifth intercostal space at the midclavicular line (apex of the heart). You may detect a palpable thrill in a client with valvular heart disease, especially a valve closure abnormality.

Using the diaphragm of the stethoscope, auscultate the heart over the aortic, pulmonic, tricuspid, and mitral areas and Erb's Point. Listen for S_1 and S_2 over each area, noting the intensity and splitting of S_1. The first heart sound signals the onset of ventricular systole. S_1 is loudest at the base of the heart.

Also listen for the extra diastolic heart sounds, S_3 and S_4, which may be detected in an older client. An S_3 (ventricular gallop) is heard between S_1 and S_2, usually at the lower sternal border, and indicates ventricular decompensation. In older clients, S_3 is not a reliable sign of congestive heart failure (CHF). An S_3 may be physiologic or may occur in response to an increased diastolic flow. An S_4 (atrial gallop) is auscultated after

S_2 and before S_1. S_4 sounds are most audible over the heart's apex.

Next, auscultate for cardiac murmurs. A murmur is an audible, prolonged vibration that may be associated with abnormalities of the heart valves, bloodstream, or cardiac chambers. Note, however, that a murmur does not necessarily indicate an abnormality. Common heart murmurs among the elderly, secondary to valvular heart disease, include aortic sclerosis, aortic stenosis, mitral regurgitation, and idiopathic hypertrophic subaortic stenosis.

Listening over the apex of the heart, count the heartbeats for 1 full minute. Note the rate and rhythm. Abnormal rates include bradycardia (fewer than 60 beats/minute) and tachycardia (more than 100 beats/minute). Widespread abnormalities of impulse formation and condition occur in elderly clients, including sinus bradycardia, chronic atrial tachycardia, tachybradycardia, and chronic atrial fibrillation. A common rhythm abnormality seen among the elderly is atrial fibrillation, which presents as an irregular rhythm.

Examination of the vascular system includes assessment of the arteries and veins that supply the head and neck, trunk, and legs. The clinical skills required to perform a thorough vascular assessment include inspection, palpation, and auscultation. The American Heart Association recommends the following grading system for pulse strength: $\uparrow$ = increased, $\downarrow$ = decreased, 0 = absent. Assist the client to a sitting position, and examine the carotid arteries one at a time. Begin by inspecting the neck for the arterial pulsation. Gently palpate one carotid artery with the pads of two fingertips. Then repeat the procedure on the other carotid artery. Press lightly to avoid obliterating the carotid pulse. Because of the increased sensitivity of the baroreceptors as well as the atherosclerotic changes of the vessels, palpation of the carotid arteries can result in narrowing of the arterial lumen. Note the rate, rhythm, strength, and equality of both pulses.

Next, using the bell of the stethoscope, auscultate over each carotid artery for bruits. Bruits represent a narrowing of either the arterial or venous lumen. Adventitious sounds produced by bruits are characteristically high-pitched. To differentiate a carotid bruit from a transmitted heart murmur, inch up the artery with the stethoscope, starting at the base of the neck. Murmurs typically are loudest at the neck base, whereas bruits become louder as you inch up the neck. Also, bruits tend to be higher-pitched than murmurs.

Assist the client to a supine position, elevating the head 30 degrees. Ask him to turn his head slightly to the left so that you can examine the right neck veins. The jugular venous pulse, particularly of the right internal jugular vein, reflects events, such as CHF, occurring in the right heart chambers.

Identify the level of venous pulsation and measure its height in relation to the sternal angle (using centimeters). A height exceeding 3 cm is considered abnormal, indicating right-sided heart failure. To assess for hepatojugular reflux, observe the level of venous pulsation while applying pressure for approximately 1 minute to the upper right quadrant of the abdomen. A positive finding exists when the height of the venous pulsation is greater than that of the baseline valve.

Palpate and auscultate the following arteries, noting the presence of bruits, as well as pulse rate, rhythm, strength, and equality: radial, ulnar, brachial, femoral, popliteal, dorsalis pedis, and posterior tibialis. In the elderly client, expect arteries to be tortuous and to appear kinked. Arteries may feel stiffer. The pulses should be symmetrical in strength. Using the fingertips, palpate the temporal arteries one at a time, noting pulse strength and equality and the presence of cords.

Inspect the legs, noting color, temperature, edema, trophic changes of the digits, and varicosities. Color variations may include pallor, erythema, or pink, red, mottled, cyanotic, or brawny discoloration. Pallor is observed in clients with arterial insufficiency; erythema may be secondary to contact dermatitis, cellulitis, lymphangitis, or superficial or deep vein phlebitis; cyanotic or mottled discoloration is found in clients with arterial occlusion; and brawny discoloration results from long-standing venous insufficiency. The older client should have no significant deterioration in color attributed to age alone.

Use the ball of the hand to assess temperature changes symmetrically in both legs. Thrombosis is usually associated with a feeling of heat, but this response may be reduced in elderly clients.

Edema, the presence of excessive amounts of fluid in body tissues, may result from CHF, lymphatic obstruction, renal failure, hypoalbuminemia, and inflammation; however, in an elderly client, lower leg edema is usually attributed to chronic venous disease. Edema is best assessed over bony prominences, such as the medial or lateral malleolus, the tibia, or the sacrum, and is typically pronounced in the most dependent areas of the body (the feet of an ambulatory client or the sacrum of a bedridden client). Edema is characterized as pitting or nonpitting; in pitting edema, a depression, or pit, forms when the examiner presses the thumb over edematous tissue. Edema is typically graded as trace, $+1$, $+2$, $+3$, or $+4$, based on the examiner's clinical judgment.

Trophic changes include the loss of hair on the distant extremities; they can be observed in arterial disease, neuropathies, and diabetes. Varicosities are twisted, swollen veins, typically in the legs.

GASTROINTESTINAL SYSTEM

The abdomen should be assessed with the client supine and the abdominal nodes relaxed. Standing on the client's right side, inspect the belly, noting shape, symmetry, scars, masses, pulsating aorta, distention, or striae. Abdominal scars from appendectomy or cholecystectomy may aid the nurse in completing the health history. The abdomen may be described as obese, scaphoid, or distended.

The abdominal cavity is divided into the right and left upper quadrants and the right and left lower quadrants. Auscultate all four quadrants for the presence of bowel sounds (recorded as absent, present, hyporeactive, hyperactive). Using the bell of the stethoscope, listen over the aorta for bruits.

Percuss the belly to determine the presence of air or fluid, the size of the liver, and the presence of bladder distention. Air in the large bowel will sound tympanic, whereas fluid will sound dull. Bowel obstruction can occur secondary to long-standing fecal impaction. On percussion, this presents as a distended and tympanic abdomen. Percuss the liver in the right upper quadrant; mark its borders if you detect a change in percussion. The normal liver size at the midclavicular line is 2¼" to 4¾" (6 to 12 cm) in diameter. Percuss over the symphysis pubis toward the umbilicus, noting any change in percussion. Dullness in this area may indicate bladder distention. (Clients may experience tenderness with this maneuver.)

Palpate the belly, noting any masses or tenderness upon light or deep palpation, and peritoneal signs, such as rigidity or rebound tenderness. Masses in the lower quadrants may be impacted stool. Palpate the lower edge by placing your left hand under the client's back and pressing upward with your right hand in the right quadrant below the rib cage. Ask the client to inhale during this procedure. The liver may not be palpable.

GENITOURINARY SYSTEM
Male genitalia

Assist the client to a supine position and drape him appropriately. Inspect the pubic hair, glans of the uncircumcised penis, penile shaft, scrotum, and inguinal canals for bulging, masses, lesions, inflammation, edema, or discoloration. The pubic hair becomes sparse and gray with age. Palpate any lesions, noting size, shape, consistency, and tenderness.

Palpate the testes between the thumb and index finger, noting size, shape, consistency, and tenderness.

Assess the inguinal canal with the client in the standing position. Gently insert one finger of a gloved hand in the right side of the scrotum, proceeding until you feel the inguinal ring in the canal. Ask the client to cough or bear down. You should feel a tightening around the finger in the absence of a hernia.

Female genitalia

Inspect the perineum for rash, lesions, or nodules. Inspect the labia majora, labia minora, clitoris, and urethral and vaginal orifices for color, size, and shape. During inspection of the vaginal orifice, separate the labia with a gloved hand and ask the client to bear down. Observe for any bulging of tissues or organs, such as cystocele or rectocele; either of these may occur in older women who have had more than one child.

An internal pelvic examination is recommended for all women, especially those over age 50. Care must be taken during this exam to maximize comfort because of the atrophic changes of the vaginal mucosa in the older female. Pap smears, which screen for cervical cancer, need to be performed routinely even if they have been negative in the past. (See "Menopause," pages 161 to 164.)

Rectum
For a rectal examination, the female client should be in a side-lying position and the male client bent over. Drape the client appropriately. After applying lubrication to a gloved hand, inspect the anus for external hemorrhoids, then insert one finger into the canal. Tell the client to take a deep breath in and out and then bear down. This will relax the anal sphincter. Palpate the canal for masses, nodules, lesions, or hemorrhoids. Ask the client to tighten the sphincter muscle around your finger so that you can note its tone. Withdraw the finger and test any stool for blood. For males, assess the prostate gland, located at the base of the bladder. Note its size, consistency (firm, hard), shape, surface (nodular, smooth), and symmetry, and record any tenderness. The gland should be round, soft, nontender, free of masses, and about ¾″ to 1½″ (2 to 4 cm) in diameter.

MUSCULOSKELETAL SYSTEM
Assessment of musculoskeletal function is vital in determining the older client's overall ability to function. Limitations in range of motion, difficulty ambulating, and diffuse or localized joint pain can be detected easily in the physical examination.

Begin by watching the client ambulate into the examination room. Observe gait (walking), posture (the position or bearing of the body), and station (the position assumed in standing). Gait is influenced by the integration of reflexes as well as motor function. Older people tend to take smaller steps, reduce the height of the steps taken, reduce their arm swing, and flex their elbows and knees. Gait disorders may occur if the client limps or drags a foot from paresis. Posture may reveal kyphotic changes of the spine (such as the head flexing forward); to avoid injury, the client with this condition must compensate by tilting the head back.

To assess static balance and station, gently push on the client's shoulders while he is standing (the client must be guarded by two persons and informed of the nudge). The normal response includes bending at the waist, knees, ankles, and shoulders to create a forward flexion of the body. An abnormal response, in which the client falls over without bending, may indicate musculoskeletal or neurologic dysfunction. Ask the client to walk heel to toe in a straight line and then turn around (tandem walking). Watch for any exaggerated ataxia, and observe the position of the head and neck in relation to shoulders and legs. Note whether the client turns quickly and whether the head, neck, and shoulders move as one unit or separately. Osteophytes may develop along the cervical spine, endangering cerebral perfusion as the client turns quickly.

To assess calf muscle or ankle muscle weakness, ask the client to walk on his toes and then heels. Observe his spine from the side. Assess the height of the hips; both hips should be equally aligned. Clients who have had hip fractures or surgery may present with shortened limbs.

Try to elicit Romberg's sign by asking the client to stand with his feet together and his eyes closed. Swaying indicates a positive Romberg's sign.

Inspect the joints of the hands, wrists, elbows, shoulders, neck, hips, knees, and ankles, noting any joint enlargement, swelling, tenderness, crepitus, temperature change, or deformity. A client with degenerative joint disease will complain of pain with motion and will have enlarged joints due to bony changes, stiffness with range of motion, tenderness, crepitus, joint deformities, and palpable osteophytes.

Common foot deformities in elderly clients include hallux valgus, prolapsed metatarsals, and hammer toes. Carry each joint through range-of-motion (ROM) exercises, and palpate for muscle tone and strength. Compare symmetrical muscles. Cupping the hand over the joint while moving the joint through ROM exercises will help detect crepitus.

Inspect each muscle group for atrophy, fasciculations, involuntary movements, and tremors. A client suffering from hemiplegia commonly develops disuse atrophy of the affected side. Fasciculations appear as rapid flickers in a muscle group—for example, in the tongue. Involuntary movements, such as those exhibited in tardive dyskinesia, can be observed in clients who have experienced adverse psychotropic drug reactions. Tremors have been observed among elderly clients who present with certain diseases. Resting tremors and pin-rolling tremors are associated with Parkinson's disease, whereas intentional tremors are associated with cerebellar disorders.

Move the joints through passive range-of-motion (PROM) exercises, and palpate the muscles for tone. Resistance to PROM indicates hypertonicity, whereas flaccidity indicates hypotonicity. Assess the client for rigidity and spasticity. Rigidity can be detected best in the wrist or elbow joint through PROM exercises. Cogwheel rigidity commonly occurs secondary to diseases involving the basal ganglia and side effects of certain neuroleptic drugs. It should not be confused with peroneal rigidity, which initially presents with little or no resistance to rapid passive movements and is followed by a gradual increase in muscle tone resulting in a final state of spasticity. This disorder is seen in frontal lobe diseases and in acute stroke with hemiplegia.

During the physical examination, ask the client to show you how he buttons or zippers his clothing. This will allow you to directly observe the client's ability to perform selected ADLs. Also ask the client to open the door of the examination room, which will demonstrate manual dexterity and hand strength. Try to determine whether the client can turn the faucet on and off and discriminate cool and warmer temperatures; this will

(Text continues on page 25.)

NORMAL PHYSIOLOGIC AGE-RELATED CHANGES

System	Age-related changes	Effects	Consequences
Sensory			
Vision	• Supporting tissue structure weakens, and elasticity of the eyelid muscle decreases	• Reduced eye movement, deviation of the eyes, jerking eye movement • Entropion (inversion of margin of lower lid) • Ectropion (eversion of margin of the lower lid)	• Wrinkling and loosening of skin around eyelids • Damage to cornea and conjunctiva from eyelid turning in or out
	• Elevator muscle degenerates and orbital fat is lost	• Enophthalmus (sinking of eyes deeper into the orbit)	• Limited upward gaze; sunken appearance of eyes
	• Pupils become smaller because of iris rigidity	• Increased sensitivity to glare and difficulty adapting to dark	• May need to give up night driving
	• Lens of the eye tends to appear yellow (opaque) and flattened, to increase in size, and to decrease in elasticity	• Altered depth perception and changes in color vision	• Distortion of colors in blue-green spectrum, resulting in red and orange becoming more pleasing
	• Lipids are deposited on periphery of cornea	• Whitish gray discoloration around limbus (arcus senilis)	• Decreased corneal sensitivity
	• Iris loses its pigment	• Tendency to have grayish or light blue eyes	• None
	• Decreased lacrimal secretions cause a decrease in tear production	• Chronic eye dryness	• Complaints of dry eyes, scratchiness, or discomfort
	• Vascular changes and decreased oxygen supply to the retina cause degenerative changes and decreased quality and intensity of the light reaching the retina; the optic disc and retina become pallid.	• Decreased visual acuity • Diminished peripheral vision	• Need to wear eyeglasses for reading or distance • Inability to locate objects or people outside range of vision
Hearing	• Ceruminous glands decrease in number and activity	• Drier cerumen (ear wax)	• Wax impaction within external auditory canal, especially in men
	• Organ of Corti atrophies	• Presbycusis (decreased ability to hear the pitch or level of a sound)	• Loss of ability to hear high-pitched sounds first, then low-pitched sounds
	• Amount of subcutaneous tissue decreases, and tissue elasticity is lost.	• Drooping auricle	• None
	• Blood supply to the neurosensory receptors is limited	• Tinnitus (ringing in the ears)	• Inability to hear horns and sirens (hearing aid will be required)
	• Eardrum becomes thickened	• Reduced speech perception	• Inability to understand fast speech
	• Cranial nerve XIII becomes impaired	• High-tone hearing loss	• Poor discrimination of consonants, such as s, t, f, and g
Smell	• Olfactory fibers in the nasal lining atrophy	• Diminished sense of smell (usually completely lost by age 80)	• Decreased ability to enjoy foods and possible decreased appetite

(continued)

NORMAL PHYSIOLOGIC AGE-RELATED CHANGES *continued*

System	Age-related changes	Effects	Consequences
Taste	• Papillae of the tongue atrophy • Saliva production drops, and number of taste buds decreases	• Smooth and balding tongue • Diminished sense of taste (exacerbated by smoking, dryness of mouth, and food quality)	• None • Loss of interest in food
Touch	• Touch receptors lose some of their ability • Skin on palms and other hairless areas becomes less sensitive	• Decreased ability to recognize fine and rough textured objects • Increased tolerance to pain	• Increased skin tears • Decrease in touching
Integumentary *Skin*	• Amount of collagen and subcutaneous fat decreases • Sweat glands diminish in number, size, and function • Number of capillaries declines • Larger vessels surface	• Skin wrinkling, furrowing, and sagging; decreased skin turgor • Inability to regulate heat • Pale skin • Purpura	• Loss of fat in face and limbs; increased fat deposits over the abdomen and hips • Less sweating; inability to maintain body temperature • Anemic appearance • Easy bruising
Hair	• Follicles produce less melanin • Unopposed adrenal androgens are produced	• Graying • Coarse facial hair around nose and chin in women	• None • None
Nails	• Vascular supply to the nailbeds is diminished • Longitudinal striations increase.	• Dull, brittle, hard, thick nails • Splitting of nail surface	• Accumulated debris under nails • Possible infection
Respiratory	• Anteroposterior chest diameter increases • Respiratory muscles weaken and atrophy, rib cage becomes calcified, and chest wall becomes stiffer • Epithelial atrophy of the cilia • Number of alveoli decreases; remaining alveoli are larger with thick elastic fibers	• Barrel-shaped chest or senile emphysema • Reduced vital capacity, reduced maximum breathing capacity, and greater residual lung volume • Poor ciliary function • Decline in PaO_2 levels	• Hyperresonance upon percussion of chest • More energy required to stretch chest wall and lungs during inspiration and expiration (diaphragm will be used to increase maximum breathing force) • Slowed cough reflex and increased chance of infection • Gradual decrease in normal activity • Shortness of breath • Dyspnea
Cardiovascular	• Increased peripheral resistance • Amount of lipofuscin, a yellow-brown lipid pigment, increases in the myocardial fibers, producing "brown heart" • Cardiac valves, especially mitral and aortic valves, become thicker and more rigid	• Blood pressure increases to compensate (increase more pronounced with systolic than diastolic pressure) • 30% to 40% drop in cardiac output • Increased stiffness at the bases of the aortic valve cusps	• Headaches • Dependent edema • Heart failure • Congestive heart failure • Systolic ejection murmur in the absence of disease

NORMAL PHYSIOLOGIC AGE-RELATED CHANGES *continued*

System	Age-related changes	Effects	Consequences
	• Baroreceptors are less sensitive	• Changes in blood pressure regulation in various positions	• Orthostatic hypotension
	• Smooth muscle of artery walls becomes less responsive to beta-adrenergic stimulation and to other vasoactive agents	• Blunted cardiovascular response to the stress of exercise	• Decrease in exercise tolerance
	• Aorta and large arteries lose elasticity, and systemic vascular resistance increases	• Greater resistance to ventricular pumping	• Hypertrophy of the heart muscle, atrial gallop (S_4), diminished peripheral pulses
	• Number of pacemaker cells in the sinoatrial node decreases, with a loss of fibers in the bundle of His	• Longer PR and QT intervals and changes in R and S wave amplitude	• Possible dysrhythmias, such as sick sinus syndrome, on electrocardiogram
Gastrointestinal			
Mouth	• Dentin production decreases, the root pulp shrinks and becomes fibrotic, the gingivae retract, and bone density decreases in the alveolar ridge	• Sharp, ragged, worn, brittle teeth • Reduced salivary flow • Thin, dehydrated mucosa	• Decreased ability to chew • Xerostomia (dry mouth) • Ill-fitting dentures
Esophagus	• Esophageal smooth muscle tone decreases	• Esophageal peristalsis decreases swallowing • Inadequate relaxation of the lower esophagus occurs	• Swallowing difficulties with heartburn after eating • Hiatal hernia
Stomach	• The gastric mucosa atrophies	• Decreased secretion of hydrochloric acid, intrinsic factor, and pepsin	• Altered absorption of iron, calcium, fat, protein, vitamin B_{12} and folic acid
Liver	• Blood flow to liver is reduced	• Diminished cholesterol synthesis and enzyme activity	• Decreased drug metabolism, decreased absorption of fats and fat-soluble vitamins • Biliary stones
	• Number of hepatic cells decreases	• Compromised hepatic protein synthesis	• Reduced liver weight and mass
Intestines	• Peristalsis and blood flow to the colon decrease	• Decrease in bowel sounds	• Chronic constipation
	• Muscle tone of the large intestine's internal sphincter decreases	• Rectocele, altered rectal sensation	• Fecal impaction, staining, and incontinence
Genitourinary			
Kidneys	• Renal mass and number of nephrons and identifiable glomeruli are decreased	• Decreased glomerular filtration rate	• Drug excretion decreases • Elevated creatinine clearance rate and serum blood urea nitrogen and creatinine levels
	• Renal blood vessels show sclerotic changes	• Decreased renal blood flow	• Decreased kidney size lowers the glomerular filtration rate
Bladder	• Fibrous connective tissue replaces smooth muscle and elastic tissue	• Weakened bladder muscles • Decrease in force of stream • Hyperreflexia of detrusor muscle • Cystocele	• Urinary incontinence • Decreased bladder capacity • Increased frequency and urgency • Urine retention
Prostate	• Gland becomes enlarged (gland feels firm and smooth and is symmetrically enlarged)	• Urethral obstruction	• Dribbling after urination, overflow incontinence, urine retention

(continued)

NORMAL PHYSIOLOGIC AGE-RELATED CHANGES *continued*

System	Age-related changes	Effects	Consequences
Female	• Production of estrogen decreases	• Atrophy of tissues of the ovaries, uterus, cervix, vagina, and vulva • Diminished and less acidic vaginal secretions • Atrophy of breast tissue • Altered pigmentation	• Vaginal stenosis, atrophic vaginitis, painful intercourse • More frequent infections • Sagging, thin breasts • Graying of pubic hair
	• Muscle tone and elasticity decrease	• Weakened pelvic musculature, uterine prolapse	• Urinary incontinence
Male	• Testosterone production decreases	• Testicular atrophy	• Fewer viable sperm
	• Penile arteries and veins become sclerotic	• Slower erection and ejaculation	• Decrease in sexual activity
Musculo-skeletal	• Intervertebral disks progressively narrow	• Exaggeration of the thoracic spine	• Kyphosis (dowager's hump), stooped posture
	• Height of individual vertebrae decreases	• Compression of the spinal column	• Decrease in height, 2″ (5 cm) for women, 1½″ (3 cm) for men
	• Number of muscle fibers decreases, and muscles atrophy	• Decreased amount of lean body mass (muscle)	• Decrease in movement, strength, and endurance
	• Amount of fat in muscle tissue increases	• Increased subcutaneous fat	• Narrow-based waddling gait in women, wide-based gait in men
	• Glycogen stores are reduced	• Loss of elasticity of ligaments, tendons, and synovial membrane	• Stiffening and mild flexion of joints (hips, knees, elbows, wrists), neck, and vertebrae
	• Articular cartilage deteriorates, resulting in formation of new bone at the joint surfaces	• Osteoarthritis (degenerative joint disease)	• Local symptoms of pain, stiffness, and joint hypertrophy
	• Bone density decreases, producing a porous-looking skeletal frame.	• Osteoporosis	• Falls, hip fractures
	• Muscles and tendons shrink and become sclerotic.	• Diminished reflex response	• Spasticity • Clonus
Neurologic	• Blood flow to the brain is reduced, and the number of neurons in the brain and spinal cord decreases	• Decreased intellectual responses and abstract thinking	• Loss of short-term memory, deteriorating learning ability
	• Lipofuscin accumulates in the neurons	• Decrease in proprioception	• Syncope, "drop attacks"
	• Number of neurotransmitters may diminish	• Slowed autonomic nervous system response	• Orthostatic hypotension, hypothermia
	• Myelin sheath degenerates	• Altered motor neuron conduction	• Decreased reaction time, reduced deep tendon reflexes (patellar and Achilles)

help you decide whether the client would benefit from assistance in bathing.

NEUROLOGIC SYSTEM

The neurologic examination includes assessment of the older client's mentation, including awareness or level of consciousness, mood and affect, orientation, speech, general knowledge, memory, reasoning, object recognition, praxis, higher cognitive functions, cranial nerves, motor and sensory systems, and reflexes.

Inspection is the primary clinical skill used in the neurologic exam; equipment used includes a flashlight, an ophthalmoscope, a reflex hammer, two cotton applicators, and mental status measurement tools, such as a mini mental examination. Studies using these tools have shown that changes in cognitive function correlate positively with changes in functional ability; that is, the loss of intellectual abilities interferes with performance of certain ADLs and IADLs.

Assessing the higher cognitive function of an older client requires a thorough mental status review of systems and the administration of a mental status measurement tool. Ask the client if he:
• has a sense of well-being
• has difficulty sleeping
• has unresolved problems or concerns
• feels sad or blue
• has lost interest in usual activities
• has thought of suicide
• forgets words, recent events, or names of people
• wanders
• gets lost
• gets confused about date or place.

Determine whether the client's symptoms have developed rapidly or progressed gradually over several years. Acute confusion usually develops rapidly, whereas dementia progresses gradually. (See "Dementia and Alzheimer's Disease," pages 188 to 199.) Classifying cognitive dysfunction is important in determining the client's prognosis and which services will best suit him. Knowing his degree of impairment can help place him in the appropriate activity groups at adult day care centers and nursing homes.

Level of consciousness

The various levels of consciousness that have been defined center on the client's level of attention.
Consciousness. State of being fully alert, aware, and oriented. A conscious client responds quickly to questions posed and reacts spontaneously to external stimuli.
Delirium (acute confusion). Acute, transient disorder of cognition and attention often accompanied by disturbances of the sleep-wake cycle and psychomotor behavior, such as insomnia, disorientation, wandering, drowsiness, and hallucinations. It is common in dementia.
Lethargy (obtundation). Reduced level of consciousness in which the client is arousable when stimuli are applied. Responses may be inappropriate or confused. A lethargic client appears drowsy and may sleep frequently when unstimulated.
Stupor. Partial or near-complete unconsciousness. The client responds only to strong stimuli, such as loud noises and bright lights, and typically groans or moans.
Semicoma. Stupor from which the client may be aroused. The client withdraws a body part in response to painful stimuli, but doesn't respond verbally.
Coma. State of unconsciousness from which the client cannot be aroused, even by powerful stimuli. The client fails to respond even to painful stimuli.

Mood and affect

Observe the client's general appearance, including mood (normal, calm, depressed, elated, anxious, agitated); affect (flat, inappropriate); and grooming (well-groomed, unkempt clothing). Note whether the client responds appropriately to questions and is appropriately dressed (winter clothes in the winter). Flat affect (failure to show emotions) is a symptom of diseases of the basal ganglia, such as Parkinson's disease. An elderly client who is depressed may require further evaluation. (See "Depression," pages 264 to 269).

Orientation

Assess the client's orientation to person, time, and place by asking him his name, address, and phone number; the day of the week, date, month, year, and season; and where he currently is—that is, hospital or clinic, room number or floor, and name of town. Changes in the environment, such as a hospital admission, can cause acute confusion in a previously alert and oriented client.

Speech

Speech disorders usually occur in response to circulatory disorders, such as acute CVA secondary to emboli or bleeding, and can readily be detected during casual conversation. The client may present with sensory aphasia or dysarthria. (See "Aphasia," pages 241 to 246.)

General knowledge

Assess the client's vocabulary and general knowledge level by discussing with him current news or family events. Vocabulary and general knowledge increase with age.

Memory

Memory consists of immediate, recent, and remote recall. To assess immediate recall, name three objects, such as tree, apple, and airplane, then ask the client to repeat them immediately; or recite six numbers and ask the client to repeat them forward and backward. To elicit recent memory, ask about events that occurred in the last 24 to 48 hours, such as what the client had for breakfast today or what television shows he watched last night. To assess remote memory, ask the client to recall significant events that occurred many years ago, such as date and place of birth, number of children, and anniversary date.

Reasoning

Ask the client questions requiring judgment, insight, and abstraction to determine reasoning abilities. For instance, ask him to tell you what he would do if he became ill or saw a house on fire. A client with intact judgment would respond by saying he would notify the doctor if he became ill or call the fire department if he saw a fire. Insight can be evaluated by asking the client why he is in the hospital. A response of "I'm not sure" indicates poor insight or lack of knowledge regarding his condition.

Abstraction, which requires both insight and judgment, is commonly assessed by asking the client to interpret a proverb, such as "People in glass houses shouldn't throw stones." An incorrect interpretation (concrete reasoning) would be, "Because the house will shatter." Another sample question is, "What do an apple and orange have in common?"

Object recognition

Point to two objects, such as a clock and a pen, and ask the client to tell you what they are. The response is graded as normal or agnosia (inability to name objects).

Praxis

Inability to perform familiar movements in the absence of motor deficits is termed apraxia. Test constructual apraxia by asking the client to construct or copy geometric designs, such as intersecting polygons. This exercise tests perception, cortical function, and motor ability.

Higher cognitive function

Higher cognitive function is evaluated by testing the client's basic knowledge and ability to use acquired knowledge, social skills, judgment, and abstract thinking. When interpreting the client's responses, consider his educational level, past occupations, and life experiences.

Cranial nerves

Cranial nerves are examined sequentially, beginning with I and progressing to XII. Few changes occur among elderly clients as a normal function of aging. The following chart can be used to assess for cranial nerve function.

Motor and sensory systems

See "Musculoskeletal System," pages 20 and 21, for assessment of muscle and joint function. Also assess for rapid, rhythmic, alternating movements, which determine coordination; for example, have the client walk across the room, turn, and sit in a chair. Observe the client for ability to repeat the manuever and smoothness in execution. The speed of the response is typically reduced in the elderly client.

ness in execution. The speed of the response is typically reduced in the elderly client.

Assessment of sensory nerve function involves checking the client's ability to perceive pain, using the sharp and dull end of a safety pin; temperature, using hot and cold test tubes; light touch of the hand; and two-point discrimination vibration and position sense.

Reflexes

The older client's reflexes are assessed in the same manner used for other age-groups. The plantar and Babinski's reflexes are important in assessing for upper motor neuron diseases. Plantar responses are graded as up- or down-going, great toe equivocal or withdrawal. Other deep-tendon reflexes are graded as 0 (absent), 1 (decreased), 2 (normal), 3 (increased), and 4 (clonus).

The following reflexes can be elicited easily during the physical examination.
• Glabellar tap. Ask the client not to blink. Tap the eyelid 10 times so as not to elicit visual threat response. Record number (0 to 10) of stimuli required for habituation of reflex (absence of significant upper lid response). A score of more than 5 is positive.
• Snout. Press firmly with index finger over philtrum of upper lip. A pouting response is positive.
• Sucking. Touch flat surface of tongue blade lightly to vermillion portion of lips. A pouting response is positive.
• Rooting. Stroke curved portion of tongue blade gently at angle of mouth. Movement of angle toward stimulus is positive.
• Jaw jerk. Place index finger on chin, and tap finger with percussion hammer. A brisk response is positive.
• Palmomental. Stroke thumbnail against thenar eminence six times, once per second. Score number of stimuli before habituation occurs. Habituation requiring four or more stimuli is positive.
• Grasp. Ask client not to grasp. Distract the client and stroke the palms. Score as positive if client grasps.

SELECTED REFERENCES

Carstensen, L., and Edelstein, B. *Handbook of Clinical Gerontology.* New York: Pergamon Press, 1987.

Eliopoulos, C. *Gerontological Nursing.* Philadelphia: J.B. Lippincott Co., 1987.

Groth, K. "Age-Related Changes in the Gastrointestinal Tract," *Geriatric Nursing* 9(5):278-80, September/October 1988.

Matteson, M.A., and McConnell, E.S. *Gerontological Nursing: Concepts and Practice.* Philadelphia: W.B. Saunders Co., 1988.

SECTION II

CLINICAL CARE PLANS

INTEGUMENTARY SYSTEM

Pressure Sores

A pressure sore is any skin opening that involves a loss of epidermis and part of the dermis. The sores can be superficial (the lesion remains confined to the outermost layers of the skin) or deep (the lesion damages all layers of skin and possibly muscle or bone). Pressure sores affect 17% to 25% of hospitalized clients and 3% to 11% of clients in extended care facilities.

ETIOLOGY
Pressure sores develop when the skin receives external pressure for extended periods. The pressure causes insufficient circulation and ischemia, which leads to localized tissue damage. Paralyzed or immobile elderly clients are at great risk for pressure sores. Other factors contributing to sore formation include incontinence, which causes skin maceration, and friction, which removes the epidermal skin layer. Shearing can distort or compress the dermal layer and vessels, and poor nutrition causes decreased levels of essential nutrients needed to protect against skin breakdown and to heal.

HEALTH HISTORY FINDINGS
In a health history interview, the client may report or the nurse may detect many of these findings:
• pain at or around sore
• incontinence
• fecal staining
• decreased mobility
• sensory deficits
• thrombophlebitis
• varicosities
• peripheral vascular disease
• arterial insufficiency
• diabetes
• cardiovascular disease
• anemia
• history of vascular surgery
• history of recent bed rest or institutionalization
• use of steroid or immunosuppressive medications
• vitamin C deficiency
• history of tobacco use

PHYSICAL FINDINGS
In a physical examination, the nurse may detect many of these findings:

Integumentary
• sores over bony prominences
• reddened, warm, firm area progressing from partial- to full-thickness skin loss
• undermining of wound edges
• granulation tissue, epithelialization, necrotic tissue
• signs or symptoms of local infection (erythema, induration, purulent drainage, malodorous drainage, crepitus)
• signs or symptoms of systemic infection (confusion, malaise, leukocytosis, fever, increased pulse rate)

DIAGNOSTIC STUDIES
The following studies may be performed to evaluate the client's health status:
• complete blood count (CBC) with differential, electrolyte, and glucose levels—to differentiate the type and possible cause of the sore
• serum cholesterol and triglyceride levels—elevated levels indicate hyperlipidemia and possible atheromas
• serum protein level—result reflects the protein available for healing
• serum and urine osmolarity—to determine fluid and electrolyte status
• angiography, oscillometry, Doppler testing—to determine the degree of vascularization around the sore
• X-rays—to rule out osteomyelitis

POTENTIAL COMPLICATIONS
• infection
• cellulitis
• sepsis
• gangrene
• electrolyte imbalance

Nursing diagnosis: *Impaired skin integrity related to pressure sore and debridement*

NURSING GOAL: To restore the client's skin integrity without complications

Signs and symptoms
• partial- or full-thickness skin loss
• necrosis
• copious drainage

Interventions

1. Relieve or reduce factors contributing to pressure sore formation, such as prolonged pressure and incontinence.

2. Reduce pressure on the affected area by establishing a turning schedule and by using a pressure-reducing device (such as an air, water, foam, or gel mattress or a low-air-loss bed or air-fluidized bed).

3. Clean the client's skin after every incontinent episode, and apply a moisture barrier ointment.

4. Keep the head of the bed at or below a 30-degree angle, or flat if not contraindicated. Apply a knee gatch or footboard when the head of the bed is elevated. Use assistive devices, such as turning sheets, a trapeze, or lifts, to facilitate client movement.

5. Consult with a dietitian to assess the client's nutritional deficiencies.

6. Evaluate the sore for possible debridement.

Rationales

1. Factors that contribute to pressure sore formation, including prolonged pressure and incontinence, impede wound healing.

2. Relief of external pressure helps reestablish blood flow.

3. Excessive moisture or contact with urine or stool can contribute to skin breakdown.

4. These measures reduce sliding, heel pressure, surface cling, and friction. Friction from sliding on the bed contributes to pressure sore development.

5. Wound healing depends on tissue hydration and positive nitrogen balance.

6. Debridement removes necrotic tissue to promote healing. Debridement techniques include application of mechanical wet-to-dry dressings or occlusive or semi-occlusive dressings, enzymatic debriding agents and ointments, and surgical debridement.

OUTCOME CRITERION
• The client will be free of wound infection, necrosis, or copious drainage.

Nursing diagnosis: *Potential for infection related to the pressure sore*

NURSING GOALS: To promote wound closure and to prevent infection

Signs and symptoms
• erythematous induration surrounding wound
• purulent and malodorous drainage

Interventions

1. Protect the wound from feces, urine, and wound drainage by covering the wound with a dressing and by changing the dressing whenever it is soiled.

2. Initiate debridement of any necrotic tissue.

3. Use clean technique when performing wound care.

4. Irrigate the wound with normal saline solution every shift.

5. Apply exudate-absorbent dressings to infected or full-thickness wounds. Avoid using occlusive dressings on infected wounds.

Rationales

1. Body waste or discharge can contaminate nearby wounds.

2. Necrotic tissue harbors infectious organisms that can delay healing.

3. Clean technique discourages the introduction of organisms into the wound.

4. Regular wound cleaning removes bacteria and debris from the wound surface. Using normal saline solution rather than iodine or hydrogen peroxide avoids harming the wound base.

5. Absorbent dressings help minimize wound drainage onto surrounding skin, fill dead space, and keep the wound surface moist. Occlusive dressings may enhance proliferation of anaerobic bacteria.

6. Use absorption dressings, such as moist gauze, co-polymer starches, and dextranomers, and follow the institution's or manufacturer's guidelines.

6. Absorption dressings absorb excess exudate, obliterate dead space, and keep the wound surface moist. Dead space impairs wound healing and promotes abscess formation.

7. Apply occlusive dressings, such as hydrocolloid dressings, to clean, partial-thickness wounds.

7. Occlusion forms a barrier between the wound and the outside environment.

8. Obtain a culture and sensitivity test after cleaning the wound base if the client exhibits signs or symptoms of infection (such as a fever or a change in mentation), if the joints or bones become involved, or if sepsis of an unknown etiology develops.

8. All dermal wounds are contaminated. A culture and sensitivity is indicated only when clinical infection or the potential for osteomyelitis exists.

9. Protect healthy skin by using Montgomery straps or taping to skin barriers to avoid tape trauma. Apply a moisture barrier ointment to the surrounding skin when using wet dressings, and apply film dressings to high-friction areas, such as elbows and heels.

9. Frequent tape removal disturbs the epidermal layer, wet dressings can macerate healthy skin, and film dressings absorb friction while protecting the skin.

OUTCOME CRITERION
• The client's wound will heal without complications.

Nursing diagnosis: *Altered nutrition: less than body requirements, related to healing sore*

NURSING GOAL: To promote wound healing and proper nutritional intake by providing a high-protein, high-carbohydrate diet

Signs and symptoms
• dietary intake less than 1,800 calories per day
• body weight 10% to 20% less than ideal
• poor skin turgor
• dry skin and mucous membranes

Interventions

1. Monitor the client's calorie count, nutritional intake, and serum albumin level.

2. Teach the client to eat high-protein, high-carbohydrate foods, such as eggs, cheese, milk, fish, meat, potatoes, peas, corn, pasta, and cereal.

3. Offer the client small, frequent meals and frequent snacks.

4. Provide the client with supplemental, high-protein feedings, such as Ensure or milkshakes.

5. Explain to the client and family the dietary goals and the reasons for increasing his calorie intake.

Rationales

1. These measures help identify nutritional deficiencies and provide dietary goals.

2. Metabolic needs vastly increase in the client with open wounds because more calories are needed to repair tissue.

3. Small, frequent meals and snacks may be more appealing to the client who cannot each much at one meal

4. The client initially may be unable to consume enough to meet his metabolic needs because of a recent acute illness.

5. The client may be more likely to comply with his new diet if he and his family understand how compliance will benefit him.

OUTCOME CRITERIA
• The client will increase his weight to within 5 lbs (2.3 kg) of his ideal weight.
• The client will accurately identify nutritious foods.
• The client will incorporate nutritious foods in his daily diet.

NURSING ACTIONS IN VARIOUS SETTINGS

Nursing actions for a client with pressure sores depend on the setting in which care is provided. This section identifies which actions are appropriate in all settings and which pertain to acute care, extended care, and home care.

All settings
• Teach the client and family about the disease and contributing factors.
• Involve the client and family in the treatment plan.
• Teach and reinforce prevention measures.
• Evaluate the need for special beds, such as Clinitron or Mark IV.
• Avoid drying the surface of a pressure sore with heat lamps.
• Caution the client and caregiver not to apply alcohol, hexachlorophene (pHisoHex), certain soaps, and hydrogen peroxide, which damage newly formed, fragile skin cells.

Acute care
• Assess the client on admission for risk factors for skin breakdown.
• Follow hospital infection control practices when caring for a client with a draining wound.
• Notify the physician if a client has a full-thickness wound, if signs and symptoms of local or systemic infection develop, or if debridement is necessary.
• Consult a dietitian for a nutritional assessment and for assistance in implementing a diet plan.
• Refer the client to home care services to ensure consistency in wound treatment after discharge.

Extended care
• Follow the institution's infection control practices when caring for a client with a draining wound.
• Perform daily skin assessments on a client at risk for skin breakdown.
• Place an incontinent client on a skin care regimen to prevent skin breakdown.
• Request that a dietitian perform a nutritional assessment of the client.

Home care
• Teach the client's family to properly dispose of dressings removed from draining wounds.
• Enlist home care services for follow-up nursing supervision.

SELECTED REFERENCES

Allman, R.M., et al. "Pressure Sores among Hospitalized Patients," *Annals of Internal Medicine* 105(3):337-42, March 1986.

Bobel, L.M. "Nutritional Implications in the Patient with Pressure Sores," *Nursing Clinics of North America* 22(2):379-90, February 1987.

Felice, P. "Wound Management and the Dermal Ulcer," *Ostomy/Wound Management* 20-27, Summer 1985.

Gosnell, D.J. "Assessment and Evaluation of Pressure Sores," *Nursing Clinics of North America* 22(2):399-416, February 1987.

Iverson-Carpenter, M.S. "Impaired Skin Integrity" *Journal of Gerontological Nursing* 14(3):25-29, March 1988.

Levine, J.M., et al. "Pressure Sores: A Plan for Primary Care Prevention," *Geriatrics* 44(4):75-87, April 1989.

Matteson, M.A. "Age-Related Changes in the Integument," in *Gerontological Nursing Concepts and Practice.* Edited by Matteson, M.A., and McConnell, E.S. Philadelphia: W.B. Saunders Co., 1988.

Schuler, J.J. "Combatting the Silent Wound: Venous Stasis Ulcers," *Advances in Wound Healing* 2:4-5, 1987.

Shannon, M.L., and Miller, B.M. "Pressure Sore Treatment: A Case in Point," *Geriatric Nursing* 154-57, May/June 1988.

Stotts, N.A. "Age-Specific Characteristics of Patients Who Develop Pressure Ulcers in the Tertiary Care Setting," *Nursing Clinics of North America* 22(2):391-98, February 1988.

"Standards of Care," in *Dermal Wounds: Pressure Sores, Dermal Wounds, Leg Ulcers.* Irvine, Calif.: International Association for Enterostomal Therapy, 1987.

INTEGUMENTARY SYSTEM

Skin Cancer

Three types of skin cancer typically occur in the elderly client: basal cell epithelioma, squamous cell carcinoma, and malignant neoplasms. *Basal cell epithelioma,* the most common and least malignant form of skin cancer, occurs almost exclusively on hair-bearing skin. Three types of lesion characterize this form of skin cancer: nodule-ulcerative, superficial, and sclerosing. Nodule-ulcerative lesions usually occur on the face and begin as small pink or translucent papules. They develop depressed centers and raised, pearly borders and eventually ulcerate if not treated. Superficial lesions typically occur on the chest and back, are oval or irregular in shape with a light pigment, and have well-defined borders. The centers may be dry and scaly. Sclerosing lesions are yellow to white with a shiny, waxy appearance. They have no distinct border and may or may not ulcerate. Basal cell epithelioma rarely metastasizes and, if treated early, has a 90% cure rate.

Squamous cell carcinoma occurs less frequently and may metastasize. The lesions usually evolve from actinic keratoses but may also arise from normal skin. Although squamous cell carcinoma usually occurs on areas exposed to the sun, such as the face and forearms, it may also develop on unexposed areas, such as mucous membranes. New lesions begin as flesh-colored nodules that become red and scaly; preexisting lesions indurate and become inflamed. Lesions ulcerate if not treated and thus may metastasize.

Malignant neoplasms, or malignant melanomas, are relatively rare. However, these lesions may metastasize rapidly, making this the most serious form of skin cancer. Of the four types of malignant melanomas, superficial-spreading melanoma accounts for 70% of the cases. These lesions appear slightly elevated with an irregular, indented margin and variegated color (shades of brown, blue, black, and red). The majority develop from preexisting, pigmented lesions on the feet, legs, hands, back, and trunk. The lesions, which may change shape, size, or color as the cancer develops, may bleed easily and itch.

ETIOLOGY

A significant correlation exists between many years of sun exposure and the development of both benign and malignant lesions. Repeated sun exposure has a cumulative effect. Skin cancer commonly occurs in sunny, warm climates, with fair-skinned individuals with blonde or red hair and blue eyes being the most susceptible. Skin cancer rarely affects blacks. People who work outdoors have the highest risk for developing skin cancer. Skin cancer may also result from X-ray therapy, burns, chronic skin irritation, exposure to local carcinogens (tar), or premalignant lesions. Clients with a history of one melanoma have an increased risk for developing a second. Skin cancer has an excellent prognosis when detected and treated during an early or premalignant stage.

HEALTH HISTORY FINDINGS

In a health history interview, the client may report or the nurse may detect many of these findings:
• a change in the size, color, or shape of a skin lesion or a tendency of a lesion to bleed or itch
• history of skin cancer or melanoma
• prolonged exposure to sunlight
• family history of albinism
• occupational exposure to carcinogenic agents (arsenic, tar, radiation)

PHYSICAL FINDINGS

In a physical examination, the nurse may detect many of these findings:

Integumentary
• actinic (solar) keratoses
• nevi (moles)
• ulcerated lesions that bleed easily

DIAGNOSTIC STUDIES

The following studies may be performed to evaluate the client's health status:
• skin biopsy—to distinguish the type of skin cancer
• complete blood count (CBC) with differential, erythrocyte sedimentation rate, and platelet count—may provide information about the likelihood of metastasis
• bone scans, chest X-rays, or CAT scans—indicated in cases of suspected metastasis

POTENTIAL COMPLICATIONS
• fear
• impaired skin integrity

Nursing diagnosis: *Potential for impaired skin integrity related to cancerous lesions*

NURSING GOALS: To promote the healing of cancerous lesions and to prevent skin infection and the development of new lesions

Signs and symptoms
• preexisting lesions with potential for malignant change
• lesions that have changed shape, color, or size
• itching or bleeding at the site of lesions
• wounds that will not heal

Interventions

1. Teach the client the signs and symptoms of cancerous lesions and how to identify normal and abnormal lesions.

2. Advise the client to avoid exposure to carcinogenic irritants, such as tar and arsenic.

3. Advise the client to avoid overexposure to the sun by wearing protective clothing (preferably dry, nonwhite cotton) and a hat with a brim or visor, by applying topical sunblock and lipscreen with the highest protection factor (SPF 15) 1 hour before sun exposure and after swimming, and by avoiding the sun between 10 a.m. and 3 p.m.

4. Advise the client to avoid clothing with seams, which can irritate preexisting nevi.

5. Teach the client with basal cell epithelioma to wash affected skin with care.

6. Teach the client to eat foods high in protein, vitamins, and nutrients.

7. Teach the client about treatment options (including surgical excision, curettage and electrodesiccation, topical chemotherapeutic agents, irradiation, and chemotherapy) and possible complications.

8. Minimize the side effects of chemotherapy, such as nausea, vomiting, fever, and chills, by administering medications, as ordered.

9. Administer analgesics as ordered by the physician.

10. Teach the client to apply cool compresses or corticosteroid ointment after treatment with 5-fluorouracil.

11. After removal of a cancerous lesion, teach the client to keep the wound clean and dry.

12. Teach the client to observe carefully for recurrences of cancerous lesions.

Rationales

1. Skin cancer has a high cure rate when identified and treated early.

2. Although sunlight is the primary factor in skin cancer development, radiation, exposure to tar and oil, and arsenic ingestion also predispose the client to skin cancer.

3. Skin cancer is directly related to exposure to intense, short-wave, ultraviolet light. White fabric, especially when wet, transmits large amounts of ultraviolet light, and polyester fabrics do not stop ultraviolet rays. A hat with a brim or visor helps deflect the light from the ears, nose, and upper cheeks. Sunscreen prevents abnormal DNA synthesis in the epidermis. Solar effects are most harmful between 10 a.m. and 3 p.m.

4. Chronic irritation and ulceration of nevi may lead to cancerous changes.

5. The crust that sometimes forms is friable, and trauma may cause bleeding.

6. Vitamins A and C and protein promote healthy skin cells and tissue healing.

7. The nurse should discuss options and complications to ensure that the client is fully informed and to help alleviate the client's fears.

8. Antiemetics and acetaminophen may be ordered to control nausea and treat fever.

9. Analgesics help relieve the pain from surgical excisions, skin grafts, and metastasis.

10. These measures help relieve possible local inflammation and irritation after treatment.

11. Keeping the wound clean and dry promotes healing and helps prevent infection.

12. Individuals with a history of skin cancer are at risk for a recurrence.

OUTCOME CRITERION
• The client will be free of skin complications secondary to skin cancer.

Nursing diagnosis: *Fear related to possible side effects and complications of treatment*

NURSING GOALS: To identify the client's fears and to help alleviate them

Signs and symptoms
• restlessness
• increased muscle tension
• expressions of dread, nervousness, or fear

Interventions

1. Teach the client and family the possible side effects of treatment, post-treatment care, and other relevant aspects of medical care.

2. Allow the client and family time to express their concerns and to ask questions.

Rationales

1. Providing such information may alleviate fear of the unknown.

2. Encouraging communication and the exchange of information allows the nurse to discover the focus of the client's and family's fears and provides the nurse with the opportunity to offer support and encouragement.

OUTCOME CRITERION
• The client will not fear skin cancer or its consequences.

NURSING ACTIONS IN VARIOUS SETTINGS
Nursing actions for a client with skin cancer depend on the setting in which care is provided. This section identifies which actions are appropriate in all settings and which pertain to acute care, extended care, or home care.

All settings
• Inform the client and family of the importance of avoiding sun exposure.
• Teach the difference between normal and abnormal skin changes.
• Instruct the client and family on proper skin care.

Acute care
• Assess the integumentary system during the initial nursing assessment.
• Notify the physician of abnormal findings.

Extended care
• Observe the client's skin regularly for abnormal changes and premalignant lesions.
• Notify the physician of abnormal skin findings.

Home care
• Instruct the client to avoid sun exposure.
• Reinforce post-treatment care.
• Instruct the client to observe for a recurrence of cancerous changes.

SELECTED REFERENCES
Bates, B. *A Guide to Physical Examination and History Taking,* 4th ed. New York: J.B. Lippincott Co., 1987.
Berliner, H. "Aging Skin—Part 1," *American Journal of Nursing* 86(10):1138-39, 1986.
Berliner, H., "Aging Skin—Part 2," *American Journal of Nursing* 86(11):1258-61, 1986.
Diseases, 2nd ed. Springhouse, Pa.: Springhouse Corp., 1987.
Gordon, M. *Manual of Nursing Diagnosis.* New York: McGraw-Hill Book Co., 1985.
Habif, T. *Clinical Dermatology: A Color Guide to Diagnosis and Therapy.* St. Louis: C.V. Mosby Co., 1985.
Macmillan, A.L. "Aging and the Skin" in *Textbook of Geriatric Medicine and Gerontology.* Edited by Brockelhurst, J.C. New York: Churchill Livingstone, 1985.
Matteson, M.A., and McConnell, E.S. *Gerontological Nursing.* Philadelphia: W.B. Saunders Co., 1988.
Silverberg, N., and Silverberg, L. "Aging and the Skin." *Postgraduate Medicine* 86(1):131-44, 1989.

INTEGUMENTARY SYSTEM
Herpes Zoster

Herpes zoster, or shingles, and postherpetic neuralgia, a serious complication of herpes zoster, predominantly affect the elderly population. Herpes zoster is an acute unilateral and segmental inflammation of the dorsal root ganglia caused by infection with the herpes virus varicella. It produces localized vesicular skin lesions and pain in the dermatome of the nerve arising in the inflamed root ganglia. Motor and sensory deficits may occur in the elderly client; for example, urine retention may result from affected sacral dermatomes. Herpes zoster ophthalmicus, a zoster infection of the ophthalmic division of the trigeminal nerve, particularly affects elderly clients.

The vesicles containing the virus crust over within 1 week and heal in about 1 month. The initial lesions may become infected and permanently scar. Herpes zoster has a good prognosis unless the infection spreads to the brain. Most clients recover completely except for possible scarring or visual impairment from corneal damage. However, postherpetic neuralgia may persist for months or years. Elderly clients over age 70 and clients with underlying leukemia, lymphoma, or myeloma are most vulnerable to postherpetic neuralgia.

ETIOLOGY
The same herpes virus that causes varicella (chicken pox) also causes herpes zoster. Reactivation of the varicella-zoster virus that has been latent in the sensory dorsal ganglia since a childhood infection may cause the outbreak. During an attack of shingles, the reactivated virus travels from the ganglia to the corresponding dermatome. The most common infection sites are the thoracic and cranial areas.

HEALTH HISTORY FINDINGS
In a health history interview, the client may report or the nurse may detect many of these findings:
• pain, tingling, or itching along a dermatome 3 to 5 days before the appearance of small groups of vesicles
• chills, fever, nausea, vomiting, or diarrhea
• pruritus, paresthesia, or hyperesthesia
• unilateral rash, usually on the trunk and face
• headache
• stiff neck
• sensory or motor deficits
• recent exposure to persons with chicken pox or viral infections
• history of leukemia or other cancers, such as Hodgkin's disease
• history of recent trauma at the site of the herpetic outbreak

• use of steroid or immunosuppressive medications
• poor diet

PHYSICAL FINDINGS
In a physical examination, the nurse may detect many of these findings:

Integumentary
• unilateral, bandlike rash on the trunk, ending at midline or midspine
• erythematous vesicles on areas supplied by sensory neurons
• lesions deeper and more confluent than those of chicken pox
• rash over brow and upper eyelid
• edematous and hemorrhagic skin adjacent to vesicles

Genitourinary
• palpable bladder

Neurologic
• confusion
• disorientation

Other
• keratitis
• uveitis
• eye redness
• orbital edema
• decreased extraocular movement on affected side

DIAGNOSTIC STUDIES
The following studies may be performed to evaluate the client's health status:
• white blood cell count—leukocytosis exists during eruption
• sedimentation rate—usually elevated because of acute inflammation
• Tzanck test—performed on a scraping from the base of an intact vesicle to confirm the diagnosis of herpes virus infection, but will not differentiate zoster from herpes simplex
• culture and sensitivity—to rule out secondary bacterial infection

POTENTIAL COMPLICATIONS
• neuralgia and chronic pain
• bacterial superinfection
• malnutrition
• depression
• acute pain
• herpes zoster ophthalmicus

Nursing diagnosis: *Potential for infection related to pruritus and herpetic rash*

NURSING GOALS: To promote healing of lesions, to avoid adjacent skin breakdown and to prevent a change in the client's mental status

Signs and symptoms
• inflamed, red, and purulent skin surrounding herpetic lesions
• fever
• change in mental status such as increased confusion or agitation
• ophthalmic redness and tearing
• pruritus

Interventions

1. Assess the client's temperature, pulse, respiratory rate, and blood pressure every 4 hours while he is awake.

2. Assess the client's mental status every 4 hours while he is awake.

3. Assess the client for ophthalmic changes (such as redness, increased tearing, and itching) every 4 hours while he is awake; notify the physician immediately of changes.

4. Assess skin lesions for redness, inflammation, and purulent drainage.

5. Discourage the client from touching, picking, scratching, or squeezing lesions.

6. Teach the client to use topical treatments, such as aluminum acetate (Burow's solution) and calamine lotion.

7. Teach the client and family the importance of thorough handwashing and of properly disposing of dressings and compresses.

8. Encourage the client to eat foods high in protein, carbohydrates, and vitamins.

9. Teach the client not to use home remedies, such as creams or ointments.

Rationales

1. Elevated temperature, pulse, and respirations and decreased blood pressure may indicate infection.

2. A change in mental status (such as increased confusion, lethargy, or agitation) may indicate cerebral involvement (herpes encephalitis).

3. Such ophthalmic changes, if left untreated, can result in corneal laceration and vision loss.

4. These signs usually indicate a superimposed bacterial infection.

5. Improperly touching the lesions may cause infection or breakdown in uninfected tissue.

6. Aluminum acetate, an antipruritic and astringent, effectively treats herpetic lesions. Calamine lotion, an astringent, relieves itching.

7. During the acute phase, herpes zoster is a communicable disease.

8. Diminished protein and carbohydrate stores contribute to tissue destruction.

9. Unprescribed topical medications can produce an adverse dermatitis reaction.

OUTCOME CRITERIA
• The client's skin surrounding the herpetic lesions will be less reddened and free from drainage.
• The client will remain oriented to time, place, and person.

Nursing diagnosis: *Pain related to an acute herpes zoster episode*

NURSING GOAL: To relieve the client's pain

Signs and symptoms
• burning or stabbing pain along the affected nerve root
• pruritus
• unilateral bandlike rash
• fever
• headache

Interventions	Rationales
1. Warn the client to avoid scratching, rubbing, or breaking the vesicles.	1. Improperly touching the vesicles can cause further injury and irritation.
2. Apply cool compresses to the lesions.	2. Cool compresses help desensitize painful lesions.
3. Teach the client to take lukewarm baths, with oatmeal or aluminum acetate (Burow's solution) added to the water.	3. Bathing in oatmeal or aluminum acetate soothes itchy skin and reduces the risk of secondary infection caused by scratching the skin.
4. Discuss the administration of analgesics with the physician, if necessary. Use narcotics cautiously in the elderly client.	4. A client with acute infection may require narcotic analgesics for pain relief. These should be used cautiously to avoid overmedication and adverse systemic effects.
5. Discuss the use of sedatives with the physician, if necessary, to help the client rest comfortably.	5. Sedatives promote rest and relaxation. Sedatives with a short half-life and a reduced dosage should be used because of the decreased renal perfusion that typically occurs with aging.
6. Apply idoxuridine as prescribed by the physician.	6. Topical idoxuridine hastens recovery and decreases pain and the severity of postherpetic neuralgia.
7. Suggest the use of acyclovir ointment and oral therapy to the physician.	7. If administered during the initial eruption of vesicles, acyclovir may hasten the course of the virus and reduce the severity of pain.
8. Closely monitor serum blood urea nitrogen and creatinine levels if administering oral acyclovir.	8. Oral acyclovir may alter renal function in the elderly client.
9. Administer steroids as prescribed by the physician.	9. The physician may prescribe steroids to prevent postherpetic neuralgia, and short-term use of prednisone can decrease inflammation. Steroid use remains controversial, however, particularly for an elderly client, and is contraindicated in herpes zoster opthalmicus.
10. Administer triamcinolone as ordered for the client with herpes zoster opthalmicus.	10. Triamcinolone helps treat ocular complications caused by herpes zoster such as herpes zoster ophthalmicus (HZO), a zoster infection of the ophthalmic division of the trigeminal nerve. Besides severe pain, HZO can cause conjunctivitis, keratitis, and iridocyclitis, which can ultimately result in loss of vision if not treated aggressively in the acute phase of the infection.

OUTCOME CRITERION
• The client's pain will be minimized during the acute outbreak of herpes zoster.

Nursing diagnosis: *Chronic pain related to postherpetic neuralgia*

NURSING GOAL: To assist the client in identifying pain-relief measures

Signs and symptoms
- phantom pain that occurs after the lesions have disappeared
- scarring
- decreased mobility of the areas with lesions
- pruritus
- changes in the pigment of the affected skin

Interventions

1. Assess the client for postherpetic neuralgia, and, if necessary, refer him to a pain clinic that uses nonpharmacologic pain-control options.

2. Teach the client to avoid pressure against the affected areas and to expose the lesions to air.

3. Teach the client to avoid temperature extremes.

4. Assess the client to determine whether he would benefit from transcutaneous electrical nerve stimulation (TENS) treatment.

5. Teach the client about cognitive therapies, such as relaxation techniques and music therapy.

6. Avoid the use of narcotics and other addictive analgesic agents.

7. Discuss with the physician the possibility of administering amitriptyline or doxepin to the client at bedtime.

8. Refer the client with intractable pain to a pain specialist.

Rationales

1. Pain from postherpetic neuralgia persists more than 4 weeks after the vesicles have healed.

2. Light tactile stimuli excite the affected nerve and may stimulate annoying sensations or increase pain.

3. Temperature extremes intensify neuralgia.

4. TENS is a safe, accessible, and inexpensive initial treatment for many chronic pain syndromes. However, benefits from TENS decrease with long-term use.

5. These activities provide distraction from pain.

6. The pain from postherpetic neuralgia does not significantly respond to analgesic medications, including narcotics, because of tissue damage.

7. Amitriptyline is the drug of choice for postherpetic neuralgia because of its analgesic effect. Doxepin may be used if side effects occur from amitriptyline.

8. Intractable pain may be relieved by second-line drugs (phenothiazines and anticonvulsants), regional sympathetic nerve blocks, and, in rare cases, surgery.

OUTCOME CRITERION
- The client will have minimal pain through identification and use of effective interventions.

Nursing diagnosis: *Altered nutrition: less than body requirements, related to loss of appetite*

NURSING GOAL: To improve the client's nutrition through increased intake of protein and complex carbohydrates

Signs and symptoms
- nausea
- malaise
- decreased body weight
- loss of appetite

Interventions

1. Weigh the client on the same scale at the same time every day.

2. Record the client's fluid intake and output each shift.

Rationales

1. Weighing the client daily can help the nurse assess the client's nutritional needs.

2. A positive fluid balance prevents dehydration.

3. Assist the client with meal selection, stressing the value of foods high in protein and carbohydrates. Document the amount and type of food eaten.

4. Suggest supplemental snacks to augment nutritional intake.

5. Assess the client for pain, and administer pain medication before meals.

3. During infectious periods, catabolism commonly occurs in the elderly client. High-protein, high-carbohydrate foods prevent rapid depletion of body stores.

4. A client usually can tolerate small, frequent meals more easily than two or three larger meals.

5. A client who is free of pain may have an enhanced appetite.

OUTCOME CRITERION
• The client will not lose any more weight and will attain his optimal weight by the end of the acute herpetic illness.

Nursing diagnosis: *Ineffective individual coping related to depression and fear*

NURSING GOAL: To provide support and understanding to the client

Signs and symptoms
• insomnia
• fatigue
• chronic depression
• irritability
• decreased verbal communication
• decreased social participation

Interventions

1. Explain the course of the disease, the treatment, and the possibility of postherpetic neuralgia to the client and the caregiver.

2. Encourage the client to express his fears and concerns.

3. Encourage the client to participate in activities of daily living.

4. Encourage the client to maintain social contacts.

Rationales

1. Understanding all aspects of the disease helps eliminate misconceptions and fears of the unknown.

2. Discussing fears and concerns can enhance communication between the client and the nurse and may increase the client's knowledge of the disease. Such discussion can also benefit a client with facial herpes, who may experience an altered body image.

3. Independently performing activities of daily living increases feelings of self-worth, maintains function during convalescence, alleviates anxiety, and prepares the client for discharge and self-care.

4. Isolation may increase depression, and spending time with others can divert the client's attention from pain.

OUTCOME CRITERION
• The client will begin to socialize with others and participate in activities of daily living.

NURSING ACTIONS IN VARIOUS SETTINGS
Nursing actions for a client with herpes zoster depend on the setting in which care is provided. This section identifies which actions are appropriate in all settings and which pertain to acute care, extended care, or home care.

All settings
• Instruct the client and caregiver on the course of acute herpes zoster and the possibility of chronic pain.
• Clarify the difference between herpes zoster and herpes simplex I and II to avoid misconceptions about transmission routes.

• Teach the client and caregiver about managing the acute phase, including the importance of handwashing and proper disposal of dressings and compresses to avoid transmission of the virus.

Acute care
• Tell the client to avoid contact with immunosuppressed clients or those with debilitating diseases.
• Have an occupational therapist and a dietitian evaluate the client.
• Assess the client's home and support systems to determine whether he will need supervision or assistance after discharge.

Extended care
• During the acute phase, confine the client to one room to avoid cross-contamination.
• Keep the client's room, clothing, and sheets clean and dry.
• Assess the client's nutritional status and provide additional supplements if needed.

Home care
• Tell the client to avoid contact with children until the virus advances to the crustation phase.
• Keep the client's clothing and linens clean and dry.
• Encourage the client to follow a nutritious diet, and provide supplemental snacks.

SELECTED REFERENCES
Cormack, D. *Geriatric Nursing.* London: Blackwell Scientific Publications, 1985.

Ebersole, P., and Hess, P. *Toward Healthy Aging.* St. Louis: C.V. Mosby Co., 1985.

Hoole, A.J., et al. *Patient Care Guidelines for Nurse Practitioners,* 3rd ed. Boston: Little, Brown & Co., 1988.

LeFort, S.M. "Herpes Zoster and Postherpetic Neuralgia: The Need for Early Intervention in the Elderly," *Nurse Practitioner* 14(31):30-41, 1989.

Loeser, J.D. "Herpes Zoster and Postherpetic Neuralgia," *Pain* 24:149-64, 1986.

Matteson, M.A., and McConnell, E.S. *Gerontological Nursing.* Philadelphia: W.B. Saunders Co., 1988.

Portenoy, R. "Postherpetic Neuralgia: A Workable Treatment Plan," *Geriatrics* 41:11, 34-48, 1986.

INTEGUMENTARY SYSTEM

Pruritus and Xerosis

Pruritus, or generalized itching, is the most common dermatologic complaint of elderly clients and frequently results from xerosis, or dry skin. Dry, scaly, itchy skin typically occurs on the lower legs, hands, and forearms but also occurs in skin folds and in the genital and anal regions. Understanding how to treat these conditions enables the nurse to prevent more serious complications, such as scaling, skin tears, pressure sores, and infections secondary to itching. Pruritus and xerosis, combined with environmental irritants, predispose an elderly client to dermatitis, which may take twice as long to heal as in a young adult.

ETIOLOGY
Pruritus may occur with or without a rash and can result from physiological, environmental, or psychological factors.

When no rash exists, consider physiological causes such as hepatic disorders, uremia, malignant tumors, anemia, polycythemia, lymphomas, or drug reactions. Other precipitating conditions may include eczema, allergic reactions, and stasis dermatitis with leg ulcers. Scabies and lice should be ruled out as a cause, especially in a client living in a nursing home.

Xerosis probably results from maturation abnormalities in the epidermis. Decreased sebaceous secretion, and reduced perspiration, both associated with aging, promote dry skin. Environmental factors, such as low humidity, harsh soaps, frequent hot baths, dry indoor heated air, and exposure to cold wind, contribute to dry skin and pruritis. Dehydration pulls additional moisture from the skin.

HEALTH HISTORY FINDINGS
In a health history interview, the client may report or the nurse may detect many of these findings:
• dry, itchy, reddened skin
• flaking skin
• leg ulcers
• rash
• diabetes mellitus
• renal insufficiency
• liver disease
• hyperthyroidism
• history of neoplasm
• family or client history of psoriasis, eczema, or other genetic or familial skin disorders
• recent burns or abrasions
• use of topical steroids
• history of poor nutrition and inadequate fluid intake
• recent exposure to plants, animals, chemicals, or other potentially irritating substances
• recent exposure to cold, dry weather
• history of sun exposure

PHYSICAL FINDINGS
In a physical examination, the nurse may detect many of these findings:

Integumentary
• dry, scaly, itchy skin on lower legs, hands, and forearms
• rough-textured skin
• poor skin turgor on chest or abdomen
• pale or flaky skin
• tears or abrasions
• wrinkling on the face, neck, hands, and other exposed areas
• allergic urticaria (hives) with maculopapular rash
• inflammation and redness in the skin folds under the breasts, in the groin, in the transverse abdominal folds, and in the axillae
• dandruff
• head lice

Cardiovascular
• stasis dermatitis with bluish ulcerations around the ankle
• hemorrhagic fissures of the legs
• crustations
• cellulitis

Psychological
• stress
• negative body image

Other
• poor personal hygiene
• offensive body odor

DIAGNOSTIC STUDIES
The following studies may be performed to evaluate the client's health status:
• complete blood count (CBC)—to rule out anemia or other blood dyscrasia
• serum blood urea nitrogen, creatinine, electrolytes, liver function studies, thyroid studies, and blood glucose—to detect underlying disease
• skin cultures—to rule out infection
• skin scrapings—to detect scabies

POTENTIAL COMPLICATIONS
• skin breakdown
• infection
• poor self-image

Nursing diagnosis: *Pain related to dry, itchy skin*

NURSING GOALS: To reduce skin dryness, to improve the client's personal hygiene, and to prevent complications

Signs and symptoms
• scrapes and lesions resulting from scratching
• shiny skin
• excessive scaling

Interventions

1. Assess the client's hydration status; encourage him to drink at least six 8-oz glasses (1,500 ml) of fluid daily.

2. Instruct the client to avoid daily bathing and harsh soaps, to bathe in tepid water, and to use a fat-based soap.

3. Add baby oil or mineral oil to the client's bath water, and be sure to assist the client in getting in and out of the tub.

4. In severe cases of pruritus, add about 1 cup of oatmeal to the bath water, and instruct the client to soak for 20 to 30 minutes.

5. Pat the client's skin dry with a towel; do not rub.

6. Teach the client to use heavy emollient creams and lotions containing urea or lactic acid, such as Eucerin or Nivea, after bathing or swimming.

7. Encourage a female client to use light-toned liquid make-up or sunscreen instead of powder.

8. Increase humidity by using a room humidifier or one connected to the central heating system, by placing bowls of water in the room, or by air-drying clothes in the room.

9. Discourage the client from wearing restrictive clothing or clothing that rubs against the skin.

10. Trim the client's nails regularly.

Rationales

1. Dehydration causes moisture loss from the skin.

2. Daily bathing dries the skin, and harsh soaps act as irritants. An elderly client need not bathe more than once or twice weekly to maintain cleanliness.

3. Oils lubricate the skin but make the tub slippery.

4. Oatmeal baths help decrease itching.

5. Rubbing the skin removes moisture.

6. These substances restore lipids and retard water loss from the skin, thus reducing itching.

7. Powders and cake foundations dry the skin.

8. Low humidity and dry heat contribute to dry skin.

9. Such clothing overstimulates the skin and can cause pruritus.

10. Neatly trimmed nails help minimize injury to dry skin from scratching.

OUTCOME CRITERION
• The client will be free from the discomfort of pruritus and xerosis.

Nursing diagnosis: *Impaired skin integrity related to dry skin*

NURSING GOAL: To prevent skin breakdown and subsequent infection

Signs and symptoms
- wrinkling
- skin that is hot to the touch
- bloody, purulent drainage from excoriated areas
- dehydration

Interventions

1. Assess the client for signs and symptoms of dermatitis, including erythema, edema, heat, and pain.

2. Assess the client's fingers, hands, and arms for signs and symptoms of eczema, such as inflammed and itchy skin.

3. Discuss measures the client can take to prevent further complications, such as wearing hats or scarves when outdoors, wearing rubber gloves when washing dishes or using cleaning agents or other chemicals, using humidifiers or pans of water on radiators, avoiding exposure to excessive heat, and using facial creams.

4. Use soft bed sheets, preferably flannel, without wrinkles. Avoid strong detergents and starches when cleaning bed sheets.

5. Protect the client's skin from dragging or pulling during transfers from or to the bed.

6. Encourage the client not to remain in one position for extended periods. If the client is confined to bed, reposition him at least every 2 hours.

7. Apply gloves to a confused or psychotic client who cannot control scratching.

Rationales

1. Excessive scratching associated with pruritus can lead to dermatitis.

2. The inflammation and itching that accompany eczema can cause the client much discomfort. Assessment helps to ensure prompt intervention and treatment.

3. Hats and scarves protect the face and neck from the drying effects of the wind; rubber gloves prevent drying and burns; humidifiers add moisture to the air; excessive heat increases the client's susceptibility to hyperthermia because of a reduced ability to sweat; and facial creams neutralize the drying effects of soap.

4. Strong detergents, starches, and wrinkles irritate the skin.

5. An elderly client's skin has decreased flexibility and strength and may tear or burn.

6. Staying in one position reduces circulation to the skin at pressure points, such as those on the buttocks, knees, and ankles, and can cause skin breakdown and pressure sores.

7. Gloves help prevent nail damage and subsequent skin breakdown and infection from scratching.

OUTCOME CRITERION
- The client will be free of skin infection and ulcers after using appropriate measures.

Nursing diagnosis: *Body image disturbance related to aging*

NURSING GOAL: To help the client regain a positive self-image

Signs and symptoms
- visible signs of aging
- verbalized negative feelings about body
- self-imposed isolation
- depression

Interventions

1. Encourage the client to express his concerns about aging and his changing body image.

2. Emphasize the client's character strengths or special skills, and refer to his age only when necessary.

Rationales

1. Verbalization allows the client to ventilate negative feelings and anxieties and encourages communication and the exchange of information.

2. Identifying positive aspects of the client's life may enhance his self-esteem.

3. Show a female client how to select and apply cosmetics properly.

4. Encourage the client to focus on achievable appearance goals, such as good personal hygiene, an attractive hairstyle, make-up, and flattering clothes.

5. Promote social interaction.

3. Proper cosmetics and facial creams help clean the skin, relieve skin problems, and cover imperfections.

4. Focusing on achievable goals is positive and prevents frustration.

5. Isolation fosters feelings of depression, whereas group interaction can be therapeutic.

OUTCOME CRITERION
• The client will identify positive aspects of his physical appearance.

NURSING ACTIONS IN VARIOUS SETTINGS
Nursing actions for a client with pruritus or xerosis depend on the setting in which care is provided. This section identifies which actions are appropriate in all settings and which pertain to acute care, extended care, and home care.

All settings
• Instruct the client and family on normal skin changes associated with aging.
• Teach the client and family proper skin care.
• Instruct the client and caregiver about aspects of the environment that may need modification to promote skin integrity, such as air humidification.
• Encourage the client and family to express their feelings about the client's changing appearance and advancing age.

Acute care
• Avoid bathing the client frequently, and don't use harsh soaps.
• Provide the client with adequate fluids and a well-balanced diet.
• Avoid activities that may traumatize the client's skin.
• Regularly reposition a client who is confined to bed.

Extended care
• Offer the client private bathing measures if he is embarrassed by his skin's appearance.
• Provide the client with opportunities to socialize and diversional activities.

Home care
• Assess the client's home for skin irritants, such as incontinence pads, detergents, or other cleaning agents.
• Encourage the client to maintain social contacts, such as with adult day care centers and senior citizen groups.

SELECTED REFERENCES
Burnside, I. *Nursing and the Aged.* New York: McGraw-Hill Book Co., 1988.
Ebersole, P., and Hess, P. *Toward Healthy Aging.* St. Louis: C.V. Mosby Co., 1985.
Esberger, K.K., and Hughes, S.T. *Nursing Care of the Aged.* Norwalk, Conn.: Appleton & Lange, 1989.
Grantz, R.A. "Variables Associated with Skin Dryness in the Elderly," *Nursing Research* 35(2): 98-100, March/April 1986.
Habif, T. *Clinical Dermatology: A Color Guide to Diagnosis and Therapy.* St. Louis: C.V. Mosby Co., 1985.
Macmillan, A.L. "Aging and the Skin," in *Textbook of Geriatric Medicine and Gerontology.* Edited by Brockelhurst, J.C. New York: Churchill Livingstone, 1985.
Matteson, M.A., and McConnell, E.S. *Gerontological Nursing.* Philadelphia: W.B. Saunders Co., 1988.
Silverberg, N., and Silverberg, L. "Aging and the Skin," *Postgraduate Medicine* 86(1): 131-43, July 1989.

INTEGUMENTARY SYSTEM

Bunions, Calluses, and Corns

Bunions are bony prominences on the medial aspect of the first metatarsal head (joint of the great toe) or on the lateral aspect of the fifth metatarsal head. Bunions cause inflammation and thickening of the bursa. The joint usually becomes enlarged, and the affected toe displaces laterally.

Calluses and corns are hyperkeratotic lesions that occur when layers of fibrous connective tissue replace subcutaneous tissue. The fibrous tissue eventually intrudes into the stratum corneum. Calluses occur primarily on the large, flat surfaces of the feet. Corns occur on smaller, protuberant surfaces and are cone shaped with a point or tip.

ETIOLOGY
Approximately 80% of people over age 50 have at least one foot problem, although elderly clients typically do not report them. Bunions, calluses, and corns, the most common complaints, result primarily because of trauma or a lack of preventive measures. Tight-fitting footwear that forces the toes together is one cause of bunions; people with flat or weak feet are particularly vulnerable. Calluses and corns result from repeated pressure and friction against the skin. Decreased sebaceous activity, decreased hydration, and the metabolic and nutritional changes associated with aging can lead to changes in pedal skin, making hyperkeratotic changes more likely. Poor eyesight and decreased mobility contribute to the problem as elderly clients are more likely to have difficulty inspecting and caring for their lower extremities.

HEALTH HISTORY FINDINGS
In a health history interview, the client may report or the nurse may detect many of these findings:
• foot pain
• discomfort
• gait disturbances
• diabetes mellitus
• peripheral vascular disease
• neurologic disorders
• history of trauma to cutaneous surfaces of the foot

PHYSICAL FINDINGS
In a physical examination, the nurse may detect many of these findings:

Integumentary
• hard corns on small, protuberant surfaces of the foot
• soft corns between toes
• calluses on large, flat surfaces of the feet

Musculoskeletal
• enlargement of the affected joint and displacement of the toe
• reduced flexibility
• pain, especially with stress on affected areas
• decreased mobility

Other
• decreased visual acuity

POTENTIAL COMPLICATIONS
• pain
• deformity
• difficulty walking
• infection
• loss of limb

Nursing diagnosis: *Potential for impaired skin integrity related to injury to affected foot*

NURSING GOALS: To promote healing of foot lesions, to prevent the development of new lesions, to alleviate discomfort, and to assist the client in proper shoe selection.

Signs and symptoms
• gait disturbances
• pain or discomfort
• small, cone-shaped lesions or large, flat, hard lesions
• lateral displacement of great or small toes
• enlargement or inflammation of first or fifth metatarsal heads
• skin discoloration of the foot

Interventions

1. Teach the client proper foot and skin care. This includes washing, but not soaking, feet in warm water daily or on alternate days and then drying them with a soft towel, paying particular attention to the interdigital spaces. Also instruct the client to apply a moisturizing lotion to the feet, including the area around the nails, daily.

2. Advise the client to wear cotton, wool, or wool-blend socks.

3. Teach the client to relieve pressure on corns by using pads cut into a "U" shape.

4. Tell the client to place lamb's wool between toes that have soft corns.

5. Advise a client with thick or hard nails to soak his feet in warm water before performing foot care.

6. Cut each toenail by making three or four separate cuts with toenail clippers rather than making only one cut. First, cut from each corner toward the middle; then, trim straight across the edge of the nail plate. Do not cut nails too short.

7. Apply moleskin to calluses. Use care when removing to prevent tearing.

8. Teach the client not to remove corns or calluses with razors or scissors.

9. Discourage the client from using over-the-counter preparations for corn removal. Instead, suggest a special foot emery file on rough areas of the heel and foot.

10. If the client is bedridden, smooth rough toenail edges with a nail file or emery board.

11. Discourage the client from walking barefoot.

12. Instruct the client in proper shoe selection. Explain the need for accurate foot measurement and the benefits of flexible leather shoes with ties or straps.

13. Advise a client with diabetes or a circulatory disorder to visit a podiatrist regularly.

Rationales

1. Foot washing promotes frequent inspection and proper foot hygiene, and careful drying prevents accumulated moisture and resultant skin breakdown. Soaking can cause excessive skin dryness; a moisturizing lotion prevents skin dryness and subsequent cracking and breakdown.

2. Synthetic fibers, such as polyester, do not allow the skin to "breathe."

3. Circular pads create greater pressure on the affected area and decrease circulation to the surrounding tissues. U-shaped pads relieve pressure without decreasing circulation.

4. Lamb's wool separates the toes and prevents skin maceration.

5. Soaking softens hard, brittle nails, making foot care easier to perform.

6. This method decreases soft tissue trauma and reduces the incidence of ingrown toenails and infection.

7. Moleskin remains in place for several days and decreases the friction that causes and exacerbates callus formation.

8. The client should not use razors or scissors to remove corns or calluses because of the potential for tissue trauma and infection.

9. Chemical agents destroy healthy tissue as well as affected areas and can cause open wounds and infection.

10. This prevents the toes from scratching the skin on the legs.

11. Walking barefoot can lead to cuts and bruises.

12. Tight-fitting shoes exert pressure and friction and do not allow the toes to spread, causing bunions, calluses, and corns. Proper measurement prevents shoe tightness. Leather molds to the foot and allows it to breathe, and ties and straps support the foot.

13. A client with peripheral vascular disease is prone to ulcers and gangrene.

OUTCOME CRITERIA
- The client will perform routine foot care.
- The client will be free of complications caused by bunions, calluses, or corns.

NURSING ACTIONS IN VARIOUS SETTINGS

Nursing actions for a client with bunions, calluses, or corns depend on the setting in which care is provided. This section identifies which actions are appropriate in all settings and which pertain to acute care, extended care, and home care.

All settings
• Instruct the client and family on the selection of proper shoes.
• Encourage the client and family to examine the client's feet regularly and to provide thorough foot care.

Acute care
• Examine the client's feet during the physical assessment.
• Provide thorough foot care.

Extended care
• Ensure that an ambulatory client wears properly fitted shoes and stockings rather than slippers.
• Refer a client with diabetes or a circulatory disorder to a podiatrist for the care of foot problems.

Home care
• Reinforce correct treatment procedures.
• Regulary observe the client's feet for the development of problems.

SELECTED REFERENCES

Bates, B. *A Guide to Physical Examination and History Taking,* 4th ed. Philadelphia: J.B. Lippincott Co., 1987.

Carnevali, D. *Nursing Management for the Elderly,* 2nd ed. Philadelphia: J.B. Lippincott Co., 1986.

Ebersole, P., and Hess, P. *Toward Healthy Aging.* St. Louis: C.V. Mosby Co., 1985.

Esberger, K.K., and Hughes, S.T. *Nursing Care of the Aged.* Norwalk, Conn.: Appleton & Lange, 1989.

Hobday, M.C. "Care of the Foot" in *Nursing Elderly People.* Edited by Redfern, S. London: Churchill Livingstone, 1986.

INTEGUMENTARY SYSTEM

Psoriasis

Psoriasis is a chronic, noninfectious skin disorder characterized by exacerbations and remissions in which round or oval pink to red lesions covered with a silvery scale appear on the skin. The scale may flake or become dense; if the scale is removed, small bleeding points (Auspitz sign) appear. The client may complain of pain or itching. The lesions may become confluent or remain well defined from neighboring, normal skin. Psoriasis can appear on any cutaneous surface, most commonly on the elbows, knees, scalp, gluteal cleft, fingernails, and toenails. It affects about 1% of the population, affecting men and women of all ages equally, but occurs more often in Caucasians than in those of other races.

Up to 30% of elderly clients with psoriasis may also have arthritis. Arthritis commonly involves the terminal interphalangeal joints, especially in clients with severe nail involvement. Psoriasis may mimic secondary infections (such as syphilis), other inflammatory skin diseases (such as seborrhea), or allergic reactions to drugs.

ETIOLOGY
Uncontrolled, accelerated replication of basal epidermal cells causes psoriasis. Normal basal cells divide every 28 days whereas psoriatic cells replicate as often as every 4 days. Its etiology is unknown, although experts believe that individuals may transmit the disease genetically. Because clients with psoriasis have higher than normal levels of some histocompatability antigens (HLA), the condition may result from an autoimmune deficiency.

Many individuals are predisposed to psoriasis, but stress factors trigger the disease. Trauma, infection, emotional stress, and endocrine changes may precipitate the onset of psoriasis in a genetically prone individual. Although no cure exists, treatment can control the symptoms and significantly improve or clear skin lesions.

HEALTH HISTORY FINDINGS
In a health history interview, the client may report or the nurse may detect many of these findings:
• pruritus
• pain
• infection
• arthritis
• history of beta-hemolytic streptococcus
• endocrine disorder
• history of skin trauma
• recent exposure to cold weather
• recent emotional stress

PHYSICAL FINDINGS
In a physical examination, the nurse may detect many of these findings:

Integumentary
• flat-topped, round to oval papules covered with a layer of silvery white scales
• bleeding points when scales are removed
• pain on touch
• pitted and discolored nail beds

Musculoskeletal
• arthritic symptoms, such as stiffness

Psychological
• anxiety
• depression

DIAGNOSTIC STUDIES
The following studies may be performed to evaluate the client's health status:
• skin biopsy—to confirm the diagnosis and to differentiate psoriasis from other skin disorders
• serum uric acid level—elevated level may indicate psoriasis
• serum tissue typing tests—presence of HLA antigens 13 and 17 indicates psoriasis

POTENTIAL COMPLICATIONS
• impaired skin integrity
• disturbed body image

Nursing diagnosis: *Impaired skin integrity related to psoriatic lesions*

NURSING GOALS: To promote healing of lesions and to prevent further skin breakdown and subsequent infection

Signs and symptoms
• pain or itching
• psoriatic lesions

Interventions	Rationales
1. Tell the client not to scratch or rub lesions.	1. Scratching or rubbing can cause bleeding, a breakdown of healthy neighboring tissue, or infection.
2. Assess the client for inflammation of lesions, and discuss the use of topical steroid creams or antibiotics with the physician if inflammation occurs.	2. Inflammation may be a sign of Koebner's phenomenon.
3. Teach the client to use oatmeal baths, antihistamines (as ordered by the physician), and lotions containing menthol and phenol.	3. Systemic and topical antipruritic medications relieve itching.
4. Recommend frequent application of emollient ointments or creams, such as Eucerin, Aquaphor, or Albolene.	4. These products moisturize the skin and minimize desquamation. Frequent application reduces pruritus and increases the efficacy of specific therapy.
5. Discuss the benefits of aspirin or acetaminophen and topical heat application.	5. These measures can alleviate pain and discomfort.
6. Explain the advantages and disadvantages of other treatments for psoriasis, such as coal tar preparations, topical corticosteroids, anthralin, and phototherapy (see *Selected treatments for psoriasis,* page 50).	6. The physician may prescribe one or more of these treatments to alleviate psoriasis. The client will be more likely to comply with treatment if he understands its purpose, method of action, and need for special precautions.
7. Recommend that the client apply Alpha Keri lotion or bath oil before having sexual intercourse.	7. Emollients soften and smooth psoriatic skin and prevent further skin breakdown.
8. Assist the client and family in identifying factors that may precipitate outbreaks of psoriasis, such as trauma, emotional stress, acute illness, or cold temperatures.	8. Identifying the factors that can precipitate psoriasis may help the client and family to prevent or minimize outbreaks.

OUTCOME CRITERION
• The client will be free of discomfort and itching during exacerbations of psoriasis.

Nursing diagnosis: *Body image disturbance related to skin lesions*

NURSING GOAL: To assist the client in identifying factors that will improve self-esteem

Signs and symptoms
• negative expressions about body or appearance
• fear of rejection by others

Interventions	Rationales
1. Encourage the client to discuss his concerns about body image.	1. Such discussion allows the client to ventilate negative feelings, enhances communication, promotes the exchange of information, and provides the nurse with opportunities to offer support and encouragement.
2. If the client has discontinued sexual activity because of skin condition, suggest that he disrobe after turning off the lights or that he have intercourse in a dimly lit or totally darkened room.	2. The client may fear rejection and so may be unwilling to appear naked before another person. These changes may help the client feel less self-conscious.
3. Discuss the benefits of dressing nicely and using appropriate makeup.	3. Wearing attractive clothes and using makeup properly can improve the client's appearance and enhance self-image.

SELECTED TREATMENTS FOR PSORIASIS

A client with psoriasis can experience pain, itching, inflammation, and other symptoms. To alleviate the client's discomfort, the physician may prescribe or recommend one or more of the following treatments:

Tars

Treatment regimens may use coal tar preparations alone or with ultraviolet light, which provides an additive effect. Tar preparations are commonly used to control scalp psoriasis but must be used at least every other day to be effective. Various over-the-counter and prescription preparations range from crude coal tar with strengths up to 10% to the more cosmetically acceptable refined tar products, including various gels, creams, oils, and emulsions. Crude coal tar is a black, thick, messy, viscous preparation used most often in hospital or office settings with ultraviolet light treatments. Tar gels, creams, and oils are more suitable for home use. Tar preparations usually do not irritate the skin, so the client need not limit its application to the lesions. However, folliculitis may develop as a side effect, especially on the legs or other hair-bearing areas. To minimize this complication, the client should apply the tar preparation in the direction of hair growth. Phototoxicity may develop with excessive ultraviolet light exposure after tar application.

Topical corticosteroids

The physician may prescribe a topical corticosteroid, such as 0.1% triamcinolone acetonide cream or ointment (Aristocort, Kenalog), to relieve inflammation and pruritus, especially of excoriated psoriatic lesions. The client may apply thin layers of strong fluorinated corticosteroid creams or ointments in the morning and again at night, thoroughly rubbing the cream into the skin and then covering the area with plastic wrap for at least 4 hours. For severely pruritic, inflamed psoriasis, the client may use topical corticosteroids on a short-term basis because such lesions do not respond well to tar or anthralin. Low-potency topical corticosteroids, such as 1% hydrocortisone cream or lotion (Cort-Dome, Dermacort), effectively control psoriasis in skin folds and on the face, locations which preclude the use of tar and anthralin.

A client should use corticosteroids for only a few months at a time to prevent systemic absorption and side effects; tolerance will occur with prolonged use. Complications include atrophy or thinning of the skin and striae (stretch marks), and lesions can worsen after discontinuation. In addition, treatment can be expensive, particularly if lesions are widespread. As a result, the physician may recommend simultaneous use of other treatments.

Anthralin

Applied in increasing concentrations from 0.1% to 1% in a petroleum-mineral oil base and used with tar baths and ultraviolet radiation, anthralin can clear psoriasis in about 3 weeks. The physician may prescribe anthralin for psoriatic plaques that are resistant to coal tar, corticosteroids, and other preparations. Anthralin slows psoriatic skin cell proliferation and is not absorbed systemically. A client with localized, plaque-type psoriasis may use a water-soluble cream (Drithocreme). The client should allow the medication to remain on the lesions for 1 to 2 hours and then remove it with soap and water. The client's response determines the strength of the cream and the length of time that the medication should remain on the lesions. To avoid skin irritation, the client should not apply anthralin to skin folds or facial lesions. Another anthralin treatment, called short-contact therapy, involves application of a 1.0% anthralin ointment in petrolatum for 30 minutes to 1 hour before thoroughly removing the medication with soap and water. Short-contact therapy may take longer to resolve psoriasis than other treatments but is nevertheless an effective home treatment method.

Phototherapy

Ultraviolet (UV) radiation from artificial sources or from natural sunlight depresses DNA synthesis and slows the rapid, uncontrolled replication of epidermal cells. Because of their photosensitizing effect, tar preparations applied before UV exposure may accelerate clearing. However, acute overexposure to UV rays can exacerbate the disease, probably because normal skin cells reproduce more quickly to repair the damaged cells.

Phototherapy is done in full-body treatment cabinets or in small cabinets used to treat hands, feet, or localized lesions. Limit the initial ultraviolet exposure to 5 to 10 minutes and slowly increase as tolerated by the client. A client taking a potentially photosensitizing drug for another problem should be particularly careful to avoid overexposure to UV rays from either natural sunlight or a sun lamp. A combination of psoralen and ultraviolet light A (known as PUVA therapy or photochemotherapy) is extremely effective but rarely used for psoriasis because it can cause squamous cell carcinoma.

OUTCOME CRITERION
• The client will develop a more positive self-image despite psoriatic episodes.

NURSING ACTIONS IN VARIOUS SETTINGS

Nursing actions for a client with psoriasis depend on the setting in which care is provided. This section identifies which actions are appropriate in all settings and which pertain to acute care, extended care, or home care.

All settings

• Instruct the client and family on possible side effects of treatment and appropriate actions to take if side effects occur.

• Inform the client that a remission has an unpredictable duration and that spontaneous remissions also may occur. Tell the client to plan on long-term follow-up care.

• Help the client and family to recognize and, when possible, to eliminate factors that may contribute to a flare-up.

• Offer the client support and encouragement during psoriatic flare-ups.

• Notify the physician immediately of any treatment side effects.

• Use gloves and proper handwashing techniques when applying topical lotions and medications.

Acute care
• Protect the client's lesions from bedsheets.
• Teach the client and family about the various treatments used for psoriasis.

Extended care
• Regularly observe the client's skin for outbreaks of psoriasis.
• Provide the client with comfort measures when pain and itching occur.

Home care
• Reinforce correct treatment procedures.

SELECTED REFERENCES
Abel, E., and Farber, E. "Managing the Patient with Psoriasis," *Modern Medicine* 55:82-95, July 1987.

Bates, B. *A Guide to Physical Examination and History Taking,* 4th ed. Philadelphia: J.B. Lippincott Co., 1987.

Berliner, H. "Aging Skin," *AJN* 86(10):1138-41, October 1986.

Diseases, 2nd ed. Springhouse, Pa.: Springhouse Corp., 1987.

Dunn, M.L., et al. "Treatment Options for Psoriasis," *AJN* 88(8):1082-87, August 1988.

Gordon, M. *Manual of Nursing Diagnosis.* New York: McGraw-Hill Book Co., 1985.

Habif, T. *Clinical Dermatology: A Color Guide to Diagnosis and Therapy.* St. Louis: C.V. Mosby Co., 1985.

Macmillan, A.L. "Aging and the Skin," in *Textbook of Geriatric Medicine and Gerontology.* Edited by Brockelhurst, J.C. New York: Churchill Livingstone, 1985.

RESPIRATORY SYSTEM

Pneumonia

Pneumonia is an acute infection of the lower respiratory tract that inflames lung tissue distal to the terminal bronchiolus, alveolar ducts, and alveoli. Elderly clients are especially prone to bronchopneumonia, which affects alveoli in contact with the bronchi. About 20% of elderly clients in an institution acquire pneumonia, compared with 3% in the community. Once treatment has begun, recovery may take up to 14 weeks in elderly clients as opposed to 6 to 8 weeks in younger clients.

Pneumonia and influenza are the fourth leading cause of death in the United States in those over age 65. Bacteremia, which occurs in 15% to 25% of elderly clients, increases the chance of fatality.

ETIOLOGY
Pneumonia may result from a bacterial or nonbacterial infection or from a noninfectious process, such as aspiration or a hypostatic condition. Pneumonia in the elderly client usually results from a bacterial infection. Unlike bacterial pneumonia in younger clients, mixed flora of two or more respiratory pathogens cause a substantial portion of pneumonia cases in elderly clients. *Streptococcus pneumoniae* and *Haemophilus influenzae* are the major bacterial causes of community-acquired pneumonia in elderly clients. Gram-negative bacilli, such as *Streptococcus pneumoniae, Staphylococcus aureus, and Legionella pneumophila,* and anaerobic bacteria are the major causes of infection in hospitalized elderly clients or residents of long-term care facilities. Viral pneumonia may follow acute influenza, and bacterial superinfection may further complicate this illness. Age, chronic illness, debility, immobility, and immunosuppression place a client at risk for developing pneumonia.

HEALTH HISTORY FINDINGS
In a health history interview, the client may report or the nurse may detect many of these findings:
• fever
• lethargy
• cough
• chest pain
• dyspnea
• tachypnea
• sputum production
• dysphagia
• vomiting
• muscle weakness
• decreased ability to ambulate
• confusion
• congestive heart failure
• pulmonary edema
• chronic obstructive pulmonary disease
• influenza

• seizure disorder
• stroke
• multiple myeloma or other cancers
• acquired immunodeficiency syndrome (AIDS)
• recent fall
• recent endotracheal intubation
• use of sedatives, steroids, or immunosuppressant medications
• poor fluid intake
• heavy alcohol or tobacco use
• diminished ability to perform activities of daily living, such as feeding self, dressing, and toileting
• recurrent urinary tract infections

PHYSICAL FINDINGS
In a physical examination, the nurse may detect many of these findings:

Respiratory
• dullness on percussion
• crackles
• rhonchi
• wheezing
• pleural friction rub
• bronchial breath sounds
• blood-flecked or rusty sputum
• increased tactile fremitus
• whispered pectoriloquy
• egophony
• cough with or without sputum production
• tachypnea

Integumentary
• pallor
• cyanosis
• poor skin turgor

Cardiovascular
• tachycardia
• elevated blood pressure

Neurologic
• disorientation
• altered mental status
• stupor
• delirium

DIAGNOSTIC STUDIES
The following studies may be performed to evaluate the client's health status:
• white blood cell (WBC) count—leukocytosis with an increased number of immature WBCs suggests a bacterial etiology

• chest X-ray—shows incomplete consolidation in one or more lobes
• Gram stain and culture—performed on lower respiratory secretions collected by expectoration or nasopharyngeal aspiration to diagnose the causative agent and determine antimicrobial therapy
• blood culture—reveals causative agent in about 20% of clients hospitalized for bacterial pneumonia and indicates the severity of the infection

POTENTIAL COMPLICATIONS
• respiratory failure
• dehydration
• delirium
• malnutrition

Nursing diagnosis: *Ineffective airway clearance related to accumulated lung secretions*

NURSING GOALS: To remove secretions and to promote optimal air movement in and out of the lungs

Signs and symptoms
• increased mental confusion
• increased shortness of breath or rapid respirations
• decreased activity tolerance
• chest pain

Interventions

1. Assess the client's vital signs every 4 hours while the client is awake or as needed.

2. Assess the client for changes in mental status, such as confusion, restlessness, or aggression.

3. Auscultate the client's lungs and assess the need for chest physiotherapy or suctioning. Discuss this with the physician if indicated.

4. Monitor arterial blood gas (ABG) levels as ordered or as indicated by increased dyspnea.

5. Teach the client to perform coughing and deep-breathing exercises every 2 hours.

6. If ordered, teach the client to use an incentive spirometer, and encourage its use every 1 to 2 hours.

7. Obtain a specimen of the client's respiratory secretions by having him inhale deeply and then cough into a sterile collection container. Send the specimen to the laboratory immediately.

8. Assess the client's hydration status.

9. Administer oxygen via nasal cannula as needed and as prescribed by the physician.

10. Reposition the client every 2 hours, keeping the head of the bed elevated. Have the client ambulate as tolerated and according to the plan of care.

Rationales

1. Tachycardia is an early sign of hypoxemia, and rapid, shallow respirations may indicate further hypoxemia. Blood pressure decreases as the disease progresses. Elevated temperature increases the metabolic rate and the need for oxygen.

2. A change in mental status may be a sign of cerebral hypoxia.

3. The client may be unable to cough efficiently and may require aid to clear the airway.

4. ABG results may indicate severe hypoxemia and the need for oxygen therapy.

5. Retained secretions create an oxygen deficit and increase the risk of infection.

6. An incentive spirometer assures deep breathing and can prevent further complications.

7. This method ensures an appropriate specimen for accurate diagnosis. Sending the specimen to the laboratory immediately prevents overgrowth of normal flora.

8. Adequate hydration thins the sputum and facilitates expectoration.

9. Adequate tissue perfusion requires a normal oxygen level.

10. Repositioning minimizes the accumulation of secretions and decreases resistance to airflow. Early ambulation can prevent the hazards of immobility.

11. Use a humidifier, a steam or cool-mist vaporizer, or a pan of water placed on a radiator to add moisture to the air.

11. Increased humidity loosens secretions and relieves coughing and bronchial spasms.

12. Instruct the client to refrain from smoking.

12. Smoking irritates the tracheal lining, increases coughing episodes and inflammation, and inhibits proper gas exchange and ciliary activity.

13. Administer antibiotics as prescribed by the physician.

13. Antibiotics interfere with the replication of bacteria and resolve infection. The physician typically orders broad-spectrum antibiotics first and, once the organism has been identified, orders bacteria-specific drugs.

14. Administer both inhaled and systemic bronchodilators as prescribed by the physician.

14. Both therapies open airways and aid oxygenation.

15. Avoid the use of cough suppressants.

15. A productive cough clears the airway.

16. Avoid the excessive use of sedatives.

16. Depressants can cause confusion, obtundation, inability to cough, and respiratory depression.

OUTCOME CRITERIA
• The client's temperature, pulse rate, and respirations will be normal within 6 hours after instituting antibiotic therapy.
• The client's respiratory function will improve within 3 days, as evidenced by decreased dyspnea and improved airway clearance.

Nursing diagnosis: *Pain related to pleuritic irritation*

NURSING GOAL: To minimize the client's pain during acute illness

Signs and symptoms
• excessive coughing
• pleuritic pain
• splinting on respiration

Interventions

1. Administer mild analgesics, such as acetaminophen, as ordered by the physician.

Rationales

1. Mild analgesics can help alleviate the client's pain, thus obviating the need for splinting on respiration, which would compromise ventilation and inhibit thoracic expansion.

2. Use caution in administering narcotics or sedatives.

2. These medications suppress respirations and coughing.

3. Apply a heating pad or hot packs to the area of chest wall discomfort, as ordered by the physician.

3. Heat reduces inflammation and promotes muscle relaxation.

OUTCOME CRITERION
• The client will be free of pain and discomfort during coughing episodes.

Nursing diagnosis: *Potential for infection related to transmission of bacteria*

NURSING GOAL: To prevent transmission of pneumonia-causing organisms to other body systems or to other persons

Signs and symptoms
- productive cough
- shaking chills
- fever

Interventions

1. Explain to the caregiver the importance of thorough hand washing after completing a task with the client.

2. Teach the client and caregiver how to dispose of sputum and tissues properly.

3. Perform oral hygiene on the client before meals and at bedtime, as needed.

4. Prevent a hospitalized client or one living in an institution from sharing a room with another client.

Rationales

1. Thorough hand washing helps prevent transmission of bacteria.

2. Respiratory secretions carry the bacteria.

3. Frequent oral hygiene helps prevent expectorated organisms from causing oral infections and removes the unpleasant taste and smell of sputum from the client's mouth.

4. Debilitated and immunosuppressed elderly clients have an increased risk of contracting the illness.

OUTCOME CRITERION
- The client and caregiver will follow measures that prevent transmission of the causative organism.

Nursing diagnosis: *Altered nutrition: less than body requirements, related to loss of appetite*

NURSING GOAL: To provide the client with adequate nutrition and hydration

Signs and symptoms
- nausea
- malaise
- decreased body weight
- loss of appetite

Interventions

1. Maintain accurate fluid intake and output records.

2. Encourage the client to drink eight to twelve 8-oz glasses (2,000 to 3,000 ml) of fluid by 6 p.m. daily.

3. Avoid administering oral fluids to an unconscious or semiconscious client.

4. Weigh the client at the same time and on the same scale every day.

5. Offer the client small, frequent meals and supplemental snacks. Be sure his diet consists of nutritious foods he can digest easily.

6. Assist the client with meal selection, stressing the need for high-protein, high-carbohydrate foods.

Rationales

1. Maintaining a positive fluid balance prevents dehydration.

2. Adequate hydration keeps mucus thin and facilitates expectoration. Stopping fluid intake at 6 p.m. helps prevent nocturia.

3. Administering oral fluids to an unconscious or semi-conscious client could cause aspiration pneumonia.

4. Accurate measurement of the client's weight will reflect his nutritional needs.

5. The client may tolerate small, frequent meals more easily than two or three larger meals. Digestion requires a tremendous amount of oxygen.

6. Adequate nutrition enables the body to combat disease.

IMMUNIZATIONS AND VACCINATIONS IN THE ELDERLY CLIENT

	Pneumococcal vaccination	Influenza vaccination	Diphtheria and tetanus toxoid
Target population	• Over age 60 • Chronic disease • Those entering long-term care facilities	• Over age 65 • Presence of chronic disease	• Over age 60
Rationale	• The risk of pneumococcal pneumonia increases directly with age • Institutionalization increases the risk	• Although incidence is higher in younger populations, elderly clients have greater morbidity and mortality because of chronic disease, institutionalization, and decreased mobility	• Many elderly clients are unsure of their immunization status • Many elderly clients attended school before immunizations were mandatory; they are less likely to have had initial immunization and booster follow-ups
Recommended dosage and route	• 23-valent vaccine • 0.5 ml I.M. or S.C. • Administer once	• Inactivated virus prepared according to prevalent strains • 0.5 ml I.M. (the deltoid muscle is the recommended site)	• If no prior immunization, 0.5 ml I.M. • Diphtheria and tetanus toxoid I.M., two doses 2 months apart, then third dose 6 to 12 months later • Booster shot, 0.5 ml I.M. every 10 years
Cost	• $5.00 per vaccine	• $5.50 to $10.50 per immunization	• Approximately $2.00 per vaccine
Side effects	• Soreness at site, erythema • Systemic symptoms (malaise, low-grade fever); usually mild hypersensitivity	• Soreness at site for 1 to 2 days • Rare flulike syndrome • Immediate allergic response may be delayed occasionally in elderly clients	• Local reactions (soreness, erythema)
Contraindications	• Allergy to any component of the vaccine	• Allergy to egg protein, chicken • Do not give if person has fever, or cold symptoms; wait until symptoms subside, then adminster	• History of allergic reaction to the vaccine in the past

Nursing implications	• Give influenza vaccine and pneumococcal injection in opposite arms if administering at the same time
	• For all immunizations:
	  —Make sure documentation on the client's record is accurate and current concerning the date administered and the type and dosage of immunization
	  —Include client and family teaching in long-term care, primary care and acute hospital visits
	  —Follow up on those who refuse
		• Never use previous year's vaccine.
		• Antibodies take approximately 2 weeks to form; be aware that clients may become infected during that period
		• See "Influenza," pages 63 to 65 regarding the use of amantadine
			• Assess risk during evaluation of all wounds; clients with neglected wounds or those at high risk of tetanus may need tetanus immune globulin before diphtheria and tetanus toxoid

---

OUTCOME CRITERION
• The client will maintain a stable body weight appropriate for his age and height.

NURSING ACTIONS IN VARIOUS SETTINGS
Nursing actions for a client with pneumonia depend on the setting in which care is provided. This section identifies which actions are appropriate in all settings and which pertain to acute care, extended care, or home care.

All settings
• Inform the client and caregiver about the course of pneumonia and the extended recovery period typical for elderly clients.
• Teach the client and caregiver the infection control measures to follow during acute illness.
• Immunize a client at high risk for pneumonia with pneumococcal vaccine. (See *Immunizations and vaccinations in the elderly client.*)
• Before starting antibiotic therapy, question the client and caregiver about possible allergies. After starting therapy, assess the client for side effects.

Acute care
• Have a dietitian evaluate the client.
• Assess the client's home to determine whether he will need supervision by a visiting nurse agency.
• Institute measures to prevent aspiration.

Extended care
• Feed the client slowly, and position him correctly after feeding.
• If the client has a nasogastric tube, check its placement before each feeding to prevent aspiration.

Home care
• Assess the client's home for factors that may predispose him to incomplete recovery or relapse, such as inadequate heat, refrigeration, or help with activities of daily living.

SELECTED REFERENCES
Andres, R., et al. *Principles of Geriatric Medicine.* New York: McGraw-Hill Book Co., 1985.
Berk, S., and Alvarez, S. "Vaccinating the Elderly: Recommendations and Rationales," *Geriatrics* 41(1):79, January 1986.
Carnevali, D. *Nursing Management for the Elderly.* Philadelphia: J.B. Lippincott Co., 1986.
Esberger, K.K., and Hughes, S.T. *Nursing Care of the Aged.* Norwalk, Conn.: Appleton & Lange, 1989.
Glickman, R.A. "Community-Acquired Pneumonia in the Geriatric Patient," *Hospital Practice* 20(3):57, March 1985.
Niederman, M., and Fein, A. "Pneumonia in the Elderly," *Geriatric Clinics of North America* 2(2):241-59, May 1986.
Musher, D.M. "A Rational Approach to Treating Pneumonia in the Elderly," *Modern Medicine* 55:108-18, March 1987.
Smith, I.M. "Pneumonia and the Aging Lung," in *Relations Between Normal Aging and Disease.* Edited by Johnson, H.A. New York: Raven Press, 1985.

Chronic Obstructive Pulmonary Disease

Chronic obstructive pulmonary disease (COPD) is a complex syndrome of decreased pulmonary function that includes emphysema, asthma, and chronic bronchitis. Irreversible destruction of the distal airspace (as in emphysema), bronchial inflammation that results in sputum production (as in bronchitis), and hyperactivity of the tracheal and bronchial smooth muscle to various stimuli (as in asthma) characterize COPD. These factors persistently obstruct airflow in the bronchial tree. Because of its slowly progressive nature, COPD presents special challenges to the client and caregiver because the disability necessitates life-style and functional adaptation.

ETIOLOGY
Although primarily caused by cigarette smoking, COPD may also result from occupational exposure to respiratory irritants, air pollution, and allergies. Age-related changes of the respiratory system (such as decreased lung elasticity, alveolar duct enlargement, increased residual volume, and decreased vital capacity) mimic the abnormalities of COPD; whether these age-related changes increase an individual's susceptibility to COPD is uncertain. A viral or bacterial infection can precipitate exacerbations of COPD.

HEALTH HISTORY FINDINGS
In a health history interview, the client may report or the nurse may detect many of these findings:
• shortness of breath, first noticeable with exertion
• dyspnea
• chronic cough and sputum production, especially in the morning
• activity intolerance
• sleep disturbance
• anorexia
• congestive heart failure
• cor pulmonale
• bronchitis
• history of respiratory infections
• use of corticosteroids, bronchodilators, tranquilizers, or expectorants
• heavy tobacco or alcohol use
• occupational exposure to respiratory irritants (such as asbestos)
• exposure to air pollution
• progressive decline in activities of daily living (ADLs)
• impotence
• decreased libido
• weight loss
• fatigue
• apprehension and anxiety
• alpha$_1$-antitrypsin deficiency (inherited form of emphysema)

PHYSICAL FINDINGS
In a physical examination, the nurse may detect many of these findings:

Respiratory
• barrel chest
• diaphragmatic flattening and decreased movement
• orthopnea
• bibasilar crackles
• hyperresonance
• pursed-lip breathing
• tachypnea
• use of accessory respiratory muscles and retraction of interspaces
• decreased breath sounds
• wheezes

Integumentary
• pallor
• clubbing of the nails

Cardiovascular
• distant heart sounds
• atrial fibrillation
• jugular vein distention
• peripheral edema

Psychological
• denial
• anger
• depression
• emotional lability

Other
• hepatomegaly

DIAGNOSTIC STUDIES
The following studies may be performed to evaluate the client's health status:
• chest X-ray—normal in earlier stages but shows a low, flat diaphragm, small midlung vessels, bullae, and long, narrow heart shadow in later stages
• pulmonary function testing (spirometry)—to distinguish between restrictive and obstructive disease, determines severity of ventilatory impairment, and demonstrates the client's response to bronchodilator therapy
• arterial blood gas analysis—to demonstrate the need for oxygen therapy
• sputum analysis—to detect infection
• theophylline level—an elevated level may indicate incorrect drug administration or dosage

POTENTIAL COMPLICATIONS
• respiratory infection
• malnutrition
• immobility
• depression
• decreased activity

Nursing diagnosis: *Ineffective breathing pattern related to persistent airflow obstruction of the bronchial tree*

NURSING GOALS: To promote optimum breathing and to prevent respiratory infection

Signs and symptoms
• anxiety
• restlessness or confusion
• shortness of breath
• rapid respirations
• abrupt decrease in activity tolerance
• increased sputum production or change in color or character of sputum

Interventions

1. Assess the client for dyspnea. Teach him to sit up and lean forward in a high-backed chair or in a bed with the head elevated (semi-Fowler's to high-Fowler's position) when dyspnea occurs. If he cannot assume this position, tell him to assume the position he finds best for breathing. Include the caregiver in your instruction.

2. Teach the client coughing and deep-breathing exercises and postural drainage and percussion, as prescribed by the physician and as tolerated by the client.

3. Encourage the client to drink eight to twelve 8-oz glasses (2,000 to 3,000 ml) of fluid daily.

4. Administer low-flow oxygen therapy with humidification as ordered.

5. Administer aerosol or oral bronchodilators, with or without corticosteroids, as prescribed.

6. Carefully administer narcotics as ordered.

7. Teach the client relaxation techniques to use at bedtime to avoid using sedatives or hypnotics.

Rationales

1. The described position increases diaphragmatic excursion and reduces the use of accessory muscles. Discomfort or disability may prevent the client from using this position, however, and the caregiver should not try to make him move.

2. Retained secretions increase the client's oxygen deficit and risk of infection. These measures mobilize secretions and reduce the risk of airway obstruction by mucus or mucus plugs.

3. Fluids help maintain proper hydration, liquefy lung secretions, and decrease the effort required to expectorate.

4. High levels of oxygen can depress the respiratory stimulus in the brain, which reduces respiration and promotes carbon dioxide retention.

5. Bronchodilators (sympathomimetics and xanthines) stimulate production of, or prevent destruction of, cyclic adenosine monophosphate (3′,5′-AMP), thereby promoting bronchodilation.

6. Narcotics relieve breathlessness by reducing anxiety, decreasing awareness of muscle exertion, suppressing ventilatory drive (thus lowering demand on the respiratory muscles), and easing vascular resistance (thus reducing pulmonary edema). However, frequent narcotic use can further depress the respiratory center of the elderly client.

7. Not only do relaxation techniques promote sleep and minimize oxygen demands, but sleeping medications may depress respirations.

8. Reduce or eliminate environmental irritants by encouraging the client to stop smoking and by instructing the caregiver not to smoke or use hair spray, deodorant, room fresheners, or strong fragrances near the client.

9. Teach the caregiver that someone must always be available to monitor the client's condition.

8. Inhaled tobacco smoke causes mucous gland hypertrophy, chronic inflammatory changes, and permanent loss of cilia. Numerous environmental substances and sprays can irritate the airway of a client with COPD and exacerbate the problem.

9. Constant monitoring is necessary to detect and respond to early indications of breathlessness.

OUTCOME CRITERION
• The client will maintain adequate breathing patterns, as evidenced by normal temperature, respiration, pulse rate, and mentation.

Nursing diagnosis: *Potential activity intolerance related to fatigue and dyspnea*

NURSING GOALS: To reduce factors that fatigue the client, to increase his activity tolerance and independence, and to develop an exercise program tailored to his needs and limitations

Signs and symptoms
• fatigue or drowsiness during the day
• increased dyspnea on exertion
• breathlessness
• muscle atrophy
• decreased normal activity

Interventions

1. Teach the client diaphragmatic breathing and pursed-lip breathing.

2. Assess the client's exercise tolerance by observing the activities he can and cannot tolerate and the breathing patterns and reactions he displays at the onset of dyspnea.

3. Caution the client to expect some breathlessness with exercise, and explain that this is normal and harmless.

4. Plan an individualized aerobic exercise program according to the client's target pulse rate.

5. Assess the need for inhaled bronchodilators before exercise and the use of oxygen during exercise. Discuss your findings with the physician.

6. Encourage the client to perform as many ADLs as he can tolerate, and teach him appropriate times to inhale and exhale when carrying out these tasks. For example, explain that he should inhale, bend down from a sitting position, and then exhale through pursed lips while tying a shoe, and tell him to inhale while pulling a vacuum cleaner toward him and to exhale while pushing it away. (For more information and illustrations of these techniques to use during instruction, contact your local chapter of the American Lung Association.)

Rationales

1. These breathing patterns can help the client gain control when distressed or while exercising.

2. A client with respiratory disease usually must limit his activity and, as a result, loses muscle mass and physical endurance. Thus, he may experience dyspnea on the slightest exertion.

3. A client with respiratory disease may panic at the first sign of dyspnea.

4. Pulse rate is a much better guide than dyspnea for evaluating the amount of energy expended during exercise.

5. Oxygen supply to the tissues may become inadequate during increased physical demands.

6. These methods help prevent breath holding and promote efficient use of respiratory muscles. They also permit the client to perform ADLs more easily, thus increasing his independence and enhancing his quality of life.

Nursing diagnosis: *Altered nutrition: less than body requirements, related to loss of appetite*

NURSING GOAL: To provide nutrition and hydration adequate for maintaining a stable body weight

Signs and symptoms
• nausea
• malaise
• decreased body weight
• loss of appetite

Interventions	Rationales
1. Monitor the client's fluid intake and output.	1. Maintaining a positive fluid balance prevents dehydration.
2. Help the client select meals high in protein and carbohydrates while eliminating gas-producing foods.	2. The client's increased respiratory needs require increased caloric consumption; foods high in protein and carbohydrates help meet daily nutritional needs and prevent depletion of body stores. Abdominal distention can cause diaphragmatic compression and increase the sensation of shortness of breath.
3. Encourage the client to eat small, frequent meals and supplemental snacks.	3. Large meals may increase pressure on the diaphragm and increase the work required to breathe. If the client tolerates smaller meals and snacks more easily, his appetite may improve.
4. Caution the client to avoid dairy products, spicy foods, and alcohol.	4. These substances may increase bronchospasm and sputum production.
5. Provide a quiet, calm environment during the meal.	5. A quiet, relaxed atmosphere helps minimize the effort needed to breathe while eating.

Nursing diagnosis: *Ineffective individual coping related to chronic respiratory disease*

NURSING GOAL: To provide the client with support and adaptive coping measures

Signs and symptoms
• insomnia
• preoccupation with self
• anorexia
• denial
• depression

Interventions

1. Assess the client's past and present coping skills.

2. Encourage the client to develop effective problem-solving and stress-reducing techniques, and assist him as needed.

3. Explain the disease and treatment plan to the client and family.

4. Assess the need for other psychosocial interventions, and refer the client to appropriate professionals, such as a social worker, a psychiatrist, or a psychologist.

Rationales

1. Identifying the client's strengths and functional behaviors assists the nurse in understanding his ability to comply with treatment.

2. This action not only promotes responsibility for goal setting and health maintenance but also may increase the client's self-esteem and compliance.

3. A thorough understanding of the disease and planned treatments may alleviate their fears and promote their participation in the treatment plan.

4. The scope of the client's needs may extend beyond the nurse's capabilities.

OUTCOME CRITERION
• The client will adapt to respiratory disease, as evidenced by exhibiting less anxiety during dyspneic episodes, using medications properly, and following a planned exercise program.

NURSING ACTIONS IN VARIOUS SETTINGS
Nursing actions for a client with COPD depend on the setting in which care is provided. This section identifies which actions are appropriate in all settings and which pertain to acute care, extended care, or home care.

All settings
• Teach the client and caregiver about COPD as a chronic disease, its management, and its impact on the client's life-style.
• Encourage the client and caregiver to participate actively in health maintenance and preventive care behaviors.
• Recommend to the client and family that he receive annual influenza and pneumococcal vaccines.

Acute care
• Assess the client for signs and symptoms of acute illness, such as respiratory infections or medication interactions.
• Determine the need for a multidisciplinary assessment, including a dietitian, a social worker, and an occupational therapist.
• Encourage self-care activities as tolerated in preparation for discharge.
• Refer the client to a visiting nurse agency if indicated.

Extended care
• Teach caregivers and housekeeping staff to prevent lung irritants, such as sprays, dust, and cold air, from entering the client's room.
• Foster an environment that enhances appropriately paced activities.
• Encourage the client to socialize with others.

• Have oxygen available in the client's room.

Home care
• Assess the client's home for factors that may predispose him to incomplete recovery or relapse, such as inadequate heat, refrigeration, or help with ADLs.
• Encourage socialization with and support from other elderly adults through senior citizen centers and nutrition sites.
• Teach the client and caregiver the signs and symptoms of acute illness so that they can initiate early intervention.
• Teach the client and caregiver how to use, care for, and clean necessary respiratory equipment.
• Review with the client and caregiver the principles of using oxygen safely.

SELECTED REFERENCES

Carnevali, D. *Nursing Management for the Elderly.* Philadelphia: J.B. Lippincott Co., 1986.

DeVito, A.J., and Kleven, M. "Dyspnea," *RN* 40-46, June 1987.

Eliopoules, C. *A Guide to the Nursing of the Aging.* Baltimore: Williams & Wilkins, 1987.

Gift, A.G., et al. "Psychologic and Physiologic Factors Related to Dyspnea in Subjects with Chronic Obstructive Pulmonary Disease," *Heart & Lung* 15(6):595-601, November 1986.

Hoffman, L.A. "Home Oxygen Transtrachial and Other Options," *RN,* 464-69, April 1988.

Mahler, D., et al. "Chronic Obstructive Pulmonary Disease," *Clinics in Geriatric Medicine* 2(2):285-307, May 1986.

Rerchel, W. *Clinical Aspects of Aging.* Baltimore: Williams & Wilkins, 1989.

RESPIRATORY SYSTEM

Influenza

Influenza (flu) is an acute infection that may produce an abrupt onset of generalized symptoms, such as headache, weakness, myalgia, fever, and anorexia, or specific manifestations of lower respiratory tract involvement, such as cough, dyspnea, wheezing, and hemoptysis. Elderly clients have a four-times greater risk of acquiring this infection than persons under age 40. In addition, elderly clients have an increased risk of morbidity and mortality from influenza. The major complications of influenza are viral pneumonia and bronchitis, both of which may be complicated by a superimposed bacterial infection.

ETIOLOGY
A ribonucleic acid virus of either Type A or B causes influenza, with Type A being the more serious. Most infections occur between the months of October and April. The incubation period is 2 to 4 days. Yearly immunizations can decrease the severity of influenza in the elderly client (see *Immunizations and vaccinations in the elderly client*, page 56).

HEALTH HISTORY FINDINGS
In a health history interview, the client may report or the nurse may detect many of these findings:
• weakness
• headache
• myalgia
• fever
• anorexia
• chills
• malaise
• sore throat
• cough
• dyspnea
• hemoptysis
• weight loss
• confusion
• disorientation
• viral pneumonia

• cardiac disease
• multiple myeloma or other cancers
• use of steroids or immunosuppressant medications
• recent exposure to persons with influenza
• inability to perform activities of daily living

PHYSICAL FINDINGS
In a physical examination, the nurse may detect many of these findings:

Respiratory
• wheezing
• decreased breath sounds in lower bases
• tachypnea

Cardiovascular
• tachycardia

Musculoskeletal
• nonspecific muscular pain
• generalized weakness

DIAGNOSTIC STUDIES
The following studies may be performed to evaluate the client's health status:
• chest X-ray—may be clear or show evidence of viral pneumonia
• sputum culture—collected to diagnose the etiologic agent and select antimicrobial therapy
• serologic studies using hemagglutination-inhibiting antibody and cultures—can confirm the presence of influenza virus
• white blood cell count—may show leukocytosis and an increased number of lymphocytes

POTENTIAL COMPLICATIONS
• viral or bacterial pneumonia
• dehydration
• delirium

Nursing diagnosis: *Ineffective breathing pattern related to respiratory infection*

NURSING GOALS: To promote an optimum breathing pattern and to prevent respiratory infection

Signs and symptoms
• mental confusion
• shortness of breath
• rapid respirations
• decreased activity tolerance
• increased sputum production
• change in color or character of sputum

Interventions

1. Assess vital signs every 4 hours while the client is awake.

2. Teach the client coughing and deep-breathing exercises.

3. Reposition the client every 2 to 4 hours, and elevate the head of the bed or place two pillows under the client's upper body.

4. Encourage the client to drink at least eight 8-oz glasses (2,000 ml) of fluid daily.

5. Have the client ambulate at least twice a day as soon as his medical condition permits.

6. Encourage rest periods throughout the day.

7. Administer amantadine as needed and prescribed by the physician.

Rationales

1. Measuring and recording vital signs helps the nurse determine the severity of the infection.

2. Retained secretions exacerbate the oxygen deficit and increase the risk of infection.

3. Proper positioning prevents the accumulation of secretions and decreases the resistance to airflow.

4. Oral fluids liquefy lung secretions and decrease the effort necessary to expel sputum.

5. Ambulation decreases the pooling of secretions and helps prevent more serious respiratory distress.

6. Viral infections decrease energy.

7. Amantadine, an antiviral agent, is effective against Type A influenza. By blocking viral replication and the release of nucleic acids, amantadine helps prevent respiratory complications and reduces symptoms.

OUTCOME CRITERION
• The client will maintain an effective breathing pattern, as evidenced by productive coughing and no shortness of breath.

Nursing diagnosis: *Anxiety related to fatigue and weakness*

NURSING GOAL: To help the client manage internal or external stressors, such as a change in physical environment, sensory overstimulation, and acute illness

Signs and symptoms
• altered mental status
• restlessness
• insomnia
• decreased appetite

Interventions

1. Assess the client's mentation, and notify the physician of any change in mental status.

2. Provide nursing care in a calm, reassuring manner.

3. Encourage the client to participate in activities of daily living (ADLs).

Rationales

1. A change in mental status, such as lethargy or agitation, may indicate worsening of the infection or a physiologic change, such as decreased respirations.

2. A perceived emotional or physical threat may increase the client's anxiety.

3. Participating in ADLs helps the client maintain activity tolerance, increases independence and self-worth, and alleviates anxiety.

OUTCOME CRITERION
• The client will be less anxious as physical well-being improves.

NURSING ACTIONS IN VARIOUS SETTINGS

Nursing actions for a client with influenza depend on the setting in which care is provided. This section identifies which actions are appropriate in all settings and which pertain to acute care, extended care, or home care.

All settings

• Instruct the client and caregiver about the physiology and course of influenza infections.
• Teach the client and caregiver about infection control during acute illness, and recommend preventive measures.
• Teach the client and family about the need for annual influenza vaccinations.

Acute care

• Ensure that the client avoids contact with other clients who are immunosuppressed or who have a debilitating disease.
• Follow proper hand-washing techniques.
• Teach the client to cover the mouth during coughing and to dispose of secretions in tissues.
• Refer the client to a visiting nursing agency for additional supervision.

Extended care

• During acute illness, confine the client to one room to avoid cross-contamination.
• Follow proper hand-washing techniques.

Home care

• Assess the home for factors that may predispose the client to an incomplete recovery or a relapse, such as inadequate heat, refrigeration, or help with ADLs.

SELECTED REFERENCES

Andres, R., et al. *Principles of Geriatric Medicine.* New York: McGraw-Hill Book Co., 1985.

Berk, S., and Alvarez, S. "Vaccinating the Elderly: Recommendations and Rationale," *Geriatrics* 41(1):79, January 1986.

Bolan, G., et al. "Pneumococcal Vaccine Efficacy in Selected Populations in the United States," *Annals of Internal Medicine* 104:1-6, January 1986.

Niederman, M., and Fein, A. "Pneumonia in the Elderly," *Clinic in Geriatric Medicine* 2(2):258-59, May 1986.

"Old and at Risk for Tetanus," *Emergency Medicine* 17(13):61, July 1985.

"Prevention and Control of Influenza," *Morbidity and Mortality Weekly Report* 35(20):317-325, May 23, 1986 (U.S. Dept. Health & Human Services, Public Health Service)

Thompson, K. "Flu: How to Protect Your High-Risk Patients," *RN* 20-23, November 1985.

Tuberculosis

Tuberculosis (TB) remains a significant health problem with 28,000 new cases developing annually in the United States. The disease has a slowly progressive onset with vague symptoms, such as malaise, weight loss, and anorexia. While TB commonly affects the lungs, it can affect the kidneys, bones and joints, and the brain. In addition, in miliary TB, the bacteria disseminate throughout the bloodstream. Overall, the incidence of and the mortality rates for TB have declined since the early 1900s. However, because many elderly clients became infected before or during the early 1900s, reactivation of dormant infections in those individuals has led to an increased number of new cases in elderly clients. The single largest group with TB in the United States are individuals over age 65; the incidence is four times higher among residents of nursing homes than among residents of the community.

ETIOLOGY

Mycobacterium tuberculosis, the tubercle bacillus, causes the TB infection. The cough or sneeze of an infected individual transmits the spore-forming organism by airborne droplet nuclei. The danger of transmission directly relates to the number of organisms infecting the respiratory secretions. The client with a high concentration of organisms is very infectious. The disease incubates for 2 to 10 weeks. After initiation of antituberculosis medications, the client's infectiousness drops rapidly until, after 10 to 14 days of proper drug administration, the client becomes noninfectious. Predisposing factors include chronic disease, age-related immune system dysfunction, poor nutrition, and institutionalization.

HEALTH HISTORY FINDINGS

In a health history interview, the client may report or the nurse may detect many of these findings:
• insidious, vague decline in functional status
• weight loss
• anorexia
• malaise
• fatigue
• cough
• hemoptysis
• shortness of breath
• pleuritic chest pain
• tachycardia
• indigestion
• behavioral changes, such as confusion, agitation, or hostility

• confusion
• disorientation
• depression
• history of TB, severe respiratory infections, thoracic surgery, long-term steroid therapy, or radiation therapy
• immunologic disease
• silicosis
• poor fluid intake
• malnutrition

PHYSICAL FINDINGS

In a physical examination, the nurse may detect many of these findings:

Respiratory
• crackles at apices
• pleuritic chest pain
• purulent, foul-smelling sputum
• tachypnea

Cardiovascular
• tachycardia

Neurologic
• change in mentation from previous baseline evaluation
• depression

Other
• temperature above 100° F (37.8° C)
• inflamed, painful lymph nodes

DIAGNOSTIC STUDIES

The following studies may be performed to evaluate the client's health status:
• purified protein derivative (PPD) test—a positive result indicates that the primary immune response has occurred (not that the disease is active)
• chest X-ray—may show patchy infiltrates in apices and posterior lung segments; consolidation suggests tuberculous pneumonia
• specimen cultures and stains—to identify the presence of the tubercle bacilli and isolate the *M. tuberculosis* organism; results take up to 6 weeks because of the slow growth of the TB bacteria

POTENTIAL COMPLICATIONS
• respiratory failure
• transmission to others
• nutritional deficit
• decreased functional status

Nursing diagnosis: *Ineffective breathing pattern related to secretions from pulmonary infection*

NURSING GOAL: To keep the client's respiratory status at an optimum level by removing secretions, keeping the client well oxygenated, treating the infection, and being alert for changes that need additional treatment

Signs and symptoms
- increased shortness of breath and dyspnea
- pleuritic chest pain
- cough
- increased secretions and hemoptysis
- fever
- tachycardia

Interventions

1. Assess vital signs and auscultate the client's lungs every 4 hours while the client is awake.

2. Teach the client to turn, cough, and deep-breathe every 2 to 4 hours while awake.

3. Encourage the client to use a nasal cannula for oxygen as ordered and as needed.

4. Instruct the client to drink eight to twelve 8-oz glasses (2,000 to 3,000 ml) of fluid daily if tolerated.

5. Collect specimens and cultures as necessary.

6. Administer anti-TB medications as ordered.

7. Teach the client and caregiver about the administration of anti-TB medications, including the dosage, frequency, and length of treatment.

8. Teach the client about the side effects of anti-TB medications.

9. Advise the client receiving isoniazid (INH) therapy to avoid using alcohol.

10. Assess the client closely for compliance with the drug regimen.

Rationales

1. Assessment findings will alert the nurse to changes or complications.

2. Frequent coughing and movement prevent the accumulation of secretions.

3. Oxygen aids in maintaining adequate tissue perfusion.

4. Adequate hydration keeps secretions moist and facilitates expectoration.

5. Cultures will identify the infecting organism.

6. The appropriate medications treat the disease and decrease infectiousness.

7. After the initial treatment phase, the client must continue medication for at least 6 months after having a negative sputum culture.

8. All of the anti-TB drugs may have significant toxic effects, especially in the elderly client with impaired hepatic and renal function.

9. Using alcohol while on INH therapy increases the risk of liver complications.

10. Long-term adherence to the drug regimen is essential to cure the disease.

OUTCOME CRITERION
- The client will be afebrile and less dyspneic and will have increased physical well-being within 1 week after starting anti-TB therapy.

Nursing diagnosis: *Potential for infection (transmission to others) related to communicability of the disease*

NURSING GOAL: To prevent the spread of TB to health care workers and family members

Signs and symptoms
• cough
• purulent sputum
• fever
• chills

Interventions

1. Place the client on respiratory isolation, which includes a private room, with the door kept closed, ultraviolet light, and noncirculated air.

2. Teach the client to turn away when coughing, to cough into tissues, and to properly dispose of used tissues.

3. Have the client wear a mask when leaving the room for procedures if he cannot follow proper hygiene procedures.

4. Keep the client away from infants and young children during the infectious period.

5. Assess the client for complications related to bed rest or isolation, including constipation, pressure sores, a decline in functional or mental status, and social isolation. Use nursing measures in collaboration with the medical regimen to treat such complications as necessary.

Rationales

1. The disease travels through the air; this system ensures that air from the client's room will not circulate throughout the hospital.

2. Good hygiene helps avoid transmission of the TB infection to others.

3. Using a mask will help prevent transmission of the disease during the infectious period in the case of a demented client or a client with acute mental status changes who cannot follow directions.

4. Infants and young children are very susceptible to the disease.

5. Complications commonly occur when the client is isolated and on prolonged bed rest. The nurse should recognize the potential for complications and institute measures to prevent them or decrease their severity.

OUTCOME CRITERION
• TB will not be transmitted to others.

Nursing diagnosis: *Altered nutrition: less than body requirements, related to inability to feed self because of fatigue*

NURSING GOALS: To prevent further weight loss and to optimize nutritional status

Signs and symptoms
• weight loss
• muscle wasting
• anorexia
• increased fatigue
• inability to feed self because of weakness

Interventions

1. Assess the client's weight on the same scale at the same time every day during the early stages of the disease, decreasing to weekly or biweekly as indicated.

2. Assess the client's blood study results, such as electrolyte, blood urea nitrogen, and albumin levels.

3. Assist the client with meals as necessary.

Rationales

1. The client's weight reflects the client's nutritional status.

2. The physician may order blood studies to assess the client's nutritional status.

3. The client may be too weak to eat independently, and encouragement and assistance may be necessary to achieve proper caloric intake.

4. Teach the client to eat a high-protein, high-calorie diet with supplemental snacks as needed.

4. The client needs extra calories and optimum nutrition to combat the effects of the disease: anorexia, malaise, and increased metabolic requirements.

5. Consult a dietitian as needed.

5. The dietitian may be able to assist by following calorie counts, helping the client with food selection, and providing favorite foods for the client.

OUTCOME CRITERION
• The client will increase food intake and have no further weight loss.

Nursing diagnosis: *Potential activity intolerance related to weakness*

NURSING GOALS: To promote an optimum level of functioning and to allow for rest periods

Signs and symptoms
• decreased activity
• decreased ability to perform usual activities of daily living (ADLs)
• need for increased rest periods

Interventions

1. Assess the client upon admission and then routinely during the course of the illness.

2. Schedule rest and exercise periods as tolerated by the client.

3. Teach the bedridden client passive and active range-of-motion exercises.

4. Consult with a physical or occupational therapist as needed.

Rationales

1. An initial objective assessment of the client's ability to function provides a baseline for later comparison to measure progress or decline.

2. Although the disease will weaken the client, the client must maintain physical function. Progressive increases in exercise time will optimize function.

3. Exercises prevent contractures and disabilities caused by immobility.

4. These therapists can assist with assessment, management, and plans for home care.

OUTCOME CRITERION
• The client will regain functional abilities within 1 week of therapy.

Nursing diagnosis: *Ineffective individual coping related to dependent role*

NURSING GOALS: To provide family education and to assist the client in adapting to new illness, changes in self-concept, and the environment

Signs and symptoms
• depression
• mental status changes
• noncompliance with treatment
• denial
• decreased communication

Interventions

1. Assess the client for changes in behavior and mental status, and notify the physician if indicated.

Rationales

1. Changes may indicate worsening of the disease process, depression, or complications that need attention.

2. Encourage the client and caregiver to express their concerns and fears about TB.

2. The client may view the diagnosis as a stigma and feel like an outcast because, in the past, physicians placed clients with TB in sanatoriums or separated them from family and friends.

3. Explain the disease to the client and the client's family.

3. Education will correct misinformed beliefs and decrease anxiety.

4. Encourage the client to participate in ADLs as tolerated.

4. Independence may increase the client's sense of self-worth and help decrease anxiety.

5. Review medications with the client and family, stress the importance of maintaining long-term therapy, and, after discharge, question the client about medication compliance.

5. Since drug therapy lasts 9 months to 1 year, noncompliance is a major problem. Education and follow-up will uncover needs and help decrease non-compliance.

6. Consult an occupational therapist as necessary.

6. Diversional activities may help the client socialize and achieve independence.

OUTCOME CRITERION
• The client will adapt to the illness and become more independent, as evidenced by participation in ADLs and compliance with treatment.

NURSING ACTIONS IN VARIOUS SETTINGS
Nursing actions for a client with tuberculosis depend on the setting in which care is provided. This section identifies which actions are appropriate in all settings and which pertain to acute care, extended care, or home care.

All settings
• Explain the disease in understandable terms.
• Teach the client to avoid crowds and individuals with upper respiratory infections.
• Stress the importance of follow-up care.
• Teach the client and caregiver the symptoms to report, such as hemoptysis, dyspnea, chest pain, and drug reactions.
• Encourage the client to check with the nurse before using over-the-counter medications.
• Teach the client and family that the disease is not contagious after it becomes encapsulated.
• Consult a visiting nurse as necessary.

Acute care
• Avoid contact with clients who are immunosuppressed or who have a debilitating disease.
• Follow isolation techniques until the client has received 10 to 14 days of medication.
• Have the nursing staff and physical and occupational therapists assist the client with maintaining function while the client is acutely ill.
• Institute teaching and consult a visiting nurse at the time of discharge.

Extended care
• Administer PPD to all new admissions and employees. Document PPD status in an accessible location.
• Follow good hand-washing techniques.
• Isolate clients as necessary. Be prepared to transfer a client to an acute-care setting if complications occur.

Home care
• Monitor compliance with medications at each visit, and reinforce its importance as necessary.
• Refer the client to a social worker if medication expense affects compliance.
• Monitor the client for side effects of medications, and reinforce the importance of not drinking alcohol during administration of isoniazid or rifampin.
• If necessary, remind the client and family to avoid unpasteurized dairy products.

SELECTED REFERENCES
Esberger, K.K., and Hughes, S.T. *Nursing Care of the Aged.* Norwalk, Conn.: Appleton & Lange, 1989.
Lancaster, E. "Tuberculosis on the Rise," *AJN* 485, April 1988.
Nagami, P., and Yoshikawa, T. "Tuberculosis in the Geriatric Patient," *Journal of the American Geriatrics Society* 31(6):356-62, June 1983.
Norman, D., et al. "Infections in the Nursing Home," *Journal of the American Geriatrics Society* 35(8):798-805, August 1987.
Snukst-Torbeck, G., et al. "Treatment of Tuberculosis in a Nurse-Managed Clinic," *Heart and Lung* 16(1):30-33, January 1987.
Stead, W., and Dutt, A. "The Changing Picture in Tuberculosis," in *Principles of Geriatric Medicine.* Edited by Andres, R., et al. New York: McGraw-Hill Book Co., 1985.

CARDIOVASCULAR SYSTEM

Angina Pectoris

Angina pectoris, a manifestation of coronary artery disease (CAD), often appears in elderly clients as a presenting symptom. CAD is the most common cause of hospitalization and death among elderly clients. Transient cardiac pain, which characterizes angina, results from an insufficient supply of oxygen to the heart (ischemia). The pressurelike pain usually occurs retrosternally and may radiate, with the location varying with the client. Angina typically occurs with exertion and resolves with rest or nitrates. The relationship of symptoms to exertion is one of the most important aspects in diagnosing angina.

Many elderly clients do not present with classic angina symptoms, making diagnosis difficult. Elderly clients may not complain of chest pain at all and may instead complain of shortness of breath, indigestion, other gastrointestinal complaints, vague paresthesia, numbness in the chest or upper arms, jaw pain, dizziness, confusion, diaphoresis, cold and clammy hands, or nausea and vomiting. Diminished pain sensation, memory defects, and symptoms of other diseases complicate the diagnosis. Regardless of the complaint, if exercise provokes and rest relieves the symptom, consider that ischemia may be the cause.

Angina is classified as stable or unstable. In *stable angina*, the onset, duration, and intensity of symptoms follow a regular pattern over an extended period. In *unstable angina*, the frequency, duration, and intensity of symptoms increase, and symptoms may occur during periods of little or no activity and without emotional provocation. Occurrence of symptoms with little provocation is called *crescendo angina*. The term *coronary insufficiency* is used when symptoms persist for at least 30 minutes in the absence of myocardial infarction. Other variations of angina include status aginosis, angina decubitus, and nocturnal, Printzmetal's, and vasospastic angina. Elderly and younger clients alike may present with these patterns.

ETIOLOGY

Angina and ischemic heart disease usually result from atherosclerosis of the coronary arteries and their branches. Atherosclerosis obstructs the coronary arteries and decreases blood flow and oxygen supply. When the oxygen demand exceeds the supply, angina pectoris occurs. Any activity that increases myocardial oxygen consumption can precipitate an attack of angina. The most common precipitating factors include physical exertion, emotional stress, anger, fright, a heavy meal, and exposure to cold.

Coronary artery spasm can also upset the supply and demand balance. The causes of spasm are unknown. Angina occurring from a spasm is unrelated to myocardial oxygen consumption. The spasm may be severe enough to create inadequate oxygen delivery even at rest.

Other conditions that may precipitate anginal symptoms include severe aortic stenosis or insufficiency, hyperthyroidism, dysrhythmias, tachycardia, transient hypotension, and low circulating blood volume. Risk factors that predispose clients to atherosclerotic cardiovascular disease include hypertension, cigarette smoking, hyperlipidemia, obesity, emotional stress, a sedentary life-style, family history of the disease, glucose intolerance, personality type, age, and sex. Obviously, some risk factors, such as cigarette smoking and a sedentary life-style, allow intervention to reduce the risk, while others do not.

HEALTH HISTORY FINDINGS

In a health history interview, the client may report or the nurse may detect many of these findings:
• discomfort, tightness, or aching behind the sternum lasting 30 seconds to 30 minutes
• discomfort radiating to shoulders, arms, neck, lower jaw, or abdomen
• discomfort caused by exertion and relieved by rest
• shortness of breath
• indigestion
• nausea
• numbness
• jaw pain
• dizziness
• diaphoresis
• transient change in vision
• history of myocardial infarction, congestive heart failure, hypertension, diabetes mellitus, hyperthyroidism, or anemia
• recent change in cardiac medications
• use of nitroglycerin
• history of noncompliance with medication regimen
• diet high in calories, cholesterol, and saturated fats
• sleep disturbances caused by chest pain while dreaming or lying flat
• tobacco use
• change in exercise tolerance
• sedentary life-style with only sporadic exercise
• recent life stressors
• recent death in the family
• Type A personality
• financial crisis
• confusion
• disorientation

PHYSICAL FINDINGS

In a physical examination, the nurse may detect many of these findings:

Cardiovascular
- S_3 and S_4 gallop rhythm
- maximal impulse
- reversed splitting of the S_2 heart sound
- atrial fibrillation
- premature ventricular contractions
- premature atrial contractions
- jugular vein distention

Integumentary
- cool, clammy skin
- pallor

Musculoskeletal
- decreased mobility

Neurologic
- anxiety
- restlessness

DIAGNOSTIC STUDIES
The following studies may be performed to evaluate the client's health status:
- electrocardiogram (ECG)—may show ST segment and T wave changes, a left bundle branch block, or Q waves from an old myocardial infarction (MI)
- Holter ECG monitor—72-hour ECG recording that is later compared to client's diary of activities and symptoms during the recording
- exercise tolerance test—to establish the diagnosis and to determine the severity of the coronary disease; may be difficult to perform in elderly clients because of decreased ability to exercise
- echocardiogram—provides useful information about cardiac structures and ventricular function although is not specific for angina
- coronary angiography—may help determine a more precise diagnosis
- complete blood count (CBC)—to assess for anemia, which predisposes the client to angina.
- chest X-ray—to evaluate heart size and rule out other causes of chest pain
- nitroglycerin (NTG) trial—prompt and consistent relief of symptoms after NTG helps establish the diagnosis of angina

POTENTIAL COMPLICATIONS
- MI
- congestive heart failure
- dysrhythmias
- pulmonary embolism
- activity intolerance
- anxiety
- discomfort or pain

Nursing diagnosis: *Pain related to insufficient coronary blood flow*

NURSING GOALS: To promote a balance between myocardial oxygen supply and demand and to reduce the frequency and severity of attacks

Signs and symptoms
- recent emotional stress
- heavy exercise
- pain or tightness radiating to arms, shoulders, neck, or jaw
- pain relieved by NTG
- indigestion
- heartburn
- nausea
- paresthesia
- diaphoresis

Interventions

1. Assess and document the client's anginal episodes, noting the location, duration, and quality of pain (based on a scale of 1 to 10). Also note the precipitating factors and any associated signs and symptoms.

Rationales

1. Assessment will differentiate angina from pain related to other causes, such as pleuritic, gastric, or musculoskeletal disorders.

2. Administer NTG as ordered by the physician, and have the client lie down or sit with the feet elevated. If the client's blood pressure is less than 100/60 mm Hg, notify the physician before giving the medication. If the client's cardiac symptoms persist longer than 15 minutes, notify the physician.

2. NTG relaxes vascular smooth muscle, resulting in generalized vasodilation, reduced venous return, and decreased cardiac output, thereby lowering myocardial oxygen demand. Reduced venous return lowers left ventricular end diastolic pressure, which improves blood flow to subendocardial layers of the myocardium. However, NTG can cause orthostatic changes, including dizziness, and can precipitate falls. Symptoms unrelieved by NTG may indicate complications requiring further treatment.

3. Teach the client and caregiver to improve myocardial oxygenation by instituting oxygen therapy, having the client sit upright and maintain bedrest, and minimizing distractions and noise.

3. These measures reduce the oxygen demand of the heart and help alleviate chest pain and ensuing anxiety.

4. Teach the caregiver to look for nonverbal signs of chest pain, such as clenched fists, facial flushing or grimacing, or rubbing the chest, arms, or neck.

4. The client may view pain as a part of aging or may deny cardiac symptoms. Such symptoms may signal increasing myocardial ischemia.

5. Stay with the client during chest pain episodes.

5. Remaining with the client decreases anxiety and promotes comfort.

6. Remain calm, reassure the client, and explain all actions and events.

6. These measures will reduce the client's anxiety and help avoid increased myocardial demands.

7. Assess the client for changes in behavior or function.

7. Symptoms of illness may present atypically in the elderly client, or the client may be unable to describe the symptoms.

8. Keep a record of the frequency and pattern of angina attacks, the number of NTG tablets required for relief, and the development of side effects. Review findings with the physician.

8. This information assists in the proper regulation of the client's medications and assesses the client's tolerance to long-acting nitrates. A worsening anginal pattern may indicate the need for more diagnostic tests or a change in management. Decreased clearance of medications predisposes the elderly client to side effects.

9. Obtain a 12-lead ECG during acute episodes of new anginal pain.

9. The ECG may show ischemic changes only during periods of actual chest pain.

10. Identify factors that precipitate cardiac symptoms.

10. Identifying precipitating factors will help to decrease angina attacks in the future.

OUTCOME CRITERION
• Within 30 minutes to 1 hour after the onset of chest pain, the client will verbalize relief of pain, have normal vital signs, and show no nonverbal signs of pain.

Nursing diagnosis: *Potential activity intolerance related to incapacitating chest pain*

NURSING GOAL: To control angina symptoms so that the client may continue desired and needed activities that foster life satisfaction

Signs and symptoms
• decline in physical activity
• anginal pain on exertion

Interventions

1. Teach the client to stop all activity at the onset of an anginal attack, to sit or lie down, and to take the prescribed sublingual NTG.

2. Tell the client he may take up to 3 tablets in sequence, 5 to 10 minutes apart. If this does not relieve the anginal pain, tell the client to call the physician and immediately go to the nearest emergency room.

3. Warn the client that NTG may cause a headache, which can be relieved by an analgesic, such as acetaminophen (Tylenol).

4. Teach the client to keep NTG accessible and to store it in an airtight, dark container. Instruct the client to obtain a fresh supply after 6 months.

5. Teach the client to recognize and alleviate anginal symptoms.

6. Teach the client to initiate an exercise program that begins with warm-up activities and ends slowly with light exercise such as walking.

Rationales

1. Nitrates relieve angina by dilating peripheral and collateral vessels and coronary arteries. Since NTG may cause hypotension or fainting, sitting or lying down prevents a fall.

2. Pain unrelieved by rest and nitrates may be caused by MI.

3. NTG dilates cerebral blood vessels, which causes headaches.

4. Sublingual forms of NTG lose potency and effectiveness quickly.

5. Living with angina successfully depends on recognition and treatment of symptoms.

6. An exercise program promotes conditioning. Warm-up activities increase deep muscle temperature, prevent muscle injuries, and allow time for the elderly client's heart rate to rise. Ending exercise slowly allows time for the heart rate to return to baseline, which may take longer in the elderly client.

OUTCOME CRITERION
• The client will exercise regularly without onset of chest pain.

Nursing diagnosis: *Anxiety related to uncertainty about symptoms and fear of impending death*

NURSING GOALS: To provide emotional support to the client and caregivers, to acknowledge their fears and anxieties, and to help them develop appropriate coping mechanisms

Signs and symptoms
• preoccupation with cardiac status
• withdrawal from activities and relationships
• denial of illness or symptoms
• verbalization of fear or anxiety by client or caregivers

Interventions

1. Assess the client's support systems.

2. Encourage the client, caregiver, and family members to verbalize fears and anxieties about angina.

3. Explore the caregiver's desire and capability to learn cardiopulmonary resuscitation (CPR).

4. Observe the client's and caregiver's response to the client's symptoms, and help them modify their behavior if necessary.

Rationales

1. A client living alone or having responsibility for others may have difficulty managing daily living.

2. Verbalization of concerns allows interventions for management and control.

3. Completion of a recognized CPR course strengthens the caregiver's support.

4. Evaluation of behavioral responses will guide further nursing interventions.

5. Review the client's access to an emergency medical system. Help the client to obtain Medic Alert identification and to prepare a thorough medical history for easy access by emergency personnel.

5. Knowing how to get emergency assistance may decrease anxiety and strengthen the support system. Health care personnel need client information to provide quick and efficient care.

6. Determine whether the client has caregiving responsibilities for others and whether the client lives alone. Consider a home health care referral if necessary.

6. A home health care nurse can assist the client with responsibilities for himself and others.

OUTCOME CRITERIA
• The client and caregiver will verbalize concerns and fears.
• The client and caregiver will cope effectively with angina, as evidenced by appropriately using medical and nursing care and controlling symptoms.

Nursing diagnosis: *Potential for injury related to complications of cardiac drugs*

NURSING GOAL: To teach the client and caregiver about medications, including interactions and side effects

Signs and symptoms
• confusion
• disorientation
• dry mouth
• constipation
• dizziness
• orthostatic hypotension
• nausea
• vomiting
• frequent falls

Interventions

1. Obtain a thorough drug history, and carefully document all prescription and nonprescription drugs.

2. Watch the client take prescribed medications to assess his ability to complete the task.

3. Teach the client and caregiver about the correct administration of medications and potential side effects.

4. Take the client's blood pressure in both arms, with the client lying, sitting, and standing.

5. Assess the client for predisposing factors to medication side effects, such as age, hepatic or renal impairment, chronic diseases such as congestive heart failure, and behavioral or hormonal changes.

Rationales

1. The elderly client may use many prescription and over-the-counter drugs, which increases the chance of drug interaction.

2. Mental status and manual dexterity affect the client's ability to take medications correctly.

3. Noncompliance often results from a client's failure to understand the medication, its use, and possible side effects.

4. Hypotension is a common side effect of many cardiac drugs. Also, orthostatic hypotension commonly occurs in the elderly client.

5. Aging delays the absorption, distribution, metabolism, and excretion of drugs by the hepatic, gastrointestinal, and renal systems. The client with multiple chronic diseases may take medications for one disease that alter the absorption or distribution of drugs prescribed for another disease. Cognitive impairment may cause poor compliance, an accidental overdose, or ingestion of the wrong drug. Age-related hormonal changes also can alter the response to a drug.

> **OUTCOME CRITERION**
> • The client and caregiver will administer medications correctly and safely, as evidenced by a decrease in anginal episodes and a lack of adverse reactions.

Nursing diagnosis: *Knowledge deficit related to care of a cardiac pacemaker*

NURSING GOAL: To teach the client proper pacemaker care

Signs and symptoms
• bradycardia
• irregular heart rhythm
• chest pain
• shortness of breath
• dyspnea

Interventions

1. Review with the client the literature accompanying the pacemaker.

2. Teach the client the importance of monitoring pacemaker function.

3. Teach the client to check his radial pulse for 60 seconds every day.

4. Teach the client to use the telephone to maintain regular checkups on pacemaker function.

5. Teach the client to turn off electrical appliances in cases of suspected electrical interference.

6. Advise the client to carry a card identifying the manufacturer of the pacemaker, its settings, and its programmable functions.

Rationales

1. Reviewing the literature will help educate the client on proper use of a pacemaker.

2. Proper monitoring will detect early sensing problems, such as premature battery depletion, random electronic component failures, and electrode dislodgment.

3. A slowing pulse should alert the client to notify the physician; the pacemaker battery, which lasts 6 to 12 years, may need replacement.

4. A client who lives far away from medical service can use a small device to transmit a single-lead ECG by telephone.

5. Certain anti-theft alarm systems and magnetic resonance imaging machines have intense magnetic fields that can temporarily alter pacemaker function. Most pacemakers contain protection against electrical interference from radios, TVs, and microwave ovens.

6. An identification card allows emergency personnel access to this important information in case of an emergency.

> **OUTCOME CRITERION**
> • The client will understand the care of the pacemaker, its potential problems, and signs of malfunction.

Nursing diagnosis: *Knowledge deficit related to physical limitations imposed by the disease*

NURSING GOAL: To enable the client and caregiver to function optimally, recognize anginal symptoms, and avoid complications

Signs and symptoms
• lack of education about the disease
• noncompliance with medication and management plan
• verbalized need for knowledge

Interventions

1. Consider changes in the elderly client's sensory, central, and motor processes that influence learning, such as decreased visual acuity, pain, weakness, and confusion.

2. Assess the client's knowledge and understanding of angina.

3. Include the client's family or caregiver in client teaching sessions.

4. Review the basic pathophysiology of coronary atherosclerosis and angina.

5. Review the differences between angina attacks and the onset of an MI.

6. If prescribed, teach the client the proper use of long-acting nitrates, such as nitroglycerin ointment. This includes instructing the client to remove previous patches before applying subsequent ones and to place the patch on the chest or inner aspect of the arm.

7. Teach the client about cardiac medications, such as beta-blockers or calcium channel antagonists, if appropriate. Instruct the client to watch for side effects, such as bradycardia, dysrhythmias, depression, excessive fatigue, and hypoglycemia (with beta-blockers) and hypotension, edema, and headaches (with calcium channel antagonists).

8. Teach the client how to avoid precipitating factors, including overexertion, extremes in temperature, large meals, overeating, emotional stress, and smoking.

Rationales

1. The quality and quantity of information absorbed through the senses influence learning. The elderly client may better comprehend information presented at a normal or slow pace. Motivation, life experiences, education, cultural background, religion, socioeconomic status, and communication and language skills influence the client's ability to learn.

2. An assessment of the client's knowledge provides the basis for an effective teaching plan.

3. A cognitively impaired client must depend on others to recognize and manage symptoms.

4. The client is more likely adhere to a management plan if he understands the problem.

5. The client must know when to contact an emergency medical service to avoid complications.

6. Long-acting nitrates, prescribed in the form of paste patches that adhere to the skin, prevent or reduce the frequency of angina. Benefits last up to 6 hours after each topical application. Removing previous patches prevents an accidental overdose. Application sites on the chest and the arm allow for maximum absorption.

7. Beta-blockers decrease myocardial oxygen consumption by reducing the heart rate, blood pressure, and myocardial contractility. However, they also lower the resting heart rate, which could be a complication in elderly clients with sinus or atrioventricular node dysfunction. Calcium channel antagonists dilate the coronary arteries and decrease coronary artery spasms to improve myocardial perfusion.

8. These factors increase the demand on the heart and can precipitate chest pain and an anginal attack. A sudden temperature change causes vasoconstriction. Overeating increases myocardial work by requiring an increased blood supply to the GI tract for digestion. Stress increases circulating catecholamine levels, which increases blood pressure and overall myocardial oxygen consumption. Nicotine, a cardiac stimulant, causes vasoconstriction and reduces oxygen availability.

OUTCOME CRITERIA
- The client will be able to identify the signs and symptoms of angina pectoris.
- The client will comply with treatment measures.

NURSING ACTIONS IN VARIOUS SETTINGS

Nursing actions for a client with angina pectoris depend on the setting in which care is provided. This section identifies which actions are appropriate in all settings and which pertain to acute care, extended care, or home care.

All settings

- Caution the client and caregiver to report symptoms of an MI promptly and to obtain prompt medical care for the client.
- Inform the family and caregiver that an MI is more likely to occur in an elderly client when he is at rest or asleep.

• Promote a diet that is low in sodium and saturated fats.
• Provide a medication schedule that coincides with the client's daily routine.
• Assist the client in maintaining his customary lifestyle rather than severely limiting his activities.

Acute care
• Provide printed information on prescribed medications.

Extended care
• Record any anginal episode in the nurse's notes, along with the date and time of the incident, measures followed, measures that were successful, client's response, physician's response, and orders.

Home care
• Assess the home for stairs or other barriers that may cause exertion and increase myocardial demands.
• Review medication storage and administration.
• Ensure that client has access to an emergency medical system.
• If the client lives alone or is alone in the home for parts of the day, have the family obtain a portable telephone that the client can access easily and quickly in an emergency.
• If appropriate, suggest that the client obtain a remote beeper that will activate the telephone to contact a medical alert system or someone who can help in an emergency.
• Encourage regular exercise, such as walking, golfing, bicycling, and stretching and limbering exercises.

SELECTED REFERENCES

Brenner, Z.R. "Nursing Elderly Cardiac Clients," *Critical Care Nursing* 7(2):78-87, February 1987.

Caird, F.I., et al. "The Cardiovascular System," in *Textbook of Geriatric Medicine and Gerontology*, 3rd ed. Edited by Brocklehurst, J.C. New York: Churchill Livingstone, 1985.

Esberger, K.K., and Hughes, S.T. *Nursing Care of the Aged.* Norwalk, Conn.: Appleton & Lange, 1989.

Hechheimer, E.F. *Health Promotion of the Elderly in the Community.* Philadelphia: W.B. Saunders Co., 1989.

Horwitz, L.D., and Grover, B.M., eds. *Signs and Symptoms in Cardiology.* Philadelphia: J.B. Lippincott Co., 1985.

Moss, A.J. "Cardiac Disease in the Elderly," in *The Practice of Geriatrics.* Edited by Calkins, E. et al. Philadelphia: W.B. Saunders Co., 1986.

National Center for Health Statistics. *Health Statistics on Older Persons, United States, 1986.* Vital and Health Statistics. Series 3, No. 25 (DHHS Publication No. PHS 87-1409). U.S. Government Printing Office, 1987.

Segal, B.L. "Managing Angina in the Elderly: An Update," *Geriatrics* 44(1):55-65, January 1989.

Wild, Lorie. "Cardiovascular Problems," in *Nursing Management for the Elderly,* edited by Doris L. Carnevali and Maxine Patrick. Philadelphia: J.B. Lippincott Co., 1986.

Congestive Heart Failure

Congestive heart failure (CHF) results when the myocardium can no longer pump blood efficiently and the circulation in the body becomes congested. Any condition that compromises cardiac function can result in CHF. Although the left ventricle is more likely to fail initially, bilateral chamber failure rapidly follows. CHF is a major complication of cardiac disease in the elderly population, and the prevalence of this disorder increases with age.

ETIOLOGY

CHF may result from conditions that increase fluid volume and lead to circulatory overload (increased preload) or conditions that increase resistance to movement of blood from the heart (increased afterload). Examples of the former include increased sodium intake and too-rapid infusion of I.V. fluids. Examples of the latter include arteriosclerotic heart disease, hypertensive heart disease, and pulmonary hypertension. The severity of CHF largely depends on the extent of myocardial damage, which in turn correlates with the amount of myofiber loss.

Numerous factors can exacerbate CHF in a client with cardiac disease. A silent myocardial infarction, increased hypertension, subclinical pulmonary emboli, and atrial fibrillation may all precipitate overt CHF. In addition, fever, infection, and anemia can aggravate the condition of elderly clients with borderline compensation CHF. Regardless of the cause of the underlying problem, dietary sodium excess is a common decompensating factor in the elderly client. CHF activates the renin-angiotensin-aldosterone system, resulting in renal salt and water retention, systemic and renal arteriolar vasoconstriction, and a secondary increase in afterload resistance. The secretion of antidiuretic hormone also increases in response to CHF, which contributes to excess fluid retention and to hyponatremia.

HEALTH HISTORY FINDINGS

In a health history interview, the client may report or the nurse may detect many of these findings:
• weakness
• generalized fatigue
• shortness of breath
• dyspnea
• orthopnea
• hemoptysis
• atypical chest pain
• palpitations
• anorexia
• nausea
• vomiting
• bloated feeling
• gradual increase in body weight
• right-sided abdominal discomfort with exercise
• increased urine output at night and decreased urine output during the day
• decreased sexual function
• decreased participation in activities of daily living
• chronic hypertension
• coronary artery disease
• valvular disease
• current use of diuretic and antihypertensive medications
• alcohol or tobacco use
• high-sodium diet
• family history of cardiac disease or peripheral vascular disease

PHYSICAL FINDINGS

In a physical examination, the nurse may detect many of these findings:

Cardiovascular
• systolic murmur (in advanced CHF)
• S_3 heart sound
• S_4 heart sound with summation gallop
• venous distention
• external jugular vein distention
• pulsations of the deep jugular veins when client sits in a 90-degree position

Integumentary
• cyanotic lips
• cold, clammy skin
• pallor
• sacral edema
• peripheral and dependent edema

Respiratory
• productive cough
• wheezes
• crackles
• diffuse absence of bilateral breath sounds beginning at bases

Musculoskeletal
• noticeable fatigue with minimal exertion

Neurologic
• anxiety and restlessness
• lethargy
• confusion
• memory lapse

Other
• vasodilation of vessels and slight hemorrhages in fundus
• periorbital edema
• abdominal pain
• hepatojugular reflux (portal hypertension)

DIAGNOSTIC STUDIES
The following studies may be performed to evaluate the client's health status:
• hematocrit and hemoglobin—anemia may contribute to the pathogenesis of CHF
• serum electrolyte levels—imbalances may result from fluid shifts, diuretic therapy, or the response of the organ systems to a decreased oxygen supply and increased congestion; results may show hyponatremia, hypokalemia, or hyperkalemia
• blood urea nitrogen (BUN) and creatinine—elevated levels reflect decreased renal function

• aspartate aminotransferase (AST), alanine aminotransferase (ALT), lactic dehydrogenase (LDH), and bilirubin—elevated levels suggest decreased liver function
• urinalysis—may reveal proteinuria and elevated specific gravity
• chest X-ray—cardiac silhouette commonly enlarged and can reveal distended pulmonary veins, which reflect redistribution of pulmonary blood flow, and interstitial and alveolar edema
• electrocardiogram (ECG)—may show rhythm disturbances
• echocardiogram—to rapidly assess heart chamber size, wall thickness, and valve shape and motion; can detect pericardial effusion, pericardial thickening, hypertrophy, and valvular abnormalities

POTENTIAL COMPLICATIONS
• fluid and electrolyte imbalances
• infection
• pulmonary edema and hypertension
• end-stage heart disease

Nursing diagnosis: *Decreased cardiac output related to fluid volume overload, decreased contractility, altered heart rhythm, and increased afterload*

NURSING GOAL: To maintain adequate ventilation

Signs and symptoms
• shortness of breath
• dyspnea on exertion or while recumbent
• orthopnea
• paroxysmal nocturnal dyspnea
• periorbital, sacral, and peripheral edema
• crackles that do not clear after coughing
• sudden weight gain
• tachycardia
• restlessness
• cyanosis

Interventions

1. Assess the client's pulse, respirations, and blood pressure every 4 hours while the client is awake during acute episodes of CHF.

2. Monitor arterial blood gas (ABG) results.

3. Assess the client for skin and nail bed color changes and for capillary refill.

Rationales

1. One of the earliest signs of worsening failure is increased heart rate. Decreased blood pressure can reflect decreased cardiac output due to diminished myocardial contractility or excessive diuresis. Diminished pulse pressure or peripheral pulse loss can indicate decreased cardiac output. Increased irregularity of heart rhythm can reflect an increased number of premature atrial or ventricular contractions, a sign of increasing failure, or medication toxicity.

2. ABG indicates blood oxygenation; regular monitoring assists in diagnosing and treating CHF.

3. Skin color and capillary refill reflect tissue perfusion and peripheral circulation.

4. Raise the head of the client's bed to semi-Fowler's position, or elevate the client on 2 to 3 pillows.

4. Raising the head of the bed decreases resistance to airflow by preventing the abdominal organs from pressing on the diaphragm and permitting freer movement. An upright position redistributes blood flow to dependent areas, decreasing the amount of blood returning to the heart.

5. Administer supplemental oxygen therapy via nasal cannula as ordered.

5. A client who has difficulty maintaining an arterial oxygen level (PaO_2) above 60 mm Hg may benefit from supplemental oxygen.

6. Administer medications (such as diuretics, inotropic agents, nitrates, and vasodilators) as ordered by the physician.

6. Diuretics aid in decreasing afterload and preload. Inotropic agents increase myocardial contractility but also increase myocardial oxygen consumption. Nitrates cause vasodilation, which reduces preload. Vasodilators reduce afterload by lowering resistance to ventricular ejection.

7. Monitor the client for side effects of medications.

7. Diuretics can cause hypovolemia or hypokalemia. Digitalis can cause toxic effects in elderly clients, with symptoms including anorexia, confusion, nausea, vomiting, visual disturbances, severe dysrhythmias and irregularity, and slowing of the heart rate to fewer than 60 beats/minute. Nitrates can cause hypovolemia, which can cause orthostasis or a reflex tachycardia. Vasodilators can cause hypotension.

8. Notify the physician if coughing becomes continual, if tachycardia occurs, or if there is a sudden increase in hemoptysis.

8. Pulmonary edema creates an emergency situation as the client can "drown" in excess secretions.

9. Teach the client to avoid large meals and to eat small, frequent meals of high-density foods that supply adequate bulk.

9. CHF decreases circulation to the stomach and small intestine so that food moves slowly through the GI tract, producing a feeling of fullness and distention.

10. Teach the client the importance of not smoking and also of avoiding exposure to cigarette smoke.

10. Tobacco smoke causes permanent loss of cilia, mucous gland hypertrophy, and chronic inflammatory changes. Smoking also can cause vasoconstriction, thereby increasing blood pressure.

OUTCOME CRITERIA
- The client will have improved cardiac output, as evidenced by improved breathing and normal vital signs.
- The client will not experience adverse reactions to cardiac medications.

Nursing diagnosis: *Fluid volume excess related to fluid and electrolyte imbalances*

NURSING GOALS: To monitor the client's fluid and electrolyte levels and to prevent increasing heart failure and further complications

Signs and symptoms
- periorbital, sacral, and peripheral edema
- crackles that do not clear after coughing
- sudden weight gain
- loss of appetite

Interventions

1. Weigh the client on the same scale and at the same time every day.

Rationales

1. A weight gain of 1 to 2 lb (0.5 to 0.9 kg) a day indicates fluid retention and the need for increased diuretics.

2. Monitor and record the client's daily fluid intake and output.

2. Accurate intake and output records can alert the caregiver to early fluid excess.

3. Assess the client for a change in mentation.

3. When cardiac output decreases, cerebral perfusion suffers and confusion results.

4. Assess the client's lung sounds for crackles, decreased sounds, or a change from vesicular to bronchial breath sounds.

4. Crackles, decreased sounds, and bronchial breath sounds indicate fluid in the lungs and signal increasing right-sided heart failure.

5. Monitor the client's serum electrolytes and sodium and potassium levels, and report abnormal values.

5. Hyponatremia causes decreased blood pressure, confusion, headaches, and convulsions. Hypokalemia causes weakness, fatigue, and ventricular fibrillation. Hyperkalemia causes bradycardia and ventricular asystole.

6. Monitor creatinine and BUN levels, and report increasing values.

6. Increasing creatinine and BUN levels reflect decreased renal perfusion from worsening failure. The BUN level rises disproportionately to the creatinine level.

7. Provide a bedside commode, bedpan, or urinal for the client. During initial diuresis, restrict the client to the bed or a chair. Elevate the client's legs when he is sitting.

7. During diuresis, the resultant increased urine output may exceed what the client can safely control. Bed or chair rest increases diuresis, renal perfusion, peripheral tissue oxygenation, and venous tone.

8. Assess the client's diet by keeping a daily record of caloric intake. Place the client on a 1.5 to 2 g sodium-restricted diet.

8. Obtaining a calorie count ensures adequate food intake in relation to the client's stage of illness, level of activity, and weight. Restricting sodium intake reduces water and sodium retention.

9. Teach the client to choose fresh or frozen foods over canned and other processed foods.

9. Canned and processed foods have a high sodium content.

OUTCOME CRITERION
• The client will exhibit signs of decreasing fluid retention, such as normal sodium, potassium, BUN, and creatinine values; a normal mental exam; and decreased body weight.

Nursing diagnosis: *Potential for infection related to compromised respiratory function*

NURSING GOALS: To prevent respiratory infection and to promote an optimal breathing pattern

Signs and symptoms
• mental status change (confusion, restlessness, memory loss)
• increased respirations and shortness of breath
• change in amount, color, and consistency of sputum
• fever
• chills, sweats, or complaints of feeling warm
• fatigue or lassitude
• loss of appetite

Interventions

1. Assess the client's vital signs and auscultate lungs every 4 hours while the client is awake.

Rationales

1. Temperature may or may not be elevated. Increased pulse and respiratory rate and elevated blood pressure can indicate pulmonary congestion.

2. Teach the client to perform coughing and deep-breathing exercises, postural drainage, and percussion if tolerated and prescribed.

2. Retained secretions and an oxygen deficit increase the risk of pulmonary infection.

3. Encourage the client to turn in bed, ambulate, and perform as many activities of daily living (ADLs) as possible.

3. Activity prevents the accumulation of pulmonary secretions and reduces pulmonary congestion.

OUTCOME CRITERION
• The client will be free from pulmonary infection.

Nursing diagnosis: *Activity intolerance related to decreased cardiac output and fatigue*

NURSING GOALS: To reduce activities that cause fatigue and shortness of breath and to promote a gradual increase in activity tolerance and independence

Signs and symptoms
• dyspnea on exertion
• fatigue and complaints of weakness
• inability to complete ADLs
• increased need for rest
• increased dependency

Interventions

1. Institute a graded pulmonary and cardiac rehabilitation program that begins with regular position changes and range-of-motion exercises and progresses to active exercises, such as ambulating, walking up steps, and riding a stationary bike.

2. Encourage the client to exercise during routine activities, such as bathing and dressing.

3. Teach the client to complete a task in stages.

4. Alternate activity with rest periods.

5. Evaluate the client's tolerance for newly introduced activities. Discontinue the activity (and possibly resume at a slower pace at a later time) if the client's pulse rate increases more than 30 beats/minute above resting level; if he develops a new or increased pulse irregularity; if the systolic blood pressure drops 15 mm Hg or more below resting level; or if he develops dyspnea or a slowed respiratory rate, loses consciousness, or becomes profoundly weak.

6. Teach the client to avoid performing Valsalva's maneuver (forced expiration against a closed glottis), such as moving in bed while holding his breath (the client should exhale when changing positions) and straining while having a stool (the client should increase dietary fiber). (See "Constipation and Fecal Incontinence," pages 97 to 104.)

7. Allow time for the client to express feelings, expectations, and fears.

Rationales

1. Position changes and exercises that involve muscle contraction and change in muscle length (such as active or passive limb flexion) improve peripheral circulation and lessen the risk of thromboembolism and other adverse effects of immobility.

2. The client may be more apt to incorporate exercise into daily routines than to follow a scheduled program.

3. Demonstrating how the client can still perform a desired task relieves depression and enables the client to complete essential tasks.

4. Bed rest and inactivity cause loss of strength and endurance. Initially, even short periods of activity can induce symptoms of cardiac compromise.

5. Resuming activity too rapidly can exacerbate heart failure, myocardial ischemia, or peripheral vascular insufficiency. It can also cause a psychological setback if the client expects to meet unrealistic standards.

6. Valsalva's maneuver increases intrathoracic pressure and blood return to the heart, the latter by causing a reflexive increase in venous return once the client releases the held breath. Valsalva's maneuver can cause syncope and premature ventricular contractions.

7. Fear, apprehension, and anxiety contribute to a poor activity level.

OUTCOME CRITERION
• The client will gradually increase activity tolerance and independence, as evidenced by an ability to complete ADLs and by returning to previous levels of exercise tolerance.

Nursing diagnosis: *Anxiety related to shortness of breath*

NURSING GOAL: To relieve the client's anxiety

Signs and symptoms
• fear and apprehension
• desire not to be left alone
• difficulty focusing on a single topic in a conversation
• agitation and restlessness
• inability to sleep
• decreased appetite

Interventions

1. Encourage the client to express his feelings after episodes of shortness of breath.

2. Spend time with the client, and encourage him to call you or another nurse during anxiety episodes.

3. Elevate the head of the bed to semi-Fowler's position during shortness-of-breath episodes.

4. Teach the client to practice breathing techniques, such as breathing through pursed lips and sitting over a bedside table or chair during shortness-of-breath episodes.

5. Use the method of oxygen administration most comfortable to the client.

6. Administer medications as ordered for anxiety; however, use caution so as not to overmedicate.

7. Explain all procedures to the client in advance.

8. Maintain a quiet and calm environment.

Rationales

1. Encouraging the client to talk about feelings after shortness-of-breath episodes helps alleviate anxiety.

2. Staying with the client during the episode helps decrease the client's feeling of helplessness.

3. Elevating the head of the bed helps minimize shortness of breath.

4. These techniques facilitate air passage and exchange and increase lung expansion.

5. The client may feel more comfortable with an oxygen cannula, as a mask or catheter may feel too invasive.

6. Antianxiety agents help the client overcome severe anxiety while reducing his activity level and decreasing cardiac demands.

7. The client may be more cooperative and may tolerate procedures more easily if he understands why they are being performed.

8. A calm environment helps prevent unnecessary stimulation.

OUTCOME CRITERIA
• The client will be less anxious and apprehensive, as evidenced by verbalizing feelings during shortness-of-breath episodes.
• The client will be free from dyspnea during activities.

NURSING ACTIONS IN VARIOUS SETTINGS
Nursing actions for a client with congestive heart failure depend on the setting in which care is provided.

This section identifies which actions are appropriate in all settings and which pertain to acute care, extended care, or home care.

All settings
• Educate the client and family about the easily identifiable signs that accompany heart failure: weight gain, swelling of ankles and feet, shortness of breath, confusion, and loss of appetite.
• Help the client and family set activity priorities and understand the client's limitations.
• Encourage the client and family to comply with low-salt diet and necessary medications.
• Teach the bedridden client to perform leg exercises to prevent phlebothrombosis.

Acute care
• Educate the client's family or caregiver on hospital routines (such as meal times, bath times, and changes of shifts) to decrease the client's anxiety level.
• Avoid exhausting the client when scheduling tests and studies.
• At the time of discharge, refer the client to a home health nurse who can supervise the client's diet, activity, and medication administration.

Extended care
• Monitor administration of medications in a client with a history of CHF.
• Weigh the client at least weekly, and more frequently if necessary, depending on the client's cardiac status.
• Assess the bedridden client for edema, especially sacral edema.
• Monitor vital signs every 4 hours, and weigh the client daily during acute episodes of CHF.
• Administer care to the client in short, complete steps to increase compliance and minimize fatigue.
• Assess the client for depression or anxiety.
• Perform a mental status examination of the client (see "Delirium," pages 225 to 229) to serve as a baseline for measuring increasing confusion, which may signal worsening heart failure.
• Consult a dietitian about initiating a low-sodium diet.
• Obtain regular blood studies as needed to assess electrolyte status and digoxin levels.

Home care
• Teach the client and family about the medication regimen and how to stage activities.
• Explain to the client and caregiver the importance of weighing the client daily to monitor weight loss and fluid retention.
• Assess the client's and family's level of knowledge about the disease; continue to teach and reassure them to decrease their anxiety and dependency.
• Evaluate the client for accessibility to a medical alert system.
• Encourage the client to keep follow-up appointments.
• Perform a baseline abbreviated mental exam as indicated.

SELECTED REFERENCES
Breitung, J.C. *Caring for Older Adults.* Philadelphia: W.B. Saunders Co., 1987.
Carnevali, D., and Patrick, M. *Nursing Management for the Elderly,* 2nd ed. Philadelphia: J.B. Lippincott Co, 1987.
Eliopoulos, C. *Gerontological Nursing.* Philadelphia: J.B. Lippincott Co. 1987.
Eliopoulos, C. *A Guide to the Nursing of the Aging.* Baltimore: Williams & Wilkins, 1987.
Esberger, K.K., and Hughes, S.T. *Nursing Care of the Aged.* Norwalk, Conn.: Appleton & Lange, 1989.
Hechheimer, E.F. *Health Promotion of the Elderly in the Community.* Philadelphia: W.B. Saunders Co., 1989.
Holloway, N.M. *Medical-Surgical Care Plans.* Springhouse, Pa.: Springhouse Corp., 1988.

CARDIOVASCULAR SYSTEM

Transient Ischemic Attack

A transient ischemic attack (TIA) is a central neurologic deficit of cerebrovascular origin that does not last longer than 24 hours. A temporary interruption in blood flow to a portion of the brain causes a sudden onset of symptoms. Most TIAs last from 5 to 20 minutes, although many clients do not recover for several hours. These episodes are an important marker for vascular disease, particularly stroke. Traditionally, physicians assumed that structural damage did not occur, but recent studies show that localized cerebral blood flow disturbances may exist months after recovery from a TIA. In addition, computerized tomography (CT) has demonstrated abnormalities of the brain following TIAs.

Cerebrovascular diseases are the third leading cause of death in persons age 55 to 84 and the second leading cause of death in those over age 84. Prevalence of TIAs in the elderly population ranges between 0.3 and 1.1 per 1,000, without affinity for a particular sex or race. TIAs are categorized as carotid or vertebrobasilar, depending on the vascular supply compromised. Signs and symptoms depend on the area involved but typically include loss of muscle control and sensory and visual disturbances. The risk for stroke increases in the first year after the initial TIA. Repetitive episodes of increasing severity and duration, called crescendo attacks, almost always signal an impending or actual major vessel occlusion. Clients with TIAs have an increased risk of mortality, primarily because of coronary artery disease and cerebral infarction. Clients with carotid TIAs also may experience disturbances in expression or comprehension of language.

ETIOLOGY
Atherosclerotic plaques or a spasm of the neck and major cerebral vessels causes the temporary ischemia associated with TIAs. The syndrome often begins when atheromatous material accumulates on the vessel wall at the bifurcation of the carotid artery. Ulcers may then form, which cause platelets and fibrin to collect and form a thrombus. Fragments of the thrombus and plaque then break free and travel to distal arteries. This occludes the artery and causes a TIA. If the thrombus continues to expand and the plaque continues to accumulate, complete occlusion eventually results, which causes a stroke. When the arterial lumen becomes 50% to 75% obstructed, perfusion decreases. A client may have a totally occluded carotid or vertebral artery without neurologic deficit because of collateral circulation through the circle of Willis and other neck vessels. TIAs may also result from cardiac conditions, such as mitral stenosis, atrial fibrillation, mural thrombus after a myocardial infarction, ventricular aneurysm, mitral valve prolapse, a prosthetic heart valve, bacterial endocarditis, atrial myxoma, and congestive cardiomyopathy.

Clients having TIAs lasting only a few minutes most likely have significant proximal lesions in the neck vessels. Clients having TIAs lasting 6 to 24 hours more commonly have a larger embolus from a cardiac source. Other, although rare, causes of TIAs include hypotension, subclavian steal syndrome, hematologic disorders associated with hypercoagulability or hyperviscosity, and severe anemia. TIAs caused by hypotension and blood disorders usually involve vessel stenosis and inadequate collateral flow. Dehydration and diabetes may also predispose a client to TIAs. Mechanical compression of the vertebral arteries related to a specific head position may produce TIA-like symptoms. A sudden position change causing an orthostatic change in blood pressure may also precipitate TIA symptoms.

HEALTH HISTORY FINDINGS
In a health history interview, the client may report or the nurse may detect many of these findings:
• symptoms that occur suddenly and resolve gradually within 24 hours
• focal cerebral symptoms occasionally followed by migraine
• transient focal neurologic deficits when hypoglycemic
• amnesia of the episode
• symptoms from head and neck movement or a change in position
• temporary blindness in one eye
• diplopia
• flashes of light in eyes
• isolated limb weakness
• ataxia
• numbness in face, arms, legs, and side
• "drop attacks" (falling without losing consciousness)
• headaches
• tinnitus
• vertigo
• hypertension
• peripheral vascular disease
• stroke
• blood disorders
• diabetes mellitus
• intracranial lesions
• history of frequent falls
• current use of antihypertensive, diuretic, hypnotic, and analgesic medications
• history of poor fluid intake

PHYSICAL FINDINGS
In a physical examination, the nurse may detect many of these findings:

Cardiovascular
• blood pressure difference between arms greater than 20 mm Hg
• transient increase in pulse
• absence of pulses and palpable thrill in the carotid arteries
• decreased strength of preauricular, superficial, temporal, and orbital pulses
• marked increase in one carotid pulse
• carotid bruits
• quality difference between brachial and radial pulses
• embolic lesions

Neurologic
• brief amnesia
• lack of comprehension
• facial weakness

Other
• decreased vision
• monocular blurring
• ipsilateral blindness

DIAGNOSTIC STUDIES
The following studies may be performed to evaluate the client's health status:
• complete blood count (CBC) with differential, coagulation panel, and platelet count—to rule out hematologic disorders

• serum glucose, sodium, potassium, and blood urea nitrogen (BUN)—to exclude hypoglycemia and fluid or electrolyte imbalance
• serum lipid levels—to help determine the degree of atherosclerotic disease
• erythrocyte sedimentation rate—to detect inflammatory disorders
• electrocardiogram (ECG)—to rule out cardiac causes
• chest X-ray—to evaluate heart size and identify other abnormalities in the chest
• computed tomography (CT) scan of the brain—to rule out other disorders
• Doppler flow studies, intravenous digital subtraction angiography (DSA)—to identify vascular abnormalities
• cerebral angiography—may delineate surgically correctable intracarotid lesions or rule out other vascular disease
• Holter ECG monitor—to assess for dysrhythmias
• echocardiogram—may identify cardiac sources of emboli
• electroencephalogram (EEG)—to rule out a focal seizure disorder

POTENTIAL COMPLICATIONS
• stroke
• injury from falls
• depression
• social withdrawal

Nursing diagnosis: *Altered cerebral tissue perfusion related to ischemia*

NURSING GOALS: To support the client during acute TIA episodes and to promote his understanding of and cooperation with procedures and treatments

Signs and symptoms
• loss of muscle control
• sensory disturbances
• communication disturbances
• impaired vision
• disequilibrium
• lack of comprehension
• personality change
• confusion

Interventions

1. Assess the signs and symptoms of TIA episodes reported by the client. Question the client directly regarding the symptoms.

2. If present during a TIA episode, observe signs and symptoms and document them on the client's record.

3. Remain with the client during an attack, if possible, and stay calm while monitoring vital signs and symptoms.

Rationales

1. An accurate history is necessary for diagnosis, as the symptoms may have resolved before the examination.

2. Thorough documentation of observed changes in status aids in diagnosis and informs others about the client's problem.

3. The client may become fearful during an attack because of the threat of stroke and permanent damage.

4. Report all TIA episodes to the physician immediately.

4. Initial episodes encountered in a home or extended care setting require hospitalization for a thorough evaluation of symptoms. A hospitalized client with prolonged attacks may warrant emergency studies, such as a CT scan.

5. Administer medications as ordered by the physician.

5. Drug therapy to prevent strokes consists of giving platelet inhibitors, such as aspirin and dipyridamole. Both of these drugs inhibit the secretion of intracellular compounds that accelerate platelet aggregation. Anticoagulants may be useful for short-term therapy.

6. Explain all tests and procedures to the client and family.

6. Education may result in enhanced cooperation and reduced stress.

7. Teach the family and caregiver to report symptoms and the frequency of the episodes.

7. The client may attribute symptoms to "old age" or may avoid reporting symptoms to health care providers. The cognitively impaired client may not recognize health, behavioral, or functional changes.

8. Teach the client techniques to prevent attacks related to head and neck positioning. Tell him to avoid hyperextending or laterally rotating the neck and to wear a soft cervical collar.

8. Mechanical compression from cervical osteoarthritic changes can lead to vertebrobasilar symptoms.

9. Provide preoperative teaching and care to the client undergoing surgical intervention for TIA.

9. Carotid endarterectomy, a commonly performed surgical procedure, helps prevent strokes and stop the emboli that cause the TIAs.

OUTCOME CRITERIA
• The client and caregiver will understand treatments for TIAs.
• The client will avoid behaviors that precipitate attacks.
• The client and caregiver will recognize the signs and symptoms of a TIA and report them immediately.

Nursing diagnosis: *Potential for injury related to loss of balance during a TIA*

NURSING GOAL: To prevent injury to the client from falls during attacks

Signs and symptoms
• loss of balance
• orthostatic hypotension
• confusion
• visual field changes

Interventions

1. Measure and document the client's blood pressure while he is lying down, sitting, and standing to assess orthostatic changes. Teach the client to avoid sudden movement or position changes.

2. Have the client wear antiembolism stockings if the client has postural hypotension.

3. Assess the client's home for safety hazards, such as small rugs and narrow passageways. If needed, suggest alterations, such as adding support bars in the bathroom and safety strips in the tub.

Rationales

1. An elderly client may have orthostatic hypotension because of impaired baroreceptor reflexes, which maintain blood pressure. Sudden position changes may cause dizziness and falls.

2. Antiembolism stockings minimize venous stasis and pooling.

3. An unsafe environment increases the risk of falling.

4. Assess the need for assistive devices, such as a cane, a walker, a bedside commode, and grab bars.

4. Assistive devices maximize mobility and safety.

5. Refer the client to the physical therapy department as indicated.

5. Other diseases, such as arthritis, may contribute to mobility problems.

OUTCOME CRITERION
• The client will be free from injury during TIAs.

Nursing diagnosis: *Knowledge deficit related to management of TIAs*

NURSING GOALS: To educate the client and caregiver about the signs and symptoms of TIAs and to facilitate management of the condition

Signs and symptoms
• verbalized need for information
• fear and anxiety over diagnosis
• new onset of TIAs

Interventions

1. Teach the client the causes of TIAs, and review the common symptoms that occur.

2. Teach the client and caregiver about the medications ordered by the physician, including the dosage, frequency, and any possible adverse reactions.

3. If the physician prescribes anticoagulants, educate the client and caregiver to watch for and report any adverse reactions.

4. Encourage the client to maintain consistent medical follow-up with a physician or nurse by keeping all appointments and by immediately reporting TIAs.

5. Identify for the client emergency medical alert systems, such as Lifeline, MedicAlert, and telephone contacts.

Rationales

1. The client may blame symptoms on aging or fail to recognize them. Recognizing TIA symptoms avoids confusing them with other problems.

2. Knowledge of medications can minimize noncompliance; early identification of adverse reactions can ensure prompt treatment.

3. Adverse reactions to anticoagulants, such as bleeding gums, increased bruising, a bloody nose, black stools, or hematuria, may indicate the need for a change or a reduction in medication.

4. A client with TIA may ignore the attack because the symptoms completely resolve. An examination is necessary to prevent a major disabling stroke.

5. A client who lives alone or who has limited contact with others may have difficulty obtaining help in an emergency.

OUTCOME CRITERION
• The client and caregiver will identify signs and symptoms of TIA.
• The client will verbalize the steps for managing TIA.

NURSING ACTIONS IN VARIOUS SETTINGS
Nursing actions for a client with TIA depend on the setting in which care is provided. This section identifies which actions are appropriate in all settings and which pertain to acute care, extended care, or home care.

All settings
• Inform the client and family about the signs and symptoms of TIA.
• Review the therapies used to manage the condition.

Acute care

• Evaluate the client's symptoms by obtaining a history and physical assessment. Do not attribute complaints to old age.

• In preparation for discharge, teach the client and caregiver about the proper administration of medications.

• Assess the need for the help of community services, and refer the client to a social worker if indicated.

Extended care

• Notify the physician of all TIAs.

• Monitor the pattern of the client's symptoms and changes in function. Report any changes.

• Observe the client for drug complications.

Home care

• Review the correct way to manage TIAs and the symptoms to report.

• Assess the client's home and intervene as needed to remove hazards.

• Check the client's medication storage area and administration techniques.

SELECTED REFERENCES

Adams, H.P. "Diagnosis and Treatment of Transient Ischemic Attacks," *Modern Medicine* 55:54-61, June 1987.

Eidelman, B.H. "Transient Ischemic Attacks: Causes, Clues, and Consequences of This Stroke Precursor," *Consultant* 28(3):193-214, March 1986.

Hachinski, V., and Norris, J. *The Acute Stroke.* Philadelphia: F.A. Davis Co., 1985.

Linde, M. "Cerebrovascular Accidents," in *Nursing Management for the Elderly.* Edited by Carnevali, D.L. and Patrick, M. Philadelphia: J.B. Lippincott Co., 1986.

Matteson, M.A., and McConnell, E.S. *Gerontological Nursing.* Philadelphia: W.B. Saunders Co., 1988.

Tyler, R.H. "Transient Ischemic Attacks: Recognition and Management," *Hospital Medicine* 22(2):17-32, February 1986.

Hypertension

Hypertension is the leading cause of heart failure, stroke, and heart disease in elderly persons. About 30% of those between ages 60 and 65 and 40% of those over age 65 are hypertensive. The Joint Committee on Detection, Evaluation and Treatment of High Blood Pressure defines hypertension in elderly clients as a systolic blood pressure over 140 mm Hg or a diastolic blood pressure over 90 mm Hg. A single high blood pressure reading signifies the need to monitor blood pressure; an elevated average of two or more readings on at least two subsequent visits confirms the diagnosis.

Two forms of hypertension primarily affect elderly clients. *Isolated systolic hypertension* is an elevated systolic pressure with a normal diastolic pressure. About 43% of those over age 75 have this condition, once thought to be a normal part of aging. Studies now show that systolic blood pressure predicts the complications of hypertension in clients over age 45 more reliably than does diastolic blood pressure. *Essential hypertension,* with elevations in systolic and diastolic pressures, usually begins in clients between ages 40 and 60 and may persist in older age-groups.

ETIOLOGY
Hypertension often has no known etiology, although it is associated with a family history of the disorder, obesity, diabetes mellitus, and race (especially blacks). Many medical experts feel that isolated systolic hypertension results when the aorta loses elasticity, thereby increasing stroke volume, left ventricular ejection rate, and systemic vascular resistance. Through its association with cardiovascular disease and stroke, isolated systolic hypertension can result in a two- to threefold increase in mortality. Risk factors include obesity (more than 15% above ideal body weight), heavy sodium intake, heavy alcohol consumption, smoking, a sedentary life-style, and stress.

HEALTH HISTORY FINDINGS
In a health history interview, the client may report or the nurse may detect many of these findings:
• headache
• elevated self blood pressure reading
• flushing
• fatigue, drowsiness, or dizziness
• vision difficulties, such as blurred vision
• breathing difficulty
• anginal pain
• nausea or vomiting
• decreased appetite
• swelling of the feet or hands
• paresthesia or paralysis
• dementia
• failing memory and concentration
• history of Paget's disease or thyrotoxicosis
• personal or family history of hypertension; renal, cerebrovascular, or cardiovascular disease; or diabetes mellitus
• history of side effects from antihypertensive therapy or of noncompliance with a medication regimen
• use of over-the-counter medications, such as cold preparations or diet pills; estrogen replacement therapy; nonsteroidal anti-inflammatory medications; or diuretics
• history of overeating or heavy use of alcohol, tobacco, or caffeine
• lack of regular exercise

PHYSICAL FINDINGS
In a physical examination, the nurse may detect many of these findings:

Cardiovascular
• S_4 heart sound (suggests heart failure)
• tachycardia
• precordial heave
• dysrhythmias
• murmurs
• aortic dilatation
• increased blood pressure with orthostatic changes
• increased pulse rate
• jugular vein distention
• carotid bruits
• diminished or absent peripheral arterial pulses
• dependent edema

Integumentary
• dependent, peripheral, facial, or sacral edema

Respiratory
• orthopnea
• crackles

Gastrointestinal
• abdominal bruits

Genitourinary
• enlarged kidneys

Neurologic
• confusion with short-term memory loss

Other
• periorbital edema
• arteriolar narrowing on fundoscopic examination
• hemorrhages
• exudates
• nicking of vessels at arteriovenous crossings

• papilledema
• impaired vision
• dry oral mucosa

DIAGNOSTIC STUDIES
The following studies may be performed to evaluate the client's health status:
• serum electrolytes, creatinine, blood urea nitrogen (BUN), glucose, complete blood count (CBC), urinalysis, and electrocardiogram (ECG)—to determine related renal function and the severity and possible cause of hypertension; an abnormal ECG may show left ventricular stain or ST-T interval changes
• uric acid, total cholesterol, and lipoprotein cholesterol—to provide baseline data for monitoring the ef-

fects of therapy; a high lipoprotein cholesterol value is a cardiovascular risk factor
• blood pressure readings—to evaluate the effectiveness of treatment
• chest X-ray—to detect changes in cardiac size or shape

POTENTIAL COMPLICATIONS
• noncompliance with medications
• accidental injury
• excess fluid volume
• altered health maintenance
• hypotension
• cerebrovascular accident

Nursing diagnosis: *Noncompliance with medication regimen related to lack of understanding and motivation*

NURSING GOAL: To promote compliance by helping the client accept the diagnosis and understand the benefits of antihypertensive medications

Signs and symptoms
• denial of diagnosis
• inability to describe or follow the medication regimen
• impotence

Interventions

1. Assess the client's and caregiver's knowledge of hypertension and antihypertensive medications.

2. Assess the client's ability to read prescription labels and to differentiate among various medications.

3. Assess the client's ability to open medication bottles. Avoid using child-proof medication caps.

4. Actively involve the client in teaching, such as asking him to graph blood pressure readings or keep a calendar of medications.

5. Develop a realistic medication regimen specific for the client, relating each medication to a specific activity, such as a meal.

6. Use written instructions and visual aids to educate the client and caregiver.

7. Tell the client he can minimize hypotensive reactions to antihypertensive drugs, such as atenolol (Temormin), by rising slowly from a sitting position and avoiding strenuous exercise for 2 hours after taking medication.

Rationales

1. Involving the client and caregiver helps decrease confusion and may enhance the client's compliance.

2. Decreased visual acuity may cause inappropriate self-medication.

3. Functional deficits, such as arthritis, may contribute to noncompliance.

4. Active participation helps the client feel responsible and in control.

5. Simplifying the medication routine promotes compliance and feelings of control.

6. Written instructions and visual aids reinforce teaching, and the client and caregiver can refer to them when the nurse is unavailable.

7. Knowing how to minimize side effects may promote compliance with drug therapy and prevent injury from a sudden drop in blood pressure.

8. Assess the client's financial status and insurance policies. If he cannot afford medication, refer him to a social worker for assistance, or ask the physician about prescribing a generic brand or a less expensive medication.

8. A limited income may keep the client from purchasing and using medications.

OUTCOME CRITERIA
• The client will take medications as scheduled.
• The client will understand the actions of the medications.
• The client will have normal blood pressure readings.

Nursing diagnosis: *Potential for injury related to side effects of antihypertensive medications*

NURSING GOAL: To initiate and monitor antihypertensive therapy while preventing injury to the client

Signs and symptoms
• fluctuations in blood pressure
• altered mobility
• sensory deficits

Interventions

1. Assess the client's and caregiver's understanding of medication side effects and which ones they should report to the physician or nurse.

2. Closely supervise the client during the initial days of medication implementation.

3. Explain that the physician initially orders less than the normal dose and then increases it slowly, as needed.

4. Teach the client to change positions slowly.

5. Assess the client's home for safety hazards, such as loose rugs and inadequate lighting.

6. Refer the client who lives alone to a visiting nurse.

Rationales

1. Determining what the client and caregiver know about side effects allows the nurse to modify the care plan or teaching strategies, if necessary, and helps ensure early identification of potential problems.

2. Close supervision allows the nurse to detect and treat side effects the client may experience and to evaluate his ability to follow the medication regimen.

3. Medication is more likely to accumulate in the elderly client, and may reach toxic levels.

4. Changing positions slowly can prevent falls and helps decrease orthostatic symptoms.

5. A thorough assessment of safety hazards can decrease the potential for injury.

6. A visiting nurse can be a welcome support person for the client who lives alone, evaluating his progress and reinforcing the benefits of the medication regimen in an environment that is familiar and comfortable to him.

OUTCOME CRITERIA
• The client will identify possible adverse reactions to medications.
• The client will use proper precautions to avoid injury.

Nursing diagnosis: *Fluid volume excess related to noncompliance with sodium-restricted diet*

NURSING GOALS: To prevent fluid overload and to help the client reach and maintain an appropriate weight

Signs and symptoms
- sacral, peripheral, and periorbital edema
- pulmonary edema
- shortness of breath
- dyspnea on exertion
- productive cough

Interventions

1. Assess the client for edema, and weigh him on the same scale at the same time each day to ensure an accurate measurement.

2. Assess the client's dietary intake for 24 hours.

3. Teach the client to follow a sodium-restricted diet, and enlist the help of the caregiver or other family members, if necessary. Tell them not to add salt to his food during cooking or eating and to avoid high-sodium foods, such as lunch meats, sauces, potato chips, and fast foods. Also explain how to read food and over-the-counter drug labels to determine sodium content.

Rationales

1. Edema and steady weight gain reflect intracellular water retention.

2. This assessment can identify high-sodium foods that the client should eliminate from his diet.

3. The client may be using too much salt in his food to compensate for the decrease in taste buds associated with aging. The client and family should also be taught that most canned and processed foods and some over-the-counter drugs have a high sodium content.

OUTCOME CRITERION
- The client will comply with a sodium-restricted diet, as evidenced by decreased edema and weight loss to within 5 lb (2.5 kg) of his ideal weight.

Nursing diagnosis: *Altered health maintenance related to noncompliance with the medication regimen*

NURSING GOALS: To reduce the client's blood pressure gradually and to prevent multi-organ involvement from hypertension

Signs and symptoms
- noncompliance with treatment
- uncontrolled high blood pressure
- tachycardia
- edema

Interventions

1. Teach the client and caregiver to take the client's blood pressure. Suggest that they keep a daily chart for the nurse to review.

2. Teach the client to follow a low-sodium, low-cholesterol diet. Advise him to post on the refrigerator a list of recommended foods that he enjoys.

3. Determine whether noncompliance is related to the high cost of medication, and find out if the client qualifies for a prescription program.

4. Caution the client to avoid drinking more than 1 ounce of alcohol a day.

Rationales

1. Monitoring blood pressure regularly helps detect fluctuations and may enhance compliance with treatment.

2. Heavy sodium intake causes the kidneys to retain body fluids, which increases blood volume and results in hypertension. Reducing cholesterol helps reduce blood pressure.

3. The client may take less medication than prescribed—or eliminate medication entirely—because he cannot afford to pay for it.

4. Alcohol contains large amounts of sodium and water and elevates blood pressure.

5. If the client smokes, encourage him to quit.

5. Smoking not only depletes the body of nutrients but also stimulates the release of catecholamines, causing blood vessels to constrict and blood pressure to rise.

6. If the client is obese, develop a weight control program.

6. Restricting calories and reducing weight help decrease blood pressure, especially in the obese client.

7. Teach the client behavioral approaches to relaxation, such as biofeedback and guided imagery.

7. Emotional and physical stress increase blood pressure. Relaxation techniques can reduce such stress—and help lower blood pressure—with regular use.

8. Distribute educational materials on hypertension to the client and caregiver.

8. Educational materials reinforce the nurse's instruction and can help the client and caregiver to cope effectively with life-style changes mandated by hypertension.

OUTCOME CRITERIA
- The client will state risk factors that contribute to cardiovascular disease.
- The client will maintain optimum health of the cardiovascular system.

Nursing diagnosis: *Potential for impaired physical mobility related to side effects of antihypertensive medications*

NURSING GOAL: To prevent reduced mobility

Signs and symptoms
- reluctance to ambulate
- progressive reduction in frequency or distance of ambulation
- joint stiffness
- reduced muscular strength
- light-headedness or dizziness with postural changes
- systolic blood pressure drop of 20 mm Hg or diastolic blood pressure drop of 10 mm Hg when moving from a supine to a standing position

Interventions

1. Evaluate the client's mobility and activity level initially and during each subsequent health assessment.

2. Teach the client to check his pulse rate during routine exercise, such as walking and bathing.

3. Assess and document the client's blood pressure and pulse rate:

- Place him in the supine position, and record pressures in both arms.

- Help him to stand and ask if he feels light-headed or dizzy.
- Have him stand for 3 to 5 minutes before rechecking his blood pressure (remember to use the arm with the higher pressure).

Rationales

1. The initial assessment provides baseline data that the nurse and other health care team members can use to monitor the client's progress. Regular monitoring helps detect any decline or advancement in mobility or activity level.

2. Tachycardia during routine exercise may indicate increased blood pressure.

3. Proper assessment and documentation of blood pressure and pulse rate can help detect potential problems, such as orthostatic hypotension.

- Blood pressure may differ in each arm because of common peripheral vascular abnormalities. The arm with the higher pressure should be used for routine blood pressure checks.

- Light-headedness or dizziness on standing may indicate orthostatic hypotension.
- With age, baroreceptor responsiveness decreases and blood tends to pool in the legs, which reduces cardiac blood volume. This check can help detect profound hypotension.

• Note any substantial drop in blood pressure, change in heart rate, or new symptoms. If he shows signs of orthostatic hypotension, advise him to get out of bed each day by rising slowly, dangling his legs off the side of the bed, avoiding sudden changes in posture, and using an assistive device, such as a walker or cane.

• The client with orthostatic hypotension should take special precautions when getting out of bed to minimize dizziness and prevent injury from a fall.

4. Evaluate the client's medication regimen for other drugs that can cause orthostatic hypotension, such as tricyclic antidepressants or antipsychotics. Notify the physician of your findings.

4. Alterations in the client's medication regimen may be necessary to prevent orthostatic hypotension.

5. Assess the client for reduced circulatory blood volume from dehydration, prolonged bed rest or immobility, and peripheral vascular disease.

5. These conditions predispose the client to orthostatic hypotension.

OUTCOME CRITERION
• The client's physical mobility will not be impaired.

NURSING ACTIONS IN VARIOUS SETTINGS
Nursing actions for a client with hypertension depend on the setting in which care is provided. This section identifies which actions are appropriate in all settings and which pertain to acute care, extended care, or home care.

All settings
• Inform the client and family that hypertension is not curable but is manageable.
• Teach them that hypertension is not a normal part of aging; it requires specific therapies.
• Remind them that the client must take his antihypertensive medication even when he feels well.
• Explain the importance of keeping regularly scheduled appointments with a health care provider.

Acute care
• Maintain a restful environment.
• Consult a dietitian when appropriate.
• Before the client is discharged, assess his need for community nursing intervention, his home for potential safety hazards, his financial status and need for community services (such as Meals On Wheels or a homemaker service), his ability to administer medication and monitor for side effects, and his accessibility to a health care provider.

Extended care
• Schedule regular exercise and rest periods.
• Intervene appropriately to prevent stressful situations.
• Consult a dietitian when appropriate.
• Monitor the cognitively impaired client closely because he may not be able to articulate symptoms of hypertension or orthostatic hypotension.

Home care
• Have the client record blood pressure readings, and review them at each visit.
• Reinforce appropriate antihypertensive behaviors.
• Help develop a realistic medication regimen based on the client's life-style and activities of daily living.

SELECTED REFERENCES
Armstrong, B.A. "Protocol: Isolated Systolic Hypertension in the Elderly," *Nurse Practitioner* 12(6):1834, June 1987.
Esberger, K.K., and Hughes, S.T. *Nursing Care of the Aged.* Norwalk, Conn.: Appleton & Lange, 1989.
Hue, M.N. "Diuretics for Mild Hypertension: Still the Best Choice?" *Nursing87* 17(9):62-64, September 1987.
Klegman, E.W., and Highee, M.S. "Drug Therapy for Hypertension in the Elderly," *Journal of Family Practice* 28(1):81-87, January 1989.
Messerli, F. "The Age Factor in Hypertension," *Hospital Practice* 1:103-12, January 1986.
Reichel, W. *Clinical Aspects of Aging,* 3rd ed. Baltimore: Williams & Wilkins, 1989.
"Report of the Joint National Committee on Detection, Evaluation and Treatment of High Blood Pressure," *Archives of Internal Medicine* 148(5):1023-38, May 1988.
Sowers, J.R., and Gualdoni, S.M. "Systolic Hypertension: Its Significance and Management in Elderly Patients," *Consultant* 12:44-61, December 1985.
Yurich, A.G., et al. *The Aged Person and the Nursing Process.* Norwalk, Conn.: Appleton & Lange, 1989.

Constipation and Fecal Incontinence

Constipation is a decrease in the normal pattern of bowel movements. The onset of constipation varies from 1 to 4 days, depending on the client's normal bowel movement pattern. If the stool mass becomes hard and dry and the client is unable to expel it, fecal impaction results. Because of prolonged mucosal irritation from a large, immovable fecal mass, mucous diarrhea or the leaking of fecal material may occur. Occasionally, fecal impaction may cause a lower bowel obstruction that requires surgery.

Fecal incontinence is the uncontrolled evacuation of fecal material. Constipation, fecal impaction, and fecal incontinence frequently occur in elderly clients undergoing long-term care.

ETIOLOGY

Constipation results from either a hypertonic or hypotonic bowel. In hypertonic or spastic constipation, the client suffers from cramping of the segmental-type abdominal muscles. These contractions mix but do not propel bowel contents, which decreases transit time and increases water reabsorption. Small, hard stools result, and the client may complain of lower abdominal pain. This type of constipation may be a life-long problem because of a genetic predisposition or an emotional disturbance.

Hypotonic or atonic constipation commonly occurs in elderly clients because of decreased peristalsis, which is a normal part of aging. Decreases in fluid intake, physical activity, fiber consumption, abdominal muscle tone, and functional ability contribute to the problem. Neurologic disease, a change in environment or daily habits, or a lack of privacy may also predispose the client to constipation.

In addition, drugs such as general anesthetics, anticholinergics, analgesics, hypnotics, sedatives, and certain antihypertensives affect colon activity and may cause constipation or fecal impaction. The overuse of laxatives, which makes the colon dependent on stimulation for evacuation, or the chronic use of enemas, which damages the bowel, also cause constipation. In these instances, a bowel regimen focusing on increased fluid and fiber intake and exercise can restore normal function.

The three main causes of fecal incontinence are fecal impaction, underlying disease, and neurologic disorders. Elderly clients, particularly those who are immobilized or who have a poor fluid or dietary intake, most commonly develop fecal incontinence because of a fecal impaction. In this instance, soft, poorly formed stool seeps around the hard fecal mass and may be mistaken for diarrhea. Fecal incontinence is a presenting symptom for many underlying diseases, such as colon or rectal cancer, diverticular disease, colitis, proctitis,

or diabetic neuropathy. Sphincter damage from anorectal trauma or surgery may also cause fecal incontinence, as can chronic or excessive laxative use and radiation therapy.

Neurogenic causes of fecal impaction may be either physiologic or cognitive. Local causes include degeneration of the myenteric plexus and lower bowel, as may occur in elderly clients. Abuse of laxatives or drugs, such as the anticholinergics and phenothiazines, over 30 years or more can damage the myenteric plexus, weakening the sphincter muscle, diminishing the sacral reflex, and decreasing puborectal muscle tone, which leads to ineffective defecation.

Elderly clients commonly lose the ability to consciously inhibit the defecation reflex. Mental impairment from stroke or dementia prevents rectal fullness and causes the inability to inhibit intrinsic rectal contraction, which leads to incontinence.

HEALTH HISTORY FINDINGS

In a health history interview, the client may report or the nurse may detect many of these findings:
- small, hard stools (constipation)
- unawareness of urge to defecate prior to incontinence
- frequent, liquid stools (incontinence)
- change in stool consistency or pattern
- occasional flecks of blood in stool
- fecal staining
- abdominal pain and discomfort
- nausea and vomiting
- flatulence
- urinary incontinence
- history of diabetes mellitus, renal failure, hypothyroidism, neurologic disorders (such as cerebrovascular accident [CVA], Parkinson's disease, or Alzheimer's disease), colitis, diverticulitis, colon resection, hemorrhoidectomy, colon polyp removal, or rectal sphincter damage from irradiation or cobalt therapy
- recent bowel studies (barium enema, sigmoidoscopy)
- long-term reliance on laxatives, enemas, or suppositories
- use of anticholinergics, analgesics, narcotics, or sedatives
- use of aluminum-containing antacids or iron supplements
- diet low in fiber and fluid
- decreased appetite
- decreased functional abilities
- stressful life situations
- depression

PHYSICAL FINDINGS

In a physical examination, the nurse may detect many of these findings:

Gastrointestinal
• abdominal distention and tenderness
• masses upon palpation
• air or gas upon palpation
• decreased bowel sounds (hypomotility)
• dry, hard, small stool in rectum
• poor rectal sphincter tone
• painful rectal lesions, such as hemorrhoids or anal fissures
• rectocele
• absence of anal wink

Cardiovascular
• decreased blood pressure (fecal impaction)

Neurologic
• irritability
• impaired memory
• agitation

Other
• lethargy (fecal impaction)

DIAGNOSTIC STUDIES
The following studies may be performed to evaluate the client's health status:
• serum electrolytes and blood urea nitrogen (BUN)—to detect electrolyte imbalances and dehydration resulting from impaction, diarrhea, or the overuse of sodium phosphate enemas
• stool cultures—to rule out bacterial causes of diarrhea
• stool specimens—analyzed for ova, cysts, parasites, and leukocytosis
• guaiac specimens—to assess for occult blood
• abdominal X-rays—to identify distention or bowel obstruction
• barium enema—to identify masses, diverticula, fistulas, mucosal abnormalities (such as ulcerations and edema), or abnormalities of the bowel lumen, such as narrowing or dilation
• anorectal manometry—to gauge anal sphincter competence
• electromyography (EMG)—to document and precisely locate anal muscle weakness
• proctosigmoidoscopy—to identify Crohn's disease, ulcerative colitis, rectal neoplasms, or laxative abuse

POTENTIAL COMPLICATIONS
• constipation
• dehydration
• laxative abuse or dependence
• fecal impaction or incontinence
• diarrhea
• embarrassment
• withdrawal and social isolation

Nursing diagnosis: *Constipation related to lack of exercise and poor fiber and fluid intake*

NURSING GOALS: To promote regular bowel habits through exercise and increased fiber and fluid intake, to assess and remove fecal impaction, and to develop a long-term bowel regimen for the client

Signs and symptoms
• abdominal distention and flatulence
• abdominal cramping
• urinary incontinence
• irritability and agitation
• mental confusion
• dry, hard, infrequent stools
• excessive straining on defecation
• painful hemorrhoids
• incomplete fecal evacuation
• nausea and vomiting
• anorexia

Interventions

1. Assess the client's bowel pattern by recording his bowel movements, questioning him about habits, and performing a rectal exam.

2. Assess the client for hemorrhoids or anal fissures.

Rationales

1. These activities help to identify potential problems and to develop a reliable bowel management program. Questioning the client about bowel function may reveal elaborate systems of belief. A rectal exam will detect any stool in the rectum.

2. Hemorrhoids or anal fissures may cause pain on straining, causing the client, consciously or unconsciously, to avoid defecation.

3. Assess the client for depression or dementia. Refer a depressed client for treatment, and institute habit training in a demented client. (Habit training consists of placing the client on the toilet after breakfast and allowing him enough time for defecation.)

3. A depressed client may not have the energy or interest to use the bathroom and may need treatment before bowel function can be managed. A demented client may not remember how or when to use the bathroom, may not feel the urge to defecate, or may not be able to communicate needs to the caregiver.

4. Obtain a medication history, including patterns of laxative and enema use.

4. Anticholinergics, narcotics, barbiturates, propoxyphene hydrochloride, tranquilizers, and antacids can cause constipation. Overuse of laxatives and enemas, common in elderly clients, can lead to constipation.

5. Obtain a history of the client's usual daily diet.

5. The elderly client may eat highly refined and easy-to-prepare foods that are low in fiber.

6. Administer oral laxatives, such as docusate (Colace, Surfak) as ordered. Institute a fluid and fiber regimen if the client has not had a bowel movement for 72 hours and if the client's rectal exam is negative. Discontinue laxatives once the client has established a regular bowel pattern.

6. Laxatives help eliminate blockages high in the colon (although long-term use is habit-forming and can decrease the sensation to defecate). Bacterial degradation of fiber enhances colonic motility. An adequate fluid intake helps produce softer stools, which are easier to pass.

7. Start the client on a bowel retraining program by encouraging ten to twelve 8-oz glasses (2,500 to 3,000 ml) of fluid intake daily, recommending foods high in fiber (such as whole grains, fruits, and vegetables), and discouraging foods with a diuretic effect (such as coffee, tea, or grapefruit juice) or foods containing refined flour and sugar. Also, recommend the addition of prunes or prune juice to the daily diet. Establish a consistent, daily evacuation time and avoid using the bedpan, if possible. Respect the client's personal habits and privacy. Encourage the client to ambulate or sit up in a chair, if indicated. Perform range-of-motion exercises, leg lifts, and abdominal massage on a client confined to bed.

7. Fluids help keep stool soft and passable. Fiber helps create a bulky stool, which passes more easily; however, increasing fiber without increasing fluid intake can exacerbate the problem. Foods with a diuretic effect decrease body fluids, while refined foods add little bulk. Prune juice produces catharsis, probably because it contains magnesium salts, and prunes are relatively high in fiber. A consistent evacuation time promotes normal defecation. Bedpans cause abdominal hyperextension, which causes undue strain if the client is not properly positioned. Also, gravity may impede the passage of stool when the client is on a bedpan. Bowel motility is propulsive only in a client who is active or who participates in active or passive exercises.

8. Provide necessary physical facilities, such as bedside commodes, toilet extenders, and footstools.

8. Necessary facilities promote comfort and assist in bowel retraining.

OUTCOME CRITERIA
• The client will develop a normal bowel pattern, as evidenced by passing formed stools at regular intervals without cramping, pain, or straining.
• The client will have bowel movements without using laxatives, suppositories, or enemas.

Nursing diagnosis: *Perceived constipation related to fecal impaction*

NURSING GOALS: To remove the fecal obstruction without causing mucosal damage and to prevent recurrence by instituting a bowel management program

Signs and symptoms
• severe abdominal pain and distention
• poor appetite
• fever
• hypotension
• inability to expel stool
• history of constipation
• abdominal masses
• lethargy

• fecal mass on digital exam
• oozing of fecal material from rectum

Interventions

1. Palpate the client's abdomen for distention, rigidity, fullness, or tenderness.

2. Perform a rectal exam, and assess the size of the impaction and the hardness of the stool.

3. If the impaction is large and hard, try to break the fecal mass into smaller particles with 30 to 60 ml of full-strength hydrogen peroxide irrigation inserted into the distal rectum through a catheter tip syringe or rectal tube. Then proceed with manual removal, as described in the next intervention.

4. If the impaction is large and soft, remove as much as possible manually. Explain the procedure to the client, position him on the left side with knees flexed, ask him to take deep breaths, and encourage him to relax. Insert 1 or 2 lubricated, gloved fingers into the rectum, using a circular motion. After removing the impaction, administer a tepid milk and molasses enema (1 cup whole milk and 1 cup molasses), using a standard enema bag with a rectal tube tip. Have the client retain the enema for 15 minutes and expel contents upright on a commode or bedpan. Allow 20 minutes for full evacuation.

5. Recommend use of suppositories and digital stimulation as alternatives to laxatives and enemas. Tell the client or caregiver to insert bisacodyl or glycerine suppositories 1 hour before breakfast, to place the suppository against the bowel wall, and to administer daily until the client establishes a consistent bowel pattern. For digital stimulation, teach the client and caregiver to insert a lubricated, gloved finger gently into the rectum and to move the finger in a circular motion against the anal sphincter wall.

6. Avoid use of large-volume enemas.

7. Initiate a bowel regimen of increased fiber, fluid, and exercise.

Rationales

1. A hard mass in the left lower abdomen indicates impacted stool in the sigmoid colon.

2. A rectal exam will provide information about the size and condition of the rectum as well as about the amount and consistency of stool in the rectum.

3. Hydrogen peroxide will gently break up an impaction that is blocking the rectal orifice and assist with digital removal.

4. Manual (digital) removal of impacted stool is essential to relieve the client's discomfort and to prepare for an effective bowel regimen. The position described in the intervention allows for easy entry into the rectum. Deep breathing provides distraction and diminishes the effect of Valsalva's maneuver. One or two fingers may be needed based on the size of the impaction. Lubrication prevents trauma and eases insertion. A milk and molasses enema is soothing, cleansing, and less hazardous than other enemas, such as soapsuds or phosphate (Fleet), which can cause mucosal injury. Retention of enema promotes stool softening.

5. Laxatives and enemas can cause motor and sensory dysfunction in the colon. Damage occurs at the cellular level of the gut's autonomic nervous system. Suppositories trigger the defecation reflex and assist in establishing a regular bowel pattern. Digital stimulation causes relaxation of the internal rectal sphincter and may benefit a client who has lost voluntary control.

6. Sudden distention of the large bowel can cause shock.

7. A proper bowel regimen promotes regular bowel movements and can prevent future impactions.

OUTCOME CRITERIA
• The client will have safe and complete removal of fecal impactions.
• The client will have normal stools on a regular basis without straining or pain.

Nursing diagnosis: *Incontinence related to decreased rectal tone*

NURSING GOAL: To help the client regain control over bowel patterns and increase rectal tone

Signs and symptoms
• increased frequency and inability to control bowel movements
• use of diapers or pads
• anal irritation
• lack of awareness of the urge to defecate
• fecal stains on clothing
• frequent episodes of diarrhea
• frequent constipation or impaction

Interventions

1. Assess rectal sphincter tone by asking the client to tighten the muscle around a finger inserted into the distal rectum and by stroking the skin near the anus with a piece of cotton to elicit local contraction (anal wink).

2. Record the client's bowel movement pattern for 3 or 4 days, indicating the times, amount of stool, and relationship to meals and activities.

3. Establish a specific time, usually after a meal, for evacuation.

4. Teach the client to perform pelvic muscle-strengthening (Kegel) exercises (see "Urinary Incontinence," pages 128 to 137).

5. Promote adequate fiber and fluid intake to add bulk and to achieve a soft, formed stool.

6. Avoid the use of diapers or bed pads for stool evacuation. Instead, tell the client to sit on the commode.

Rationales

1. Failure of the anal capsule to contract on digital rectal examination indicates sphincter denervation. Absence of anal wink indicates loss of sensation in the anal area, which may cause fecal incontinence.

2. Such documentation helps identify the problem and associated causes, which assists the nurse in planning a bowel training program.

3. Bowel motility increases during and after ingestion of food. Attempting to defecate after a meal capitalizes on gastrocolic reflex action. Establishing a specific time helps the client to develop the habit of evacuation, thus preventing incontinence.

4. Kegel exercises help strengthen the pubococcygeus muscle. Control over stool expulsion is maintained voluntarily by contracting this muscle, which surrounds the external anal sphincter.

5. A soft, formed stool can be better felt and controlled.

6. When the client sits upright, gravity helps the bowel to empty. Not using diapers helps reinforce continence.

OUTCOME CRITERIA
• The client will have a decrease in the number of episodes of fecal incontinence.
• The client will develop control over bowel elimination.

Nursing diagnosis: *Diarrhea related to laxative use, medications, and bacterial infection*

NURSING GOALS: To reestablish normal bowel movements by decreasing the number and frequency of stools passed and to prevent dehydration, weakness, or anal excoriation

Signs and symptoms
• thin, watery stool
• abdominal cramping
• frequent elimination
• change in color and odor of stool
• nausea and vomiting
• malaise, sometimes accompanied by fever
• dehydration and fluid and electrolyte imbalances
• positive stool culture
• altered mental status or confusion

Interventions	**Rationales**
1. Assess the client's diarrhea for amount, consistency, and color. Perform a rectal examination to assess for fecal impaction.	1. A watery or mucoidal stool can pass around the impacted stool mass and may present as diarrhea.
2. Assess the anal area for skin irritation and breakdown. After each bowel movement, clean the area with mild soap and water, pat it dry, and apply petrolatum or a skin barrier cream (Sween cream).	2. Frequent diarrheal stool can irritate the anal mucosa. Skin care protects the skin and helps relieve discomfort.
3. Assess for exposure to flu, virus, or food poisoning.	3. Flu, virus, or food poisoning can cause diarrhea.
4. Assess the client for signs of dehydration, such as postural hypotension, sunken eyes, and rapid pulse. Obtain serum electrolyte levels.	4. Diarrhea can cause rapid development of dehydration.
5. Send a stool culture to the laboratory if indicated. If the culture is positive, follow enteric precautions: wash hands before and after contact with the client, and administer medications as ordered.	5. Infection can cause diarrhea, which is of particular concern in an institutional setting, where an infection can easily spread throughout the resident population. The usual causative bacteria, *Clostridium difficile*, is treated effectively with cholestryamin and metronidazole.
6. Assess the client for laxative abuse. Inform him that laxatives and enemas are not part of a bowel management program and should be used only for emergencies, such as an extended period without a bowel movement. Avoid using mineral oil.	6. Laxatives are a common cause of diarrhea in elderly clients. Regular use of stimulant laxatives disrupts the intrinsic innervation of the colon and thus dulls sensation for bowel elimination. Natural emptying mechanisms fail to work as the body becomes dependent on laxatives and enemas. Mineral oil interferes with absorption of fat-soluble vitamins, may precipitate hydrocarbon pnuemonitis if aspirated, and may cause fecal soiling.
7. Promote increased fiber and fluid intake to add bulk and produce regular bowel function.	7. Fiber binds with water in the intestine and forms a gel. This prevents overabsorption of water from the large intestine and ensures that its fecal content is bulky and soft. Fiber adds weight to the stool and promotes its passage through the intestine.
8. Instruct the client to avoid beverages and foods that contain caffeine, such as tea, coffee, and chocolate.	8. Caffeine increases fluid secretion in the intestine, thus increasing the amount of diarrhea.
9. Review the client's medications.	9. Magnesium-containing antacids and antibiotics may cause diarrhea.

OUTCOME CRITERIA
• The client will pass formed stools after institution of recommended measures.
• The client will reestablish normal bowel function without dependence on laxatives.

Nursing diagnosis: *Knowledge deficit related to constipation and laxative and enema use*

NURSING GOAL: To restore normal bowel function without the use of laxatives or bulk agents

Signs and symptoms
• chronic constipation or diarrhea
• need for laxatives to achieve bowel function
• unrealistic defecation goals

Interventions

1. Question the client and family about their definition of constipation and concerns about bowel function.

2. Educate the client about normal age-related changes in bowel function, such as decreased colonic motility and decreased rectal tone.

3. Teach the client and family to monitor bowel function by keeping daily records while increasing the client's intake of fiber and fluids and promoting exercise.

4. Teach the client the importance of having a regular bowel pattern. Tell him to sit on the toilet or bedside commode within 15 minutes after eating breakfast, to allow 20 to 30 minutes for evacuation, to elevate the feet on a foot stool while thrusting the body slightly forward, and to massage the abdomen along the natural progression of the colon.

5. Teach the client to heed the urge to defecate.

6. Suggest a bowel regimen centering on increased fiber, fluid, and exercise.

7. Teach the client and caregiver to increase the client's intake of bulk by slowly adding unprocessed wheat bran to the diet. Tell them to add bran to such foods as applesauce, cereals, puddings, and muffins. If the client cannot tolerate bran, tell him to mix 1 to 2 tbs of psyllium (Metamucil) with water or juice. Promote fluid intake of at least eight 8-oz glasses (2,000 ml) daily.

8. Educate the client about problems associated with chronic laxative abuse, such as dependency, frequent impaction, pain from constipation, and the need to change laxatives as tolerance develops.

Rationales

1. The client and family, because of cultural norms, may consider the lack of a daily bowel movement as constipation despite absence of clinical signs.

2. This information will increase the client's understanding of natural causes of bowel problems.

3. Weaning from laxatives takes time and requires reinforcement and reassurance.

4. Defecation may be easier for the client within 15 minutes after breakfast because eating increases colonic motility. Allowing sufficient time for evacuation is necessary because interruptions may cause voluntary contraction of the external and internal sphincters; repeated blunting of the normal defecation stimulus will cause it to be lost. Correct positioning places the body in alignment and relieves pressure on the lower back. Massaging induces the gastrocolic reflex.

5. Repeated inhibition of the defecation reflex weakens the stimulus over time.

6. Sound bowel management is based on these activities.

7. Bran is more effective than fiber in increasing bulk and colon transit time. Slowly adding bran to the diet minimizes initial gastrointestinal distress; bloating, gas, and cramps should subside within a few days. Because unprocessed wheat bran looks and tastes like sawdust, it is more palatable if mixed with food. Bran absorbs water from the gut, making adequate fluid intake necessary for stool softening. Psyllium, a high-bulk product, distends the intestines and increases peristalsis.

8. Regular use of stimulant laxatives disrupts intrinsic innervation of the colon. The chronically constipated client becomes dependent on laxatives to stimulate bowel evacuation. Besides dependence, prolonged use can lead to altered blood chemistry, physical defects, and dehydration.

OUTCOME CRITERIA
- The client and caregiver will state and understand measures to improve bowel elimination.
- The client will become less dependent on laxatives to stimulate bowel evacuation.

NURSING ACTIONS IN VARIOUS SETTINGS
Nursing actions for a client with constipation or fecal incontinence depend on the setting in which care is provided. This section identifies which actions are appropriate in all settings and which pertain to acute care, extended care, or home care.

All settings
- Develop mutually attainable goals with the client and caregiver before planning a bowel management program.
- Replace the use of laxatives with a bowel regimen consisting of increased fluid and fiber intake and regular exercise.

• Encourage the client to practice Kegel exercises regularly to increase bowel function and tone.
• Provide the client and family with information on a high-fiber diet.
• Review the interactions of laxatives with other drugs and foods, and educate the client and caregiver about these interactions.
• Teach the client about common misconceptions, myths, and realistic goals concerning bowel function.
• Assist the client to the toilet after breakfast.

Acute care
• Identify a client who is at high risk for developing constipation in order to prevent fecal impaction.
• Start a client with a spinal cord injury or other neurologic dysfunction on a bowel management program as soon as possible.
• Assess the need for intravenous fluid replacement in the client with frequent diarrhea.
• Teach the client an appropriate bowel regimen for use at home.

Extended care
• Record the client's bowel movements, noting the amount, color, consistency, time, and date.
• Provide in-service programs on proper bowel hygiene to all nursing personnel.
• Assess the need for fluid replacement therapy in the client with diarrhea.
• Consult the dietitian about palatable ways to increase the fiber content of the institutional diet.

Home care
• Teach the client and family about an appropriate bowel regimen.
• Have the client or family keep a record of bowel movements and fluid intake.
• Teach families the symptoms of fecal impaction and a method of relief.
• Perform an environmental assessment to determine deterrents to bowel retraining and the types of laxatives present in the home. Evaluate improper use of laxatives and enemas.
• Provide the client with a written bowel regimen.
• Teach the caregiver how to assist the immobile client to the bedside commode.

SELECTED REFERENCES
Behm, R.M. "A Special Recipe to Banish Constipation," *Geriatric Nursing* 216-17, July/August 1985.
Cerrato, P.L. "What to Tell Your Patients about Dietary Fiber," *RN* 63-64, January 1986.
Davis, A., et al. "Bowel Management: A Quality Assurance Approach to Upgrading Programs," *Journal of Gerontological Nursing* 12(5):13-17, May 1986.
Dodge, J., et al. "Fecal Incontinence in Elderly Patients," *Postgraduate Medicine* 83(8):258-70, June 1988.

Ellickson, E.B. "Bowel Management Plan for the Homebound Elderly," *Journal of Gerontological Nursing* 14(1):16-17, January 1988.
McShane, R.E., and McLane, A.M. "Constipation: Impact of Etiological Factors," *Journal of Gerontological Nursing* 14(4):31-34, April 1988.
Miller, J. "Helping the Aged Manage Bowel Function," *Journal of Gerontological Nursing* 11(2):37-41, February 1985.
Smith, D.A., and Newman, D.K. "Beating the Cycle of Constipation, Laxative Use, and Fecal Incontinence," *Today's Nursing Home* 10(9):12, September 1989.
Whitehead, W.E., et al. "Biofeedback Treatment of Fecal Incontinence in Geriatric Patients," *Journal of the American Geriatrics Society* 33(5):320-24, May 1985.
Wright, B.A., and Stoats, D.O. "The Geriatric Implications of Fecal Impaction," *Nurse Practitioner* 11(10):53-64, October 1986.

GASTROINTESTINAL SYSTEM

Malnutrition

Malnutrition refers to improper food intake or ineffective absorption or utilization of nutrients. Pathological malnutrition is common among hospitalized elderly persons, since those with generalized illness typically are frail and anorexic before and during hospitalization. Hospital-acquired malnutrition may result from low-calorie liquid diets prescribed before diagnostic testing. Among elderly persons residing in the community, malnutrition usually is not overt, although many older people consume foods of minimal nutritional value, which places them at risk for infections, falls, and other problems.

Age-related changes also affect proper nutrition. After age 50, the client experiences a 10% to 15% reduction in basal metabolism and often a concomitant reduction in physical activity. Thus, the client must reduce his caloric intake to maintain optimal weight. The client also experiences a loss of lean body mass and a decrease in total body protein and water. Some evidence suggests that elderly persons use protein from food intake less effectively for protein synthesis, thus depleting protein reserves. Thermoregulation changes affect the absorption and use of nutrients.

ETIOLOGY
Malnutrition can result from physical or psychosocial factors. Physical factors that can affect the client's desire to eat or ability to absorb nutrients effectively include dental problems (decayed or missing teeth or poorly fitting dentures), constipation, sensory deficits, lack of mobility, decreased strength, arthritis, physical handicaps, neurologic deficits, chronic illness, and use of multiple medications.

Psychosocial factors that may diminish the client's desire to eat or ability to prepare nutritious meals include depression, loneliness, recent bereavement, disorientation, removal from usual cultural environment and diet, abuse of alcohol and central nervous system depressants, intentional or subintentional death desires, and low income.

HEALTH HISTORY FINDINGS
In a health history interview, the client may report or the nurse may detect many of these findings:
• loss of appetite
• fatigue and generalized weakness
• lethargy
• history of chronic obstructive pulmonary disease, cancer, cerebrovascular accident, rheumatoid arthritis, or depression
• recent surgery or hospitalization
• use of diuretics or vitamin supplements, long-term laxative use, or multiple medication regimen
• food allergies, such as lactose intolerance

• prescribed restrictive diets
• inadequate knowledge of nutrition
• heavy use of alcohol or mind-altering drugs
• religious or ethnic beliefs that prevent adequate food intake
• decreased participation in normal daily activities
• recent loss, change in residence, or change in income

PHYSICAL FINDINGS
In a physical examination, the nurse may detect many of these findings:

Gastrointestinal
• nausea
• vomiting
• diarrhea
• constipation
• decreased esophageal peristalsis
• heartburn due to decreased stomach motility

Integumentary
• xerosis
• lack of fat under skin
• brittle, ridged, or spoon-shaped nails
• follicular hyperkeratosis
• thin, sparse, dry, dull hair
• angular stomatitis

Cardiovascular
• rapid heart rate
• abnormal rhythm
• elevated blood pressure

Musculoskeletal
• decreased mobility
• "wasted" appearance of muscle
• difficulty with ambulation
• epiphyseal enlargement

Neurologic
• decreased sense of taste and smell
• weakened gag reflex
• decrease in ankle and knee reflexes
• paresthesia of hands and feet

Psychological
• confusion
• disorientation
• depression

Other
• pale conjunctiva
• decreased vision
• red ocular membranes

- conjunctival xerosis (dryness)
- corneal xerosis (dullness)
- missing teeth
- multiple caries
- ill-fitting dentures
- swollen tongue
- poor oral hygiene
- poor color or condition of oral mucosa
- receding gums
- presbycusis

DIAGNOSTIC STUDIES
The following studies may be performed to evaluate the client's health status:
- complete blood count (CBC) with differential—to detect anemia
- serum iron and iron binding capacity—to detect iron deficiency
- total protein and serum albumin—decreased levels may indicate inadequate protein intake
- serum glucose—may be elevated
- folate levels—may be reduced
- percentage transferrin saturation—to detect iron deficiency
- vitamin B_{12} level—may be reduced
- serum lipids and cholesterol—may be reduced
- serum vitamin A, carotene—may be reduced
- thiamine, riboflavin, ascorbic acid—ususally decreased
- electrocardiogram (ECG)—to detect dysrhythmias
- urine specimen—for analysis and detection of glucose, blood, and ketones
- guaiac test—to assess for possible gastrointestinal hemorrhaging

POTENTIAL COMPLICATIONS
- generalized weakness and frailty
- obesity
- infection

Nursing diagnosis: *Altered nutrition: less than body requirements, related to loss of appetite, poor dentition, and lack of knowledge about proper nutrition*

NURSING GOALS: To provide a balanced nutritional diet and to maintain a stable body weight

Signs and symptoms
- weakness
- fatigue
- confusion
- insomnia
- frailty
- weight loss

Interventions

1. Assess the client for chewing problems by assessing the need for dentures, ensuring properly fitting dentures, and modifying food consistency (avoiding pureed food whenever possible).

2. Obtain a calorie count and fluid intake for 48 hours.

3. Advise the client and caregiver of deficient areas in diet, and provide suggestions for well-balanced meals based on the client's cultural background and financial status.

4. Tailor the client's diet to personal preferences and food intolerances.

5. Encourage the client to eat small, frequent meals.

6. Consider using high-calorie supplements (Ensure) or complete meal replacement formulas.

Rationales

1. Malnutrition has been correlated with the loss of natural teeth. Ill-fitting dentures may cause difficulty in chewing and swallowing or may increase the possibility of contracting or exacerbating periodontal disease. Few clients prefer foods pureed together.

2. This information is needed to assess the client's present habits and calorie intake and to determine nutritional needs.

3. The client and caregiver may lack the skills to select and prepare well-balanced meals. Cultural background and financial status may affect the client's food preferences.

4. Tailoring the diet to the client's preferences may enhance compliance.

5. The elderly client may feel full earlier and hungry sooner.

6. The client who is malnourished may need supplements to increase caloric intake.

7. Keep food warm by using heat-retaining dishes or by reheating meals in a microwave oven.

7. Warm foods are more palatable and will promote eating.

8. Avoid giving medications at mealtime, unless the medication is prescribed to be given with food.

8. Many medications interfere with the absorption of nutrients.

9. Promote the client's independence by providing self-feeding devices, placing foam rubber over utensil handles, placing the food tray where the client can easily see and reach it, removing lids, and opening packaged items.

9. A sense of independence will improve the client's general outlook and discourage depression. A physically impaired client may have difficulty eating; special feeding devices and thoughtful assistance from the nurse can make mealtimes more enjoyable.

10. Teach the caregiver to keep the client's eyeglasses, hearing aid, and dentures nearby and to prepare food based on the client's ability to chew and swallow. Explain the importance of varying the texture and consistency of food.

10. Sensory deficits affect the client's ability to eat and enjoy food.

11. Ensure a slow pace at mealtime.

11. The elderly client may have a slower reaction time. A pace that is too rapid may lead to choking or refusal to eat.

12. Assess the client for dysphagia (difficulty swallowing). If the client has difficulty swallowing, suction excess saliva before meals, and allow the sight and smell of food to stimulate salivation and prepare the swallowing reflex. Sit the client in an upright position with the head flexed slightly forward. Encourage thorough chewing, and offer solid, full-bodied foods rather than pureed, sticky, or dry foods. Inspect the client's mouth after meals for pocketed food by using a gloved finger; ask the client to sweep the inside of his mouth with his tongue and to spit out or swallow any remaining food.

12. A client with dysphagia is at risk for nutritional deficiency because of difficulty ingesting sufficient amounts of essential nutrients. Failure to clean the mouth after meals places the client at risk for aspiration.

13. Assess the client's need for oral supplementation, enteral feeding, or parenteral feeding. If any of these therapies is administered, monitor the client for complications, and document and report your findings. Provide teaching to the client and family if the client is to receive nutritional support measures at home.

13. The client may need oral supplements to improve nutritional intake. Diarrhea and aspiration are common complications in elderly clients with enteral feeding.

14. Consult with the physician if an extensive medication regimen or alcohol or drug abuse is present.

14. Certain medications interact adversely with foods; alcohol may impair effective use of nutrients.

15. Assess the client for anemia and, if present, encourage intake of iron-rich foods, such as beans, dark green vegetables, fortified cereals, and red meat.

15. Inadequate intake of iron-rich foods can lead to anemia.

16. Question the client and caregiver about any recent crisis or change in life-style.

16. Reaction to a family crisis or a change in life-style can influence dietary intake.

17. Explore precipitating factors of malnutrition, and encourage the use of community resources, such as home-delivered meals, congregate meal sites, and food stamps.

17. Limited income is a common cause of inadequate nutrition in the elderly client.

OUTCOME CRITERIA
• The client will increase his food intake.
• The client will gain 10 lb (4.5 kg) within 6 months.

Nursing diagnosis: *Altered nutrition: potential for more than body requirements, related to lack of knowledge about calorie content of foods*

NURSING GOALS: To promote a balanced diet and to help the client achieve and maintain a stable body weight

Signs and symptoms
• increased body weight
• poor nutrition from a diet consisting chiefly of "fast food" and prepackaged "instant" meals

Interventions

1. Discuss the relationship between normal weight and an increased quality of life and sense of well-being.

2. Teach general concepts about the calorie content of foods and daily nutritional needs. Discuss low-fat, low-sodium, and reduced-calorie diets as appropriate.

3. Emphasize realistic weight loss goals (12 lb [5.4 kg] per month). Divide the total desired weight loss into short-term, attainable goals. Recommend weekly recording of weight.

4. Teach the caregiver about the weight-reduction program if needed.

5. Provide the client with samples of daily menus that include nutrient-dense foods, and encourage him to avoid foods with "empty" calories.

6. Recommend the use of herbs and mild spices to enhance the flavor of foods.

7. Encourage increased physical activity, if not contraindicated.

8. Encourage the client to participate in activities, such as dancing or volunteering, where food is not the focus.

9. Inform the client of community weight-loss support groups.

Rationales

1. Such discussion may help the client realize the benefits of weight loss.

2. The client needs basic knowledge and skills to begin a successful weight-reduction program.

3. Setting realistic weight loss goals promotes good health and helps prevent the client from feeling overwhelmed by a seemingly impossible task.

4. The client may depend on others for food shopping and meal preparation.

5. Obesity does not necessarily preclude malnourishment. An obese client whose diet consists primarily of junk foods and empty calories may need examples of appropriate foods and regular reinforcement from the nurse.

6. Low-calorie and low-sodium diets with little flavor may discourage compliance.

7. Increasing physical activity will increase energy expenditure, aiding weight loss.

8. The client's previous social activities may have centered on food.

9. Social support systems can have a positive influence on the client's desire and ability to lose weight.

OUTCOME CRITERIA
• The client will monitor the number of calories he consumes daily and will eliminate high-fat foods from his diet.
• The client will lose about 12 lb (5.4 kg) per month until he attains his optimal weight.

Nursing diagnosis: *Potential for infection related to inadequate protein intake*

NURSING GOAL: To prevent skin, respiratory, and kidney infections

Signs and symptoms
• elevated temperature
• inflamed areas on skin
• difficulty breathing, productive cough, fatigue
• frequency, burning, and urgency on urination
• elevated white blood cell count

Interventions

1. Assess the client's temperature, pulse, respirations, and blood pressure daily or at each nursing visit.

2. Teach the client to recognize and report the early signs of infection (malaise, fever, loss of appetite).

3. Encourage adequate nutrition.

4. Encourage regular rest periods during the day and 7 to 8 hours of sleep nightly.

5. Promote regular physical activity, such as daily walks, and breathing exercises to improve lung capacity.

6. Discuss stress management in relation to recent and potential life-style changes.

Rationales

1. Changes from normal readings may indicate infection.

2. Early detection helps to ensure prompt treatment and a quick recovery.

3. Inadequate intake of protein and other nutrients decreases immune function.

4. Sleep deprivation can lower the client's resistance to infection.

5. Adequate physical activity helps maintain circulation and resistance to infection.

6. Knowing how to manage stress by using appropriate coping skills can help the client resist illness.

OUTCOME CRITERIA
• The client will follow a life-style that promotes better health.
• The client will be free of infection.

NURSING ACTIONS IN VARIOUS SETTINGS

Nursing actions for a client with malnutrition depend on the setting in which care is provided. This section identifies which actions are appropriate in all settings and which pertain to acute care, extended care, or home care.

All settings

• Inform the client and caregiver that malnutrition can be prevented by following a well-balanced diet and by detecting and reporting its warning signs.
• Teach the client and caregiver about low-budget meal planning when appropriate.
• Monitor the client at risk for malnutrition by assessing for signs and symptoms of the condition.

Acute care

• Assess the client for signs and symptoms of malnutrition on admission. Document and report relevant findings.
• Monitor nutritional support therapies as ordered.
• During discharge planning, assess the client's nutritional knowledge base and environmental and economic factors. If the client is to receive nutritional support therapy at home, teach the caregiver the methods for providing therapy.

Extended care

• Assess the client's food preferences, and discuss appropriate interventions with the dietary department and nursing staff.
• Encourage social interaction during meals.
• Encourage independence in meal choice and consumption.

Home care

• Teach the client and family to prepare well-balanced, economical meals.
• Inform the client of available community resources, such as Meals On Wheels, agencies on aging, and congregate meal centers.
• Assess the client's home environment, including access to shopping, ability to prepare foods, and social resources.
• Assess the availability of gas and electricity for cooking.
• Assist the client in arranging for a neighborhood store to deliver groceries if the client is unable to shop.

SELECTED REFERENCES

Bailey, L.B., and Certa, J.J. "Diagnosis and Treatment of Nutritional Disorders in Older Patients," *Geriatrics* 39(8):67-74, August 1986.

Bernard, M.A., and Rombeau, J.L. "Nutritional Support for the Elderly Patient," in *Nutrition, Aging and Health.* Edited by Young, E.A. New York: Alan R. Liss, Inc., 1986.

Breitung, J.C. *Caring for Older Adults.* Philadelphia: W.B. Saunders Co., 1987.

Drugay, M. "Nutritional Evaluation: Who Needs It?" *Journal of Gerontological Nursing* 12(4):14-18, April 1986.

Ebersole, P., and Hess, P. *Toward Healthy Aging.* St. Louis: C.V. Mosby Co., 1985.

Freedman, M.L., and Ahronheim, J.C. "Nutritional Needs of the Elderly: Debate and Recommendation," *Geriatrics* 40(8):45-62, August 1985.

Roe, D.A. *Geriatric Nutrition,* 2nd ed. Englewood Cliffs, N.J.: Prentice-Hall, 1987.

Dehydration

Dehydration is a condition in which the body is deprived of water. Older adults are more susceptible to rapid depletion of fluid and electrolytes; they have a lower water content and decreased physiologic capacity to respond to such stressors as fasting, exposure to extreme heat, strenuous exercise, diuretics, and disease. They commonly have a decreased capacity to adapt to changes in temperature and a decreased ability to maintain homeostasis. Additionally, urine concentration in older adults is typically less than three times that of plasma, instead of the usual four times. This means that elderly persons are slower to adapt to the need to conserve fluid.

ETIOLOGY
Dehydration can result from various causes and typically involves one or more of the following:
• difficulty in obtaining and drinking fluid
• vomiting
• diarrhea
• dysphagia
• increased urine production, as in uncontrolled diabetes mellitus or with diuretic use
• diaphoresis from fever or hot, dry weather
• increased respiratory rate
• upper respiratory infections
• exudates from skin affected by burns, infection, or trauma
• increased salt intake because of decreased sense of taste
• concentrated tube feedings without supplemental water
• deliberate restriction of fluid intake in the false belief that it will alleviate urinary incontinence.

HEALTH HISTORY FINDINGS
In a health history interview, the client may report or the nurse may detect many of these findings:
• thirst
• dry, warm skin
• acute confusion
• history of diabetes insipidus, pneumonia, urinary tract infection, gastrointestinal hemorrhage, cerebrovascular accident (CVA), or adrenal insufficiency
• recent major abdominal surgery, prolonged hospitalization, or acute illness
• use of diuretics and cardiac glycosides
• use of multiple enemas or laxatives
• high-protein tube feedings administered for more than 9 days
• poor dietary habits, including a high-sodium diet
• fluid intake of less than 800 ml/day
• signs of elder abuse or neglect

PHYSICAL FINDINGS
In a physical examination, the nurse may detect many of these findings:

Gastrointestinal
• dry mouth
• thirst
• reduced saliva production
• shrunken, furrowed tongue
• vomiting
• diarrhea
• nausea
• constipation
• decreased esophageal peristalsis
• hard, dry stool in lower rectum

Integumentary
• burns
• draining wounds or ulcers
• dry, warm skin
• poor color
• poor skin turgor
• abnormal perspiration

Respiratory
• increased respiratory rate

Cardiovascular
• weak, rapid pulse
• orthostatic blood pressure changes
• dysrhythmia

Genitourinary
• incontinence
• urinary frequency
• decreased urine output

Musculoskeletal
• weakness
• poor muscle tone

Neurologic
• weakened gag reflex
• decrease in ankle and knee reflexes

Psychological
• hallucinations
• irritability
• disorientation
• confusion
• restlessness
• personality changes

Other
- lethargy
- sudden weight loss
- fever or hypothermia
- dull corneas
- sunken eyes

DIAGNOSTIC STUDIES
The following studies may be performed to evaluate the client's health status:
- serum electrolytes—to indicate imbalances
- hematocrit—to indicate hydration status; levels are increased during dehydration
- serum albumin—to determine hydration status; levels are increased when body fluids are low

- serum sodium concentration—to indicate hydration status; levels are increased during dehydration
- blood urea nitrogen (BUN) and creatinine ratios—elevated levels indicate sodium and water depletion
- urinalysis—to determine hydration status; increased specific gravity and high osmolality indicate dehydration

POTENTIAL COMPLICATIONS
- hypovolemia
- infection
- constipation

Nursing diagnosis: *Fluid volume deficit related to decreased fluid intake and decreased mobility*

NURSING GOAL: To restore and maintain fluid and electrolyte balance

Signs and symptoms
- thirst
- dry tongue
- increased and irregular pulse rate
- dry skin and mucous membranes
- decreased urinary output

Interventions	**Rationales**
1. Monitor the client's pulse rate, respirations, temperature, blood pressure, and weight.	1. Rapid heart rate, elevated blood pressure, or fever may indicate dehydration or a complication that can lead to dehydration. Weight loss may signify inadequate fluid intake.
2. Encourage a gradual increase in fluid intake over 3 to 4 days.	2. Inadequate fluid intake eventually causes a deficit in the body's fluid volume. Gradually increasing fluid intake helps restore fluid balance, which takes longer to achieve in elderly clients. A sudden, substantial increase in fluid intake would place elderly clients with limited cardiac reserve at risk for congestive heart failure.
3. Promote fluid intake of at least 5 oz/hour (150 ml/hour) while awake. Offer a variety of fluids, such as fruit juices, and a variety of foods containing a high water content, such as fruit salad, gelatin, ice cream, sherbet, and popsicles.	3. An adult typically needs about 85 oz (2,500 ml) of fluid daily; 50 oz (1,500 ml) from liquids, 24 oz (700 ml) from solid foods, and 10 oz (300 ml) from oxidation of foods during metabolism.
4. Monitor the client's fluid intake and output.	4. After adequate hydration has been established, the client's fluid intake should nearly equal urine output. Careful and regular monitoring helps confirm whether this goal has been achieved.
5. Leave a water pitcher near the client's bed or chair where he can easily reach it, and refreshen the water regularly. Be sure to provide cups, glasses, and pitchers that the client can easily handle.	5. The client will be more likely to drink an adequate amount of water if it is fresh and if he can easily obtain it himself.

6. Assess the client for vomiting, diarrhea, and dysphagia, and teach the client to report these conditions immediately.

6. Dehydration can occur rapidly in an elderly client with decreased kidney mass and renal perfusion.

7. Weigh the client daily during the initial period of fluid replacement and weekly thereafter.

7. Regularly assessing the client's weight helps the nurse monitor the effectiveness of fluid replacement therapy and can prevent future episodes of dehydration.

8. Review the client's medication regimen. If the client is taking diuretics, confirm that he is taking them correctly and as indicated.

8. Misuse of diuretics is a common cause of dehydration.

9. Discourage the use of excess salt in food.

9. Increased salt intake without adequate fluid intake can cause dehydration.

10. Provide or encourage good oral hygiene.

10. Mucous membranes become dry in the dehydrated client.

11. Consult the physician on the use of hypodermoclysis if the client cannot eat and I.V. therapy or nasogastric intubation is contraindicated.

11. Hypodermoclysis, a means of fluid administration by the subcutaneous route, can be an effective means of parenteral therapy for many elderly clients. It offers several distinct advantages over I.V. and nasogastric fluid administration. For example, the client does not need to be immobilized and is at decreased risk for aspiration, thrombophlebitis, air embolism, and circulatory overload. Also, the procedure, which does not require a physician's supervision, can be started by any staff nurse familiar with subcutaneous injections and can be easily stopped at any time by closing the clamps on the clysis tubing.

12. Monitor the need for additional fluids above the maintenance volume in the client receiving high-protein tube feedings; watch for decreased urine output.

12. High-protein tube feedings given for more than 9 days are associated with dehydration because of the nitrogen load and resulting osmotic diuresis.

13. Assess the client for nocturia.

13. The client may avoid drinking fluids after the evening meal to prevent urinating at night, thus reducing his total fluid intake.

14. Use thirst as an indicator of dehydration.

14. Aging can cause a decrease in thirst sensations, resulting in dehydration.

OUTCOME CRITERION
• The client will exhibit normal vital signs and good skin turgor and will produce an adequate amount (1,200 ml/day) of amber-colored urine.

Nursing diagnosis: *Constipation related to inadequate fluid intake, lack of fiber in diet, and lack of exercise*

NURSING GOALS: To restore a normal pattern of bowel evacuation and to prevent constipation from recurring

Signs and symptoms
• straining during defecation
• hard, dry stools
• lower abdominal pain or discomfort
• abdominal masses

Interventions

1. Auscultate bowel sounds, noting any changes in activity, such as absence of bowel sounds or hypermotility.

2. Perform a rectal examination and assess the client's bowel pattern for abnormally soft, loose, or hard stools.

3. Teach the client to attempt to evacuate his bowels every morning after breakfast by sitting on the toilet, propping his feet, leaning forward slightly, and massaging his abdomen.

4. Encourage the client to exercise and to increase his intake of caffeine-free fluids. Advise the client to drink a warm beverage in the morning.

5. Teach the client and caregiver about foods that will help correct and prevent constipation, such as raw fruits and vegetables, dried fruit, and whole grain breads and cereals.

6. Tell the client to add unprocessed wheat bran to foods. Explain that bran can be used as an herb or spice and can be mixed easily into cereal, meatloaves, and casseroles.

7. Discuss the dangers of laxative and enema abuse.

8. Encourage the ambulatory client to take a brisk 1- to 2-mile (1.6- to 3.2-km) walk before breakfast, ride a stationary bicycle, or engage in other exercise on a daily basis. Encourage the bed-bound client to perform range-of-motion exercises, leg lifts, and abdominal massage.

Rationales

1. GI symptoms, such as abdominal pain, bloating, constipation, or increased flatulence, may indicate pathological problems.

2. Fecal impaction may cause constipation. A client with loose stools is losing water; a client with hard stools may be dehydrated.

3. These techniques help induce the urge to defecate (gastrocolic reflex), which is often initiated by ingesting food or warm fluids.

4. Fluids and exercise facilitate bowel evacuation. The client should be discouraged from drinking caffeine-containing beverages, as caffeine is a bladder stimulant and may cause or precipitate urinary frequency or incontinence. Warm fluids are an effective peristaltic stimulant.

5. Adding fiber and high-residue foods to the diet promotes regular bowel evacuation.

6. Bran is a high-fiber food that adds bulk to the diet and promotes bowel evacuation.

7. Laxative abuse interferes with nutrient absorption. Enemas can cause fluid and electrolyte depletion.

8. Exercise, both active and passive, can stimulate colonic peristalsis.

OUTCOME CRITERION
• The client will follow dietary recommendations to prevent further constipation.

NURSING ACTIONS IN VARIOUS SETTINGS
Nursing actions for a client with dehydration depend on the setting in which care is provided. This section identifies which sections are appropriate in all settings and which pertain to acute care, extended care, or home care.

All settings
• Teach the client and caregiver the importance of preventing dehydration.
• Explain the need for adequate fluid intake (six to eight 8-oz glasses [1,500 to 2,000 ml]) daily, unless contraindicated).

Acute care
• Assess the client for signs and symptoms of dehydration on admission and throughout hospitalization.
• Document and report relevant findings.
• If a scheduled procedure prohibits anything by mouth for a period of time, encourage the client to increase fluid intake after the procedure.

Extended care
• If the client cannot regulate fluid intake independently, keep a schedule to indicate when and how much the client should drink.
• If the evening meal is served early, be sure the client drinks some fluids during the evening to prevent dehy-

dration; keep a bedside commode or bedpan nearby for episodes of nocturia.
• Assess the client for signs and symptoms of dehydration daily; report positive signs immediately.

Home care
• Instruct the client to record fluid intake for 1 week.
• Review the client's food preferences, and encourage him to consume those with a high water content.
• Teach the client and caregiver signs and symptoms of dehydration, and stress the need for medical intervention.
• Develop a "fluid chart" for the client to follow on a daily basis.

SELECTED REFERENCES
Adams, F. "How Much Do Elders Drink?" *Geriatric Nursing* 9(9):218-21, July/August 1988.
Bernard, M.A., and Rombeau, J.L. "Nutritional Support for the Elderly Patient," in *Nutrition, Aging, and Health.* Edited by Young, E.A. New York: Alan R. Liss, Inc., 1986.
Breitung, J.C. *Caring for Older Adults.* Philadelphia: W.B. Saunders Co., 1987.
Drugay, M. "Nutritional Evaluation: Who Needs It?" *Journal of Gerontological Nursing* 12(4):14-18, April 1986.
Gaspar, P.M. "What Determines How Much Patients Drink?" *Geriatric Nursing* 9(9):221-24, July/August 1988.
Kohrs, M.B., and Czajka-Narine, D.M. "Assessing the Nutritional Status of the Elderly," in *Nutrition, Aging, and Health.* Edited by Young, E.A. New York: Alan R. Liss, Inc., 1986.
Lavizzo-Mourey, R. "Dehydration in the Elderly: A Short Review," *Journal of the National Medical Association* 79(10):1033-38, October 1987.
Lavizzo-Mourey, R., et al. "Risk Factors for Dehydration Among Elderly Nursing Home Residents," *JAGS* 36(3):213-18, March 1988.
Reedy, D.F. "How Can You Prevent Dehydration?" *Geriatric Nursing* 9(9):224-26, July/August 1988.
Roe, D.A. *Geriatric Nutrition,* 2nd ed. Englewood Cliffs, N.J.: Prentice-Hall, 1987.
Wisinger, M.W. "Hypodermoclysis in the Elderly: A Means of Hydration," *Nursing Homes* 32-33, May/June 1987.

GASTROINTESTINAL SYSTEM

Hiatal Hernia

Hiatal hernia (also called esophageal or diaphragmatic hernia) is characterized by the protrusion of part of the upper stomach into the thoracic cavity as a result of the enlargement of the diaphragmatic opening through which the esophagus passes. Most common in middle-aged and elderly clients, this type of hernia occurs more frequently in women.

Most hiatal hernias fall into one of three major categories: sliding (type 1), rolling (also called paraesophageal, or type 2), or esophagogastric (mixed). In a *sliding* hernia, the most common type, a portion of the stomach and the entire gastroesophageal junction "slide" through the weakened diaphragmatic wall into the thoracic cavity. In a *rolling* hernia, the fundus of the stomach "rolls" into the thorax through a peritoneal sac, anterior to the esophagus and posterior to the pericardium. Because of numerous and potentially life-threatening complications associated with this type, surgical correction is indicated whenever the client's health permits. In an *esophagogastric* hernia, the rarest of the three types, the protrusion characteristically includes features of both the sliding and rolling varities. It is usually treated surgically.

Only about 5% of clients with hiatal hernias are symptomatic. Gastric reflux, the most common symptom, typically manifests only when the cardioesophageal sphincter becomes incompetent. Between 85% and 90% of clients with reflux can be managed medically, such as with antacids.

ETIOLOGY
Although the cause of sliding hiatal hernia is unknown, certain conditions that lead to increased intra-abdominal pressure (such as obesity and ascites) may contribute to its development. In some cases, this type of hernia occurs secondary to a hypotensive lower esophageal sphincter (LES) caused by preexisting reflux esophagitis and spasm.

Rolling hiatal hernia, which may be a congenitally acquired condition, is usually associated with increased intra-abdominal pressure resulting from such conditions as obesity and ascites. In clients with this type of hernia, LES function and location are usually normal and reflux symptoms are rare.

The cause of esophagogastric hiatal hernia is unknown; however, some physicians believe that all large hernias through the esophageal hiatus begin as sliding hernias that ultimately evolve into massive, mixed-type hernias.

HEALTH HISTORY FINDINGS
In a health history interview, the client may report or the nurse may detect many of these findings:
• regurgitation or nocturnal aspiration of gastric reflux
• sour taste (from regurgitation of reflux)
• increasing difficulty in swallowing liquids or solids
• heartburn or epigastric pain (substernal pressure) typically occurring 30 to 60 minutes after a meal or during the night
• fullness, belching, and nausea
• discomfort accentuated by tight or constricting garments
• vomiting and retching several hours after meals (associated with rolling hernia)
• dysphagia associated with extremely hot or cold beverages or with alcoholic beverages (associated with rolling hernia)
• documented congenital abnormality
• recent ingestion of lye or another corrosive chemical
• recent trauma to the thoracic cavity
• frequent use of antacids
• long-term consumption of spicy foods, carbonated beverages, caffeine, or alcohol

PHYSICAL FINDINGS
In a physical examination, the nurse may detect many of these findings:

Gastrointestinal
• flatulence
• increased abdominal size or girth
• increased bloating
• ascites

Integumentary
• decreased skin turgor

Respiratory
• coughing
• bibasilar decreased breath sounds (secondary to aspiration of reflux)
• wheezing

Cardiovascular
• tachycardia

Other
• obesity

DIAGNOSTIC STUDIES
The following studies may be performed to evaluate the client's health status:
• complete blood count (CBC)—to detect anemia or a bleeding gastric ulcer
• guaiac test—to dectect GI bleeding
• electrocardiogram (ECG)—to determine origin of chest pain

• chest X-ray—to detect characteristic intrathoracic pressure in the retrocardiac position or to either side of the cardiac silhouette
• upper GI series—to visualize hernia (may not show reflux)
• barium esophagography—to confirm diagnosis of sliding hiatal hernia and detect strictures or ulcers
• esophageal manometry—to measure LES pressure and assess esophageal motility

POTENTIAL COMPLICATIONS
• strangulation and necrosis of a portion of the stomach, possibly leading to peritonitis
• aspiration
• anemia
• chronic pain
• dehydration
• gastrointestinal bleeding

Nursing diagnosis: *Pain related to gastroesophageal reflux*

NURSING GOALS: To eliminate pain associated with gastric reflux and to identify measures that will alleviate pain of hiatal hernia

Signs and symptoms
• heartburn
• belching
• nausea and vomiting
• pain exacerbated by lying down
• occasional regurgitation

Interventions

1. Encourage the client to eat small, frequent meals.

2. Teach the client to avoid foods that increase pain, such as spicy foods and extrememly hot or cold beverages.

3. Teach the client to avoid saturated and polyunsaturated fats, chocolate, alcohol, and carminative agents.

4. Instruct the client to remain upright for 2 to 3 hours after meals and to elevate the head of the bed 8″ to 10″ (20.3 to 25.4 cm).

5. Tell the client to avoid bending forward, straining, lifting heavy objects, and wearing tight-fitting clothing (including corsets and girdles).

6. Recommend an appropriate weight loss plan and consultation with a dietitian, if indicated.

7. Encourage the client to stop smoking, if appropriate.

Rationales

1. Because large meals overextend the stomach and promote gastroesophageal reflux, eating small, frequent meals should decrease the number of reflux episodes.

2. Spicy foods and extremely hot or cold beverages increase acid secretion in the stomach, which can lead to gastroesophageal reflux.

3. Fatty foods, chocolate, alcohol, and carminative agents can lower LES pressure, thereby causing gastroesophageal reflux.

4. Such positioning works with gravity to prevent reflux and promote esophageal clearance.

5. Increased intrathoracic pressure, caused by bending, straining, lifting, and wearing constrictive clothing, promotes gastroesophageal reflux.

6. Obesity increases intrathoracic pressure, promoting reflux.

7. Nicotine stimulates gastric acid production and lowers LES pressure, thereby promoting gastroesophageal reflux.

8. Administer antacid, cholinergic, or H_2-receptor inhibiting medications as ordered.

8. Antacids buffer acidic gastric contents and increase LES pressure by stimulating gastric secretion in response to alkalinization within the stomach. Cholinergic agents (such as bethanechol chloride and metoclopramide hydrochloride) increase LES pressure, esophageal acid clearance, and gastric emptying. H_2-receptor inhibitors (such as cimetidine and ranitidine) are sometimes indicated when symptoms persist despite medical management. These agents help to decrease the production of gastric acid, thereby relieving heartburn and other symptoms.

9. Review the client's medication regimen for drugs that may exacerbate the problem, and discuss their continued use with the client's physician.

9. Anticholinergics, theophylline, beta-adrenergic agents, diazepam, meperidine, and calium channel blocking agents may exacerbate gastric reflux.

OUTCOME CRITERION
• The client will report decreasing frequency and severity of epigastric distress.

Nursing diagnosis: *Impaired swallowing related to esophageal reflux*

NURSING GOALS: To improve swallowing ability and to prevent aspiration

Signs and symptoms
• increasing difficulty in swallowing
• frequent choking episodes
• avoidance of hot, spicy foods
• dehydration

Interventions

1. Assess the client during meals to determine the degree of dysphagia.

2. Review the client's diet, and encourage him to eliminate foods any that are difficult to swallow.

3. Encourage the client to eat soft foods, such as pudding or mashed potatoes, if necessary.

4. Instruct the client to remain upright for 2 to 3 hours after meals.

5. Encourage the client to avoid eating or drinking for 1 to 2 hours before bedtime.

Rationales

1. Such assessment is necessary because the client may be unaware of degree of swallowing difficulty. It also serves as a baseline on which to plan nursing interventions.

2. Foods that are difficult to swallow may cause choking and subsequent aspiration.

3. Soft foods are typically easier to swallow.

4. An upright position helps to prevent reflux and aspiration.

5. Avoiding food or drink for 1 to 2 hours before bedtime helps to decrease the risk of nocturnal aspiration.

OUTCOME CRITERION
• The client will experience no significant swallowing problems or aspiration.

Nursing diagnosis: *Altered nutrition: less than body requirements, related to gastroesophageal reflux*

NURSING GOAL: To provide adequate nutrition and hydration without causing gastoesophageal reflux

Signs and symptoms
- decreased intake of food and fluids
- frequent antacid use
- dehydration
- weight loss
- malnutrition
- flatulence

Interventions

1. Assess the client's nutritional status, and encourage him to eat small, frequent meals.

2. Encourage the client to decrease his intake of saturated and polyunsaturated fats, alcohol, citrus juices, caffeine, and carbonated beverages.

3. Encourage the client to increase his intake of nonirritating fluids, such as noncarbonated or nonacidic beverages.

4. Administer cholinergic agents (bethanechol chloride or metoclopramide) before meals, as ordered.

5. Help the client and his caregiver to select appropriate foods and beverages at mealtimes.

Rationales

1. A nutritional assessment may reveal malnourishment or dehydration from decreased food intake. Large meals overextend the stomach and promote gastroesophageal reflux, and should therefore be avoided.

2. These foods promote reflux by decreasing esophageal tone.

3. Adequate fluid intake prevents dehydration.

4. Administering these medications before meals helps to neutralize gastric contents and decrease acid production, thereby reducing discomfort and enhancing the client's appetite.

5. Helping the client to choose appropriate foods and beverages ensures a well-balanced diet and promotes adequate nutrition and hydration.

OUTCOME CRITERIA
- The client will achieve his optimal weight.
- The client will follow dietary recommendations.

Nursing diagnosis: *Knowledge deficit related to the disorder and management of symptoms*

NURSING GOAL: To educate the client about the disorder and factors that contribute to symptoms

Signs and symptoms
- verbalization of lack of knowledge concerning the condition
- frequent episodes of reflux and pain
- caregiver frustration over the client's meal selections or refusal to eat
- pain and discomfort after eating
- refusal to eat

Interventions

1. Assess the client's and caregiver's knowledge of hiatal hernia and its symptoms and treatment.

2. Explain to the client and caregiver that hiatal hernia is a chronic condition that may require long-term medication or sugery.

Rationales

1. Such assessment serves as a baseline on which to build nursing interventions.

2. The client and caregiver are more likely to comply with treatment if they fully understand the disorder.

3. Teach the client and caregiver to recognize the signs and symptoms of such potential complications as esophagitis (symptoms include substernal pain or heartburn precipitated by straining), esophageal erosion with hemorrhage (indicated by bleeding), aspiration (signs and symptoms include chest pain, dyspnea, and fever), and esophageal strictures (indicated by progressive dysphagia without pain).

3. Early recognition of complications can ensure prompt treatment, thereby helping to prevent serious health problems.

4. Allow opportunities for discussion, and provide appropriate feedback when necessary.

4. Such discussion helps to assess the client's understanding of the condition and how it affects him.

OUTCOME CRITERIA
• The client will demonstrate a basic understanding of the condition and its potential complications.
• The client and caregiver will identify measures to reduce the risk of potential complications.

NURSING ACTIONS IN VARIOUS SETTINGS

Nursing actions for a client with hiatal hernia depend on the setting in which care is provided. This section identifies which sections are appropriate in all settings and which pertain to acute care, extended care, or home care.

All settings
• Reinforce the importance of dietary and activity changes to control symptoms.
• Provide written instructions on suggested interventions.
• Inform the client that surgery may be required if symptoms cannot be controlled medically.
• Teach the client to take antacids only in response to symptoms and not to take them routinely.
• Keep prescribed antacids within the client's reach.

Acute care
• Assess the client for signs and symptoms of acute bleeding, swallowing difficulties, and dehydration.
• Arrange for a dietitian to evaluate the client's nutritional status and to teach him about necessary dietary changes.
• Teach the client about his condition and activity limitations and about potential complications.

Extended care
• Teach the client about necessary activity limitations to decrease reflux and pain.
• If the client is cognitively impaired, provide small, frequent, bland meals; feed the client in an upright position and instruct him to remain upright for 2 to 3 hours after meals; and elevate head of the bed 8″ to 10″ (20.3 to 25.4 cm).
• Observe the client for signs and symptoms of complications, which should be reported to the physician.

Home care
• Teach the client the correct way to use medications, if appropriate.
• Assess the client's activity level, and suggest changes to minimize bending and lifting.
• Instruct the client to elevate the head of the bed 8″ to 10″.

SELECTED REFERENCES
Burggrof, V., and Stanley, M. *Nursing the Elderly: A Care Plan Approach.* Philadelphia: J.B. Lippincott Co., 1989.
Carnevali, D.L. *Nursing Management for the Elderly.* Philadelphia: J.B. Lippincott Co., 1986.
Carroll, M., and Brue, L.J. *A Nurse's Guide to Caring for Elders.* New York: Springer Publishing Co., 1988.
Gastrointestinal Disorders. Nurse's Clinical Library. Springhouse, Pa.: Springhouse Corp., 1985.
Gray-Vickrey, M. "Color Them Special: A Sensible Guide to Caring for Elderly Patients," *Nursing '87* 17(5):59-62, May 1987.
Luckmann, J., and Sorensen, K. *Medical Surgical Nursing: A Psychologic Approach,* 3rd ed. Philadelphia: W.B. Saunders Co., 1987.

GASTROINTESTINAL SYSTEM

Dysphagia

Dysphagia is the loss or impairment of the ability to swallow, typically resulting from a head injury or degenerative neurologic disease. Although dysphagia can affect any age-group, it most commonly occurs among older adults. Estimates suggest that 40% of nursing home residents suffer from some degree of dysphagia, the most serious of which can cause severe eating and nutritional deficits.

Dysphagia can be classified according to two types: oropharyngeal (pre-esophageal), involving the oral and pharyngeal phases of swallowing, and esophageal, involving the esophageal phase of swallowing. *Oropharyngeal* dysphagia is characterized by difficulty in initiating swallowing and in transferring food from the mouth to the upper esophagus. *Esophageal* dysphagia is characterized by difficulty in the passage of food through the smooth muscle of the esophagus. The difficulty may be caused by weak or discoordinated muscles in the mouth or throat, reduced sensation in the mouth or throat, or motor sensory deficits.

Symptoms vary depending on the type of dysphagia. Oropharyngeal dysphagia is frequently associated with drooling, retention of food in the mouth, nasal regurgitation, aspiration, choking, coughing, and gagging. Esophageal dysphagia commonly involves pain behind the sternum, in the neck, or between the scapulae.

ETIOLOGY
Dysphagia can result from any process that decreases blood supply to the brain stem or damages cranial nerves. In older adults, it most commonly occurs after a cerebrovascular accident (CVA). Other common neurologic causes include head or spinal cord injury, brain tumors, anoxia, and such degenerative neurologic diseases as Parkinson's disease, amyotrophic lateral sclerosis, multiple sclerosis, and Alzheimer's disease.

Physical damage to the mouth, pharynx, or esophagus—such as narrowing of the upper GI tract, head or neck trauma, extended nasogastric intubation, tracheotomy, vocal cord paralysis, smoke inhalation, and ingestion of corrosive or caustic chemicals—can also precipitate dysphagia. Radiation therapy and treatments for cancers of the mouth, throat, and neck may damage the swallowing mechanism. Dysphagia may also occur in connection with hiatal hernia, esophageal cancer, Zenker's diverticulum, and such psychological disorders as depression and isolation.

HEALTH HISTORY FINDINGS
In a health history interview, the client may report or the nurse may detect many of these findings:
• heartburn
• sour taste

• sensation of food "sticking" in the neck or upper chest (associated with esophageal dysphagia)
• difficulty initiating swallowing, especially under stress (associated with oropharyngeal dysphagia)
• pain behind the sternum, in the neck, or between the scapulae after eating
• drooling, choking, or coughing during meals
• recurrent vomiting
• regurgitation of food through the nose
• aspiration pneumonia
• bronchitis
• asthma
• documented degenerative neurologic disease
• documented CVA
• head or neck surgery
• use of benzodiazepines or other central nervous system depressants
• use of anticholinergics
• sudden onset of snoring
• sleep apnea
• change in voice (hoarseness, gurgling, or nasalization)
• occupational exposure to dust or chemicals

PHYSICAL FINDINGS
In a physical examination, the nurse may detect many of these findings:

Gastrointestinal
• sensation of a lump in the throat
• dry mucous membranes
• paresis of the tongue, palate, or pharynx (from CVA)
• tooth loss
• delayed or absent swallow mechanism
• uncoordinated chewing or swallowing
• excessive salivation and drooling

Integumentary
• dry, warm skin
• poor skin turgor

Respiratory
• postnasal drip
• abnormal breath sounds related to aspiration

Musculoskeletal
• facial muscle weakness

Neurologic
• inability to move the mandible
• decreased sensation in face, teeth, gums, and tongue
• inability to position food for chewing
• deviation of the uvula
• irregular movement or asymmetry of the tongue
• diminished or absent gag reflex

- increased salivation
- pouching of food in the cheeks
- dysarthria

Psychological
- confusion

Other
- weight loss

DIAGNOSTIC STUDIES
The following studies may be performed to evaluate the client's health status:
- bedside dysphagia evaluation—to assess the client's ability to swallow and chew while eating
- chest X-ray—to assess for aspirated material

- pulmonary function tests—to assess the client's aspiration tolerance
- electromyography (EMG)—to study the client's oral musculature during swallowing
- ultrasound imaging—to assess oral motor functioning
- manometry and fluoroscopy—to identify motility disorders, disruptions in peristaltic waves, and esophageal sphincter disorders
- standard videofluoroscopy (cookie swallow test)—to examine the oral cavity and pharynx during swallowing

POTENTIAL COMPLICATIONS
- dehydration
- malnutrition
- aspiration
- pneumonia

Nursing diagnosis: *Potential for impaired swallowing related to physiologic dysfunction*

NURSING GOALS: To promote easy swallowing during meals and to decrease the risk of aspiration

Signs and symptoms
- drooling
- coughing while eating or drinking
- poor gag reflex
- poor suck reflex
- poor tongue mobility
- inadequate saliva production
- inability to swallow voluntarily
- inability to open mouth voluntarily
- poor control of head or neck muscles

Interventions	Rationales
1. Assess the client's overall facial muscle tone, noting any drooping or flaccidity.	1. Weak facial muscles decrease the ability to control food or fluid in the mouth, chew properly, or swallow.
2. Assess the client for speech problems.	2. Speech problems can signal a potential for dysphagia.
3. Assess the swallowing reflex by placing a finger along the client's thyroid notch and asking him to swallow.	3. Such assessment helps to determine risk for dysphagia.
4. Assess the client's ability to swallow while eating.	4. Early detection of dysphagia is imperative to prevent an obstructed airway or aspiration pneumonia.
5. Encourage the client to tilt his head forward 15 to 30 degrees and to keep his head and body aligned while eating.	5. This position keeps the epiglottis properly folded over the larynx, forcing the trachea to close and the esophagus to open, thereby easing swallowing and reducing the risk for aspiration.
6. Use pillows to elevate and support the client's upper body, if necessary, during meals.	6. The client may have reduced control over head and neck muscles and may need support for effective swallowing.
7. Face the client when feeding or assisting him during meals.	7. Food should remain in the client's visual field to stimulate salivation.

8. When the client is eating, minimize distractions, discourage him from talking with food in his mouth, and keep him focused on swallowing voluntarily.

9. Encourage the client to think or talk about food before meals.

10. Use a thickening agent to thicken fluids, such as milk, juice, soda, tea, or cocoa.

11. Encourage the client to take small bites (about one-third teaspoonful) and to eat slowly.

12. Limit the amount of food on the client's plate.

13. Offer the client bolus-forming foods, such as potatoes and pudding.

14. Instruct the client to use his tongue or finger to move food lodged between his cheek and gum to the back of his throat.

15. Keep the client's drinking cup three-quarters full, replenishing the supply as needed.

16. Give the client with a poor suck reflex a short straw, and fill his cup with a small amount of fluid.

17. Give the client fluids separately from solids, and encourage him to clear his mouth and pharynx of solid food before drinking.

18. Encourage the client to take sips of fluid between bites of food during meals (for example, tell him to take two bites of food, followed by one sip of fluid), but to avoid swallowing them simultaneously.

19. Encourage the hemiplegic client to place food in the unaffected side of his mouth and to manipulate the food with his tongue on that side.

20. Blot, rather than wipe, the client's mouth during mealtimes to remove excess food and secretions.

21. Teach the client to use his upper lip instead of his upper teeth to scrape food from utensils.

22. Instruct the client on the three phases of swallowing: the oral phase (in which the tongue and palate push food to the back of the mouth and down the throat), the pharyngeal phase (in which the food bolus is pushed into the pharynx), and the esophageal phase (in which the food is propelled into the stomach). Have him feel his throat when swallowing fluids or food.

8. The client needs to concentrate on each task involved in chewing and swallowing to minimize difficulties.

9. These activities promote saliva production, which aids chewing and swallowing.

10. Thicker fluids are typically easier to swallow.

11. Ingesting too much food too quickly increases the risk of aspiration.

12. A client with a neurologic disorder, such as dementia, may be impulsive and try to eat too quickly.

13. Foods that break apart in the mouth can easily become "lost," frustrating the client and increasing the chance of aspiration.

14. Moving food that becomes lodged in the mouth to the back of the throat helps to ease swallowing.

15. Keeping the cup three-quarters full eliminates the need to tilt the head backward, which could lead to aspiration.

16. A client with a poor suck reflex typically has trouble drawing fluid into his mouth. Using a short straw and filling the cup slightly require minimal force when sucking.

17. Because fluids do not provide as strong a stimulus for swallowing as solids do, drinking is typically more difficult for the dysphagic client. Clearing the mouth and pharynx of solid food is necessary to prevent choking or gagging.

18. Alternating fluids with solids helps to wash residual food out of the mouth and pharynx. However, swallowing fluids and solids simultaneously is more difficult than swallowing them separately and increases the risk of choking.

19. Placing food on the unaffected side of the mouth enables the client to use the unaffected portion of his mouth and tongue to manipulate the food into a bolus, thereby making the food easier to swallow.

20. Wiping stimulates the rooting reflex, which opens the mouth, making swallowing more difficult.

21. Scraping with teeth stimulates the bite reflex, which interferes with chewing.

22. The client should be aware of the phases involved in swallowing so that he can better understand his dysphagia in relation to normal physiologic mechanisms. Having the client feel his throat while swallowing forces him to be aware of the swallow reflex, which may improve voluntary swallowing.

23. Teach the client the specific swallowing sequence most appropriate for him, based on the results of diagnostic tests or other clinical analysis (for example, have the client place fluid or food in his mouth, hold his breath, move his tongue up and back, then swallow).

23. Diagnostic testing, such as a modified barium swallow, may reveal physiologic problems with the client's swallow mechanism that can be bypassed by following an individualized swallowing sequence.

OUTCOME CRITERION
• The client will be able to swallow fluids and soft foods without difficulty.

Nursing diagnosis: *Potential for aspiration related to difficulty with chewing or swallowing*

NURSING GOALS: To promote the retention of feedings and to prevent aspiration

Signs and symptoms
• choking
• pouching of food in cheeks
• excessive secretions
• inability to take food by mouth

Interventions

1. Assess the client's risk of aspiration by asking him to cough.

2. Examine the client's mouth for secretions.

3. Assess the adequacy of the client's swallow reflex by observing for the normal rise and fall of the larynx during swallowing.

4. Make sure that the client remains upright 30 minutes before to 30 minutes after meals.

5. Inspect the client's mouth between bites of food to ensure that he has swallowed all of the food.

6. Allow adequate time for meals, and encourage the client to eat slowly.

7. Encourage the client to cough and clear his throat frequently while eating.

8. Inspect the client's mouth for food at the end of the meal.

9. Advise the client to avoid dairy products.

Rationales

1. A client who cannot cough voluntarily or enough to move secretions to the front of his mouth should not be fed orally because of the risk of aspiration.

2. Thick, sticky secretions can cause the client to choke or gag; a lack of secretions can cause him to choke on food.

3. An adequate swallow reflex is essential to moving food and fluid through the pharynx and into the larnyx. Assessing the adequacy of this reflex is important because the client with a neurologic deficit may report that he has swallowed even though the reflex was not triggered. Material remaining in the pharynx may then be aspirated.

4. Maintaining the client in an upright position allows gravity to help with passing food into the stomach, thereby reducing the chance of aspiration.

5. Food remaining in the mouth and pharynx increases the risk of aspiration.

6. Eating quickly increases the risk of aspiration.

7. Coughing and clearing the throat help to remove food from the pharynx and laryngeal vestibule.

8. Food remaining in the mouth may fall into the pharynx, possibly resulting in aspiration if the client has a slow or absent swallow reflex.

9. Dairy products increase the production of saliva and mucus, possibly resulting in aspiration and lipid pneumonia.

10. Encourage the client to keep a list of specific foods (tastes and textures) that he finds difficult to swallow. Instruct him to avoid such foods when possible.

10. By avoiding foods that are difficult to swallow, the client can decrease his risk for gagging, choking, or aspiration.

11. Advise the client to avoid soft, sticky foods such as white bread, bananas, and peanut butter.

11. Such foods can adhere to the palate, making swallowing more difficult.

12. Demonstrate to the client with left hemisphere CVA the most effective way to bite, chew, and swallow.

12. A client with left hemisphere CVA will benefit more from a demonstration than spoken instructions because damage to the left cerebral hemisphere typically diminishes the ability to understand verbal instructions.

13. Provide cues, such as "Take a bite, now chew, hold your breath, now swallow," to the client with right hemisphere CVA.

13. Such cues are necessary for a client with right hemisphere CVA because damage to the right cerebral hemisphere typically causes spatial and perceptual deficits.

OUTCOME CRITERION
• The client will not aspirate food.

Nursing diagnosis: *Potential for aspiration related to enteral tube feeding*

NURSING GOALS: To promote the retention of feedings and to prevent aspiration

Signs and symptoms
• choking
• excessive secretions
• inability to take food by mouth
• dyspnea
• fever

Interventions

1. Use a small-bore weighted feeding tube when feeding the client.

2. Before each intermittent feeding, aspirate the client's stomach contents or inject 5 to 10 cc of air into the feeding tube while auscultating the stomach for air.

3. Assess the client's gastric residual volume before intermittent tube feedings or every 2 to 4 hours during continuous feedings.

4. Position the client upright during and at least 1 hour after intermittent feedings; maintain this position throughout continuous feedings.

5. Encourage the client to ambulate periodically during feedings, if appropriate.

6. Administer tube feedings at room temperature using an infusion pump.

Rationales

1. A small-bore weighted tube, which is typically more comfortable than a large-bore tube, makes swallowing secretions, food, and fluid easier. It also helps to decrease the risk of pneumonia, aspiration, and tube displacement.

2. This is done to check the placement and patency of the feeding tube.

3. Such assessment is necessary to prevent vomiting and to detect gastric retention.

4. An upright position helps prevent regurgitation and aspiration of feeding.

5. Walking aids gastric emptying.

6. Administering feedings at room temperature prevents cramping and gas formation. Maintaining a constant flow rate with an infusion pump decreases the risk of tube blockage; minimizes such adverse effects as hyperglycemia, glycosuria, and diarrhea; and maximizes absorption.

7. Assess the client for abdominal distention, bowel sounds, and esophageal regurgitation after each feeding.

7. Such assessment is necessary to determine how well the client is tolerating the feedings.

8. If the client vomits or has excessive diarrhea, discontinue the feeding and notify the physician.

8. Vomiting gastric contents can lead to aspiration pneumonia; excessive diarrhea indicates feeding intolerance.

9. Keep a suctioning device available during all meals.

9. Suctioning may be necessary to prevent the aspiration of food particles.

10. Teach the client to bend his waist or neck, if possible, during coughing or choking episodes.

10. Coughing or choking is a natural protective mechanism for the client with swallowing difficulty. Waist or neck flexion during a coughing or choking episode promotes effective airway clearance.

11. If food becomes lodged in the client's larynx, thereby compromising breathing, administer sharp blows between the scapulae. If the food does not become dislodged with this technique, use abdominal thrusts. Be sure to teach the caregiver both techniques.

11. Administering blows between the scapulae or using abdominal thrusts clears the airway and prevents aspiration.

OUTCOME CRITERIA
- The client will not aspirate tube feedings.
- The client will not develop aspiration pneumonia as a result of the tube feedings.
- The client and caregiver will be able to perform emergency interventions for choking.

Nursing diagnosis: *Altered nutrition: less than body requirements related to impaired oral intake*

NURSING GOALS: To compensate for impaired swallowing and to provide adequate nutrition and hydration

Signs and symptoms
- decreased urine output or concentrated urine
- poor skin turgor
- dry mucous membranes
- thirst
- sunken eyeballs
- weight loss
- electrolyte imbalance
- swallowing difficulty caused by physiologic dysfunctioning or emotional problems

Interventions

1. Record the client's daily food and fluid intake and output. Also record his daily weight, making sure to weigh him at the same time each day, using the same scale.

2. Review the client's laboratory values for serum electrolytes, blood urea nitrogen, and albumin studies, as indicated.

3. Administer enteral or parenteral feedings, as ordered, during the acute phase of dysphagia.

Rationales

1. Accurate recording of intake, output, and weight helps to determine the adequacy of the client's nutrition and hydration.

2. Laboratory values can help identify fluid and electrolyte imbalances that can lead to nutritional deficiencies.

3. Such feedings may be necessary to ensure adequate nutrition, which prevents muscle wasting, maintains the body's defenses against infection, and promotes wound healing.

4. Encourage the client to eat small, frequent meals.

4. Small, frequent meals are less tiring for the client and encourage thorough chewing, thereby decreasing the risk of choking and aspiration.

5. Enlist the aid of a dietitian to plan and serve meals consisting of a variety of hot and cold food and beverages.

5. Incorporating a variety of textures and temperatures into the meal plan helps to stimulate salivation, chewing, and swallowing, especially in an elderly client with a diminished sense of taste or smell.

6. Encourage the client who has trouble swallowing fluids to eat foods with a high water content, such as ice cream, gelatin, and fruit.

6. Such foods help to compensate for inadequate fluid consumption and ensure hydration.

7. Advise the client with a dry mouth to perform oral hygiene or place a slice of lemon or dill pickle on his tongue before meals.

7. Performing oral hygiene before meals helps to stimulate salivation and enhance taste perception. Tart or sour foods, such as lemons and dill pickles, can also stimulate salivation.

8. Record how much time the client spends eating during each meal.

8. Such information can help in gauging the client's progress and providing positive reinforcement. It can also help in planning schedules for activities, such as bathing or physical therapy, and determining the client's special needs, including special utensils, supervision, or assistance with feeding.

OUTCOME CRITERION
• The client will consume an appropriate number of calories to maintain adequate body weight.

Nursing diagnosis: *Self-esteem disturbance related to coughing, drooling, or choking episodes*

NURSING GOALS: To help the client accept his condition and to improve his self-esteem

Signs and symptoms
• embarrassment
• anxiety
• anger
• refusal to eat
• weight loss
• depression

Interventions

1. Offer encouragement and reinforcement regarding the client's swallowing therapy, dietary plan, and overall progress.

2. Promote a calm, leisurely environment, and encourage the client to eat at his own pace.

3. Be sure to remove any smeared or spilled food from the client's face or clothing during and after meals.

4. Teach the client how to manage choking episodes; for example, teach him to take sips of water or to try to cough to dislodge food particles.

Rationales

1. Encouragement and reinforcement help to improve self-esteem. They can also foster trust and motivate the client to adhere to the treatment regimen.

2. A calm, leisurely environment helps to reduce tension and anxiety. Eating at a controlled pace allows the client to feel more in control, which can help improve his self-esteem.

3. Residual food on the client's face or clothing may draw attention to the dysphagia, thereby contributing to the client's low self-esteem.

4. Having a specific plan to manage choking should help to reduce the client's anxiety.

OUTCOME CRITERION
• The client will demonstrate increased self-esteem by joining others for meals

---

NURSING ACTIONS IN VARIOUS SETTINGS

Nursing actions for a client with dysphagia depend on the setting in which care is provided. This section identifies which actions are appropriate in all settings and which pertain to acute care, extended care, or home care.

All settings
• Help the client and caregiver to understand the need for dietary and feeding strategies, emphasizing safety and nutrition.
• Teach client and caregiver how to perform abdominal thrusts in case of choking.

Acute care
• Assess the client's need for supervision during meals.
• Assess the client's nutritional status, and provide dietary supplements as recommended by the dietitian.

Extended care
• Assess the client's nutritional status, including his food and fluid intake and output.
• Implement safety procedures during oral feedings, and encourage the client to use techniques that promote safe swallowing.

Home care
• Compile a list of foods that the client cannot tolerate, and eliminate them from his diet.
• Reduce distracting stimuli during mealtime to help the client concentrate on chewing and swallowing.
• Change menu items as often as possible to avoid boredom and reliance on certain foods.
• Encourage the client to discuss problems or successes with his caregiver and family.

SELECTED REFERENCES
Cherney, L.R. *Evaluation of Dysphagia.* Rockville, Md.: Aspen Systems Corp., 1986.
Hufler, D.R. "Helping Your Dysphagic Patient Eat," *RN* 50(9):36-38, September 1987.
Kramer, P. "Dysphagia—Etiologic Differentiation and Therapy," *Hospital Practice* 23(3):125-49, March 30, 1988.
Logemann, J.A. *Manual for the Videofluorographic Study of Swallowing.* Boston: College-Hill Press, 1986.
Loustau, A., and Lee, K.A. "Dealing with the Dangers of Dysphagia," *Nursing 85* 15(2):47-50, February 1985.
Marshall, J. "Dysphagia," *Postgraduate Medicine* 77(5):58-68, April 1985.
Matthews, L.E. "Techniques for Feeding the Person with Dysphagia," *Journal of Nutrition for the Elderly* 8(1):59-63, June 1988.
Pritchard, V. "Tube Feeding-related Pneumonias," *Journal of Gerontological Nursing* 14(6):32-36, 1988.
Yankelson, S., et al. "Dysphagia: A Unique Interdisciplinary Treatment Approach," *Topics in Clinical Nutrition* 4(1):43-47, 1989.

Urinary Incontinence

Urinary incontinence, the inability to control urination, occurs whenever bladder pressure equals or overcomes the resistance of the urethral sphincter. An acute or a chronic condition that occurs in all age-groups, urinary incontinence affects up to 55% of all older adults living in the United States. Typically, those affected urinate at inappropriate times or places and consequently suffer embarrassment, shame, or fear over their inability to control elimination.

ETIOLOGY
In older adults, acute urinary incontinence (also called transient incontinence) typically results from any of the acute, episodic, and conventionally treated medical conditions detailed by the acronym DRIP: *dehydration* and *delirium; retention* (of urine) and *restricted mobility; infection, inflammation* (especially atrophic vaginitis and urethritis), and *impaction* (fecal); and *polypharmacy* (multiple use of diuretics, sedative-hypnotics, or antihypertensives) and *polyuria.*

Chronic urinary incontinence commonly results from persistence of any condition or combination of conditions mentioned above after treatment with conventional medical therapies. This type of incontinece can be classified into to four major categories: stress, urge, overflow, and functional.

Stress incontinence refers to the involuntary loss of small amounts of urine during activities that increase intra-abdominal pressure, such as coughing, running, laughing, or lifting heavy objects. Typically caused by weakened pelvic floor muscles or a weakened or damaged urethral sphincter, stress incontinence is most common in women but may affect men following prostate surgery.

Urge incontinence refers to the involuntary loss of urine because of the inability to reach a bathroom in time. Most common in older adults, this type of incontinence usually is caused by weakened pelvic floor muscles, detrusor hyperreflexia, sphincter incompetency, tumors, kidney or bladder stones, or diverticula. Detrusor instability (unstable bladder) is associated with disorders of the lower urinary tract or neurologic system, including multiple sclerosis and diabetes.

Overflow incontinence refers to the continuous or periodic dribbling of urine because of an atonic bladder or an anatomic obstruction, such as an enlarged prostate or a urethral stricture. This type of incontinence accounts for 10% to 15% of all incontinent clients.

Functional incontinence refers to involuntary urination because of the inability to reach a bathroom due to a specific disability, such as a physical or cognitive impairment, an inaccessible toilet, inattentive or inaccessible caregivers, or an unwillingness to move. This type of incontinence, which accounts for 25% of all incontinent clients, is common after admission to an acute care hospital.

HEALTH HISTORY FINDINGS
In a health history interview, the client may report or the nurse may detect many of these findings:
• leakage of urine when laughing, walking, or coughing (stress incontinence)
• leakage of urine when on the way to the bathroom (urge incontinence)
• dribbling of urine (overflow incontinence)
• urinary urgency and frequency
• pain on starting or stopping urination (overflow incontinence)
• weak, interrupted urine stream (overflow incontinence)
• loss of urine during sexual intercourse (stress incontinence)
• diminished sensation of bladder fullness (overflow incontinence)
• odor of urine on clothing
• nocturia
• enuresis
• perineal soreness and burning
• constipation or diarrhea
• hematuria
• bladder cancer or frequent urinary tract infections (UTIs)
• urethral dilatations
• bladder suspension or repair
• vaginal hysterectomy
• multiple difficult childbirths involving forceps and episiotomies
• surgery or radiation treatment of prostate
• radiation treatment of pelvis
• fever
• malaise
• obesity
• sacral pressure sores
• Parkinson's disease, arthritis, multiple sclerosis, or cerebrovascular accident
• current use of anticholinergic, alpha-adrenergic, antidepressant, sedative-hypnotic, diuretic, or analgesic medications
• long-term laxative use
• decreased fluid intake (because of fear of incontinence)
• heavy caffeine or alcohol consumption
• impaired mobility
• decreased cognitive ability or confusion
• depression

PHYSICAL FINDINGS

In a physical examination, the nurse may detect many of these findings:

Genitourinary
• palpable or percussable bladder
• hernia (male)
• enlarged or irregular prostate gland
• painful or swollen testes
• vaginal stenosis, atrophic vaginitis, or vaginal discharge
• cystocele or urethrocele
• foul-smelling urine
• prolapsed uterus

Integumentary
• raw, swollen perineal tissue
• perineal rash

Gastrointestinal
• hypoactive bowel sounds
• palpable masses along the colon
• abdominal tenderness or pain
• diminished anal sphincter tone
• rectocele
• fecal impaction
• absence of anal wink
• diminished rectal sensation

Musculoskeletal
• joint deformities
• difficulty in ambulation
• inability to self-toilet

Neurologic
• neuropathy

Psychological
• cognitive impairment
• depression

DIAGNOSTIC STUDIES

The following studies may be performed to evaluate the client's health status:
• urinalysis—to determine the specific gravity, pH, and color of urine and to detect the amount of glucose, blood, protein, ketones, and leukocytes in urine; abnormal findings include hematuria (which may indicate bladder cancer) and leukocytosis (which may indicate an infection)
• urine culture—to rule out infection; usually involves a clean-catch specimen to ensure that pyuria and bacteriuria do not result from contamination
• urethral catheterization—to detect urine retention and overflow incontinence; abnormal findings include a residual urine volume greater than 100 ml
• uroflowmetry—to detect obstructions, such as an enlarged prostate or urethral stricture
• urodynamic studies—to document bladder pressure and capacity, muscle contractibility, urethral length and sphincter control, and detrusor muscle stability; abnormal findings include kidney and bladder tumors and stones, obstruction of the lower urinary tract, and an enlarged prostate
• mental status testing—to evaluate cognitive function (see "Delirium," pages 225 to 229).

POTENTIAL COMPLICATIONS
• impaired skin integrity
• infection
• social isolation

Nursing diagnosis: *Altered patterns of urinary elimination related to acute illness*

NURSING GOALS: To treat and to reverse the underlying illness

Signs and symptoms
• delirium
• dehydration
• urine retention
• fecal impaction, diarrhea, or chronic constipation
• dysuria, urinary frequency, or incontinence
• atrophic vaginitis
• multiple drug use
• polyuria

Interventions

1. Assess the client for acute delirium.

Rationales

1. Acute delirium impairs sensory perception and the need to void, thereby leading to incontinence.

2. Assess for signs and symptoms of dehydration, including poor skin turgor and dry mucous membranes. Encourage fluids, if necessary, to rehydrate the client.

2. Dehydration results in the concentration of urine, which can irritate the bladder wall and precipitate incontinence.

3. Catheterize the client, as ordered, for residual urine.

3. Overflow of residual urine (greater than 100 ml) from fecal impaction, neurologic disease, or medication use can lead to incontinence. Catheterization drains residual urine from the bladder, thereby preventing incontinence.

4. Assess the client's functional status, and recommend assistive devices (such as a bedside commode or urinal), if needed.

4. A client who is recovering from surgery or an illness may be functionally disabled and require a bedside commode or urinal.

5. Perform a rectal examination to check for fecal impaction. After removing any impacted feces, institute a bowel regimen. (See "Constipation and Fecal Incontinence," pages 97 to 104).

5. Fecal impaction or chronic constipation can obstruct urine flow, thereby causing incontinence. A bowel regimen can help the client to avoid constipation and impaction.

6. Perform a dipstick urinalysis, and notify the physician if leukocytes or red blood cells appear in the urine.

6. An increased number of white and red blood cells in urine may indicate UTI, which can lead to inflammation of the bladder wall, urinary frequency, incontinence, and dysuria.

7. Assess the female client for symptoms of atrophic vaginitis, including dyspareunia, vaginal burning and itching, urinary frequency, and urine leakage. Notify the physician of the symptoms and discuss the possibility of estrogen treatment.

7. Atrophic vaginitis, common among postmenopausal women, results from estrogen deficiency. The inflammation and its resultant incontinence typically resolve with estrogen treatment.

8. Assess the client's use of medications that can cause incontinence, including diruetics, sedative-hypnotics, anticholinergics, and antihypertensives. Consult the physician about medication changes or dosage adjustments, if indicated.

8. Diuretics increase urine production and bladder pressure, thereby causing urgency and incontinence. Sedative-hypnotics dull the client's awareness of the urge to void. Anticholinergics cause incomplete bladder emptying, which precipitates retention and overflow incontinence. Antihypertensives relax the smooth muscle at the bladder neck, inducing incontinence.

9. Assess the client for polyuria and glucosuria. If the client has either of these conditions, notify the physician.

9. Polyuria and glycosuria may indicate uncontrolled diabetes, a disorder associated with urge incontinence.

10. Assess the client for Paget's disease or hypercalcemia, and notify the physician if indicated.

10. Paget's disease causes hypercalcemia, which can cause hypertonicity of the bladder muscle and increase contractibility, thereby resulting in incontinence.

11. Explain to the client that his incontinence is a temporary complication associated with his primary illness and that the incontinence should resolve with treatment. Be sure to establish a bowel and bladder regimen as soon as possible and to review all treatment recommendations with the client and caregiver.

11. Aggressive treatment of the primary illness usually resolves acute incontinence. Establishing a toileting regimen for the client helps to prevent habitual incontinence. Reviewing treatment recommendations with the client and caregiver enhances understanding and compliance.

12. Provide urinary sheaths, condom catheters, sanitary pads, adult briefs, and bedpads as needed.

12. These devices protect the client's clothing and linens until the primary illness resolves.

OUTCOME CRITERIA
- The client will follow the recommended treatment for acute urinary incontinence.
- The client will follow a bowel and bladder regimen and increase his fluid intake, as indicated.
- The client will regain partial to full bladder control.

Nursing diagnosis: *Stress incontinence related to decreased outlet resistance*

NURSING GOAL: To promote continence during activities that increase intra-abdominal pressure

Signs and symptoms
• urine leakage that occurs with increased intra-abdominal pressure (such as with lifting heavy objects, coughing, or laughing)
• history of multiple childbirths
• recent catheter removal
• recent urethral dilatation
• history of prostate surgery
• previous bladder suspension surgery (female)

Interventions

1. Teach the client how to perform pelvic muscle-strengthening (Kegel) exercises: First, have him locate his pelvic floor muscle by voluntarily stopping his urine flow in midstream or by pulling in his rectum. Next, instruct him to tighten the muscle, holding it for 10 seconds, then relaxing it for 10 seconds. Instruct him to perform the exercise for 10 minutes three times each day.

2. Instruct the client to contract his pelvic muscles before coughing, walking, or otherwise increasing intra-abdominal or thoracic pressure (such as lifting).

3. Confer with the female client's physician about the possibility of estrogen therapy.

4. Suggest the use of a pessary device to the female client with significant uterine prolapse.

5. Refer the client for biofeedback, if indicated.

Rationales

1. Exercising pelvic muscles, specifically the urogenital diaphragm, increases sphincter tone and urethral resistance.

2. Contracting the pelvic muscles before sneezing, coughing, or lifting may eliminate incontinence.

3. Estrogen therapy can restore the integrity of the urethral mucosa, thereby increasing resistance to urine leakage.

4. A pessary device, which is vaginally inserted to rest against the cervix, increases pressure on the urethra and stabilizes the ureterovesical junction under stressful conditions (such as laughing, coughing, and sneezing).

5. Biofeedback is a form of behavioral therapy that can teach the client to voluntarily inhibit bladder contractions or control sphincter muscles while relaxing abdominal muscles. It can also help remotivate the noncompliant client who is frustrated with slow progress.

OUTCOME CRITERION
• The client will eliminate or reduce incontinence within 3 months.

Nursing diagnosis: *Urge incontinence related to detrusor instability or irritation*

NURSING GOALS: To restore continence and normal patterns of urinary elimination and to teach bladder retraining measures

Signs and symptoms
• urinary frequency
• urine or ammonia body odor
• nocturia or enuresis
• social withdrawal

Interventions

1. Assess the client's voiding patterns and maintain careful bladder records. Be sure to document the time of each planned voiding, the time of each unintentional voiding, and the reason for the incontinence (such as the inability to get to a bathroom in time).

2. Assess the client's use of bladder-irritating substances (such as caffeine, aspartame, or alcohol), and encourage him to eliminate them from his diet or to minimize their use.

3. Assess the client for chronic constipation, and institute a bowel regimen, if necessary.

4. Encourage the client to drink six to eight 8-oz glasses (1,500 to 2,000 ml) of fluid during the day and to limit or eliminate his fluid intake after 6:00 p.m.

5. Instruct the client on voiding habitually if he does not void regularly (every 2 to 4 hours). Keep him on a rigid schedule (such as every 2 hours), based on his bladder record and usual continent interval.

6. Implement a bladder-retraining program once the client has successfully adapted to an every-2-hour voiding schedule. Gradually increase the voiding intervals by 30 minutes until a normal 3-to-4-hour voiding pattern is achieved.

7. Teach the client relaxation techniques, such as deep-breathing exercises and imagery, to alleviate anxiety and inhibit the urge to void. For example, teach him to relax, then to take three slow, deep breaths as soon as the initial urge to void occurs; then instruct him to wait 5 minutes before walking unhurriedly to the bathroom.

8. Teach the client Kegel exercises.

Rationales

1. Such assessment is necessary to establish a baseline. Bladder records reveal voiding patterns and help the nurse in developing a bladder retraining program.

2. Eliminating bladder irritants helps to decrease urgency, thereby helping to prevent incontinence.

3. Chronic constipation may cause urgency and increased incontinence.

4. Adequate fluids are necessary to produce sufficient urine to maintain the micturition reflex. However, drinking after 6:00 p.m. promotes nighttime urination.

5. By maintaining a habitual voiding pattern, such as every 2 hours, the client will become accustomed to voiding regularly and remaining continent.

6. Bladder retraining restores normal voiding patterns and improves bladder capacity and functioning.

7. Relaxation training helps control the urge to void, allowing the client enough time to reach a toilet.

8. Such exercises improve pelvic muscle tone, which helps to decrease urinary urgency and prevent incontinence.

OUTCOME CRITERIA
• The client will void every 3 to 4 hours during the day and only once or twice during the night and have fewer incontinence episodes within 3 months.
• The client will reduce constipation-related uregency by achieving normal bowel functioning within 1 month.

Nursing diagnosis: *Urine retention related to prostate enlargement and medication use*

NURSING GOALS: To alleviate urine retention and to restore continence

Signs and symptoms
• impaired sensation of bladder fullness
• abdominal discomfort
• inability to empty bladder despite fluid intake
• chronic bladder distention
• residual urine in excess of 100 ml
• dribbling incontinence

Interventions

1. Assess the client for fecal impaction, and take corrective measures as necessary.

2. Teach the client specific techniques to encourage complete bladder emptying, including Credé's maneuver (manually squeezing the bladder to empty the urine), bearing down with the abdominal muscles, and following a rigid (every-2-hours) voiding schedule.

3. Evaluate the client's medication regimen for drugs known to cause urine retention. If necessary, consult the physician about medication changes or dosage adjustments.

4. Perform a rectal examination and a urethral catheterization. Refer the client with an enlarged prostate or a post-voided residual of greater than 100 ml to a urologist.

5. Teach the client to perform intermittent self-catheterizations every 4 to 6 hours.

6. Insert an indwelling catheter, as ordered, providing proper catheter care and weekly reevaluations.

Rationales

1. A fecal mass in the rectosigmoid colon may compress the bladder and produce either urine retention or incontinence.

2. A client, especially one with nerve damage or paralysis, may require specific bladder-emptying techniques to ensure complete emptying and prevent incontinence.

3. The elderly client may use over-the-counter drugs, such as cold medicines and antihistamines, that can cause urine retention.

4. Prostatism and urethral strictures often cause obstructive uropathy in the male client, which may require a prostatectomy (see "Benign Prostatic Hypertrophy and Prostate Cancer," pages 138 to 146) or surgery to release the stricture.

5. Clean, intermittent catheterizations are a safe and effective long-term treatment for bladder emptying dysfunction, such as incontinence.

6. An indwelling catheter may be necessary for the client who lacks the manual dexterity to perform intermittent catheterizations, who has skin breakdown from frequent contact with urine, who is terminally ill, or who does not have a caregiver who can perform intermittent catheterizations. Providing proper catheter care decreases the risk of bladder obstruction, leakage, and spasms. Weekly evaluations help to monitor the catheter's functioning and effectiveness.

OUTCOME CRITERIA
- The client will be able to perform an appropriate bladder-emptying technique within 2 weeks.
- The client will have no signs of fecal impaction or urine retention.

Nursing diagnosis: *Functional incontinence related to decreased physical or cognitive capability*

NURSING GOAL: To enhance continence through nursing interventions and assistive devices

Signs and symptoms
- memory deficit
- anger and frustration
- recent illness or hospitalization
- impaired mobility
- inaccessible toilets or caregivers

Interventions

1. Assess the client's home and physical and mental capabilities.

2. Encourage the client to drink six to eight 8-oz glasses (1,500 to 2,000 ml) of caffeine-free fluid a day.

3. Review the client's bowel patterns, promoting good bowel function, such as regular bowel movements and no straining upon defecation.

4. Encourage the caregiver and nursing staff to respond promptly to the client's calls for assistance.

5. Instruct the client on voiding habitually if he does not void regularly (every 2 to 4 hours). Keep him on a rigid schedule (such as every 2 hours) based on his bladder record and usual continent interval, shortening the voiding interval if incontinence persists and lengthening the interval when the client remains consistently dry.

6. Place a commode near the client's bed, and leave a night-light on in the room. Keep the bed side rails down, when possible.

7. Suggest the use of other assistive devices, such as male and female urinals and fracture bedpans.

8. Advise the client to wear less restrictive clothing, such as clothing with hook and loop (Velcro) fasteners, and encourage him to ambulate regularly.

9. Recommend the use of an external urine collection device, such as a condom catheter, for the male client to wear at night or when leaving the house.

10. Advise the client to avoid using mechanical devices, such as penile clamps.

11. Encourage the client to use protective pads only as a last resort.

12. Develop a contingency management program, if necessary.

Rationales

1. Such assessment is necessary to determine whether any physical or mental barriers may be contributing to the client's incontinence. For example, the nurse may discover that the client has a severe physical disability, such as arthritis, that prevents him from walking to the bathroom; or the pathway to the client's bathroom may be cluttered, blocking its entrance.

2. Adequate fluid prevents dehydration, which causes urine concentration and bladder irritation that can precipitate incontinence.

3. Constipation and fecal impaction cause chronic incontinence.

4. Unresponsiveness or tardiness may result in an incontinence episode or the client's attempt to ambulate alone, which could lead to a fall or serious injury.

5. By maintaining a habitual voiding pattern, such as every 2 hours, the client will become accustomed to voiding regularly and remaining continent. Such a program is especially helpful for those who do not feel the need to void or who cannot communicate the imminence of voiding.

6. Placing a commode near the bed and keeping the room adequately lit facilitates toileting. Keeping the bed side rails down enables the client to have unrestricted access to the bathroom.

7. Such devices facilitate toileting, thereby alleviating or eliminating urinary incontinence.

8. Restrictive clothing and immobility prevent the client from responding promptly to the urge to urinate.

9. An external urine collection device, used for short-term therapy, is effective for controlling incontinence. However, because long-term use can cause UTIs from irritation and penile constriction, the client should be assessed daily for penile maceration, ischemia, pain, and discomfort.

10. These devices traumatize the urethra and penis and cause skin necrosis and urine retention. They are difficult to apply and can be embarrassing to the client, lowering his self-esteem.

11. Protective pads encourage dependency and incontinence.

12. Contingency management, a method of habit training that incorporates positive reinforcement, helps to promote continence in clients who are institutionalized or who require the help of a caregiver.

Nursing diagnosis: *Potential for impaired skin integrity related to urinary incontinence*

NURSING GOAL: To prevent skin breakdown caused by exposure to urine leakage

Signs and symptoms
• frequent incontinence
• itching and burning in the groin or on the upper thighs and buttocks
• excoriated epidermis
• pain over the entire affected area
• ammonia body odor

Interventions

1. Assess the client's perineum for signs of skin breakdown, rash, or infection.

2. Wash the affected area with mild soap and warm water whenever the client's clothing or pad is changed.

3. Apply a moisture barrier cream to the affected area.

4. Apply vitamin E oil from capsules to reddened areas.

5. Instruct the client or caregiver to change saturated pads or diapers promptly.

6. Dry the client's skin thoroughly and apply corn starch to the affected area.

7. Inspect the client's skin frequently.

8. Advise the female client to avoid using feminine hygiene deodorants on the affected area.

9. Review incontinence management methods, such as condom catheters, external drainage systems, and behavioral interventions, with the client and caregiver.

Rationales

1. Constant moisture in the perineal area can cause skin maceration and infection.

2. Cleaning the skin of urine prevents odor and the breakdown of the epidermal layer.

3. Moisture barrier creams help protect sensitive skin from irritation and possible breakdown.

4. Vitamin E soothes rashes and excoriated areas.

5. Heavy, wet pads or diapers promote chafing and excoriation.

6. Thorough drying and corn starch applications protect the skin from maceration.

7. Frequent inspection is necessary to ensure early detection of skin breakdown, which can lead to pressure sores, UTIs, and systemic sepsis.

8. Certain ingredients, such as alcohol, in commercial products may cause an allergic response—for example, a rash, that can lead to skin breakdown.

9. Such methods may be necessary to ensure continence and prevent the possibility of skin breakdown.

Nursing diagnosis: *Potential for infection related to urine leakage, use of perineal pads, and external or internal catheters*

NURSING GOAL: To prevent urosepsis and systemic infection

Signs and symptoms
• foul-smelling, cloudy urine
• open, red sores with possible drainage
• fever
• dysuria
• perineal itching
• worsened incontinence

Interventions

1. Instruct the client to drink at least six 8-oz glasses (1,500 ml) of caffeine-free fluid a day.

2. Obtain a urine specimen for urinalysis and urine culture, as ordered.

3. Notify the physician if the client experiences any changes in the amount or color of perineal drainage or if he develops a fever.

4. Administer antibiotics as prescribed.

5. Teach the client and caregiver the signs and symptoms of UTI.

6. Reevaluate the client's use of internal and external catheters weekly, and teach the client appropriate behavioral interventions, as needed.

Rationales

1. Increasing fluid intake dilutes urine, thereby decreasing the bacterial count and risk of infection.

2. These tests identify pathogens, ensuring effective treatment for infection.

3. Increased drainage, fever, and dark brown, amber, or reddish urine, and fever usually indicate a worsening of the infection.

4. Antibiotics interfere with the replication of bacteria and resolve infection.

5. Early recognition of infection ensures prompt intervention and medical management, thereby reducing the risk of repeated infections, which can cause chronic cystitis and urosepsis.

6. Long-term use of internal and external catheters increase the client's risk of infection. Behavioral interventions, such as habitual voiding, bladder retraining, and Kegel exercises, can help chronic incontinence sufferers to avoid infection.

OUTCOME CRITERIA
• The client will have no signs of a UTI.
• The client and caregiver will learn to recognize the signs and symptoms of UTI.
• The client and caregiver will implement necessary self-care measures to decrease the risk of UTI.

Nursing diagnosis: *Social isolation related to embarrassment about urinary incontinence*

NURSING GOAL: To prevent the client's withdrawal from family, friends, and social events because of embarrassment about incontinence

Signs and symptoms
• verbalized fear of leaving the house
• lack of interest in socialization
• self-imposed isolation
• depression

Interventions

1. Question the client about his usual social activities.

2. Instruct the client on appropriate methods for dealing with incontinence such as bladder retraining, assistive devices, or incontinence pads.

Rationales

1. Such questioning helps to reveal the extent of the client's isolation.

2. Learning about methods for dealing with incontinence can provide the client with hope for improvement, which can help him to feel less isolated.

3. Encourage the client to express his concerns about his incontinence and how it affects him socially.

3. Because incontinence is not a socially acceptable topic of conversation, the client may welcome the chance to express his concerns about his condition and social situation.

4. Refer the client to an incontinence support group, such as Help for Incontinent People.

4. An incontinence support group can help the client to identify treatment options, provide general information about normal and abnormal urinary patterns, and provide a means of socialization.

OUTCOME CRITERIA
• The client will feel less isolated and more aware of methods to treat and control incontinence.
• The client will demonstrate improved self-esteem and dignity.

NURSING ACTIONS IN VARIOUS SETTINGS

Nursing actions for a client with urinary incontinence depend on the setting in which care is provided. This section identifies which actions are appropriate in all settings and which pertain to acute care, extended care, or home care settings.

All settings
• Inform the client and caregiver that incontinence is a symptom, not a disease.
• Teach the client and caregiver that incontinence is not a natural result of aging.
• Instruct the client about normal voiding patterns and behaviors.
• Reinforce behavioral interventions, such as Kegel exercises, relaxation methods, and habitual voiding.

Acute care
• Assess the client for signs and symptoms of acute incontinence.
• Refer the client to the physician for treatment, when indicated.
• Consider temporary catheterization in clients who have significant perineal and sacral skin breakdown.
• Assess the need for follow-up nursing supervision when planning the client's discharge.

Extended care
• Teach the client relaxation techniques to use in response to his urge to void.
• Teach the client Kegel exercises, and help him to maintain accurate bladder records.
• Institute a habitual voiding schedule, and ensure that the nursing staff consistently implements the plan.
• Implement necessary alternative measures, such as intermittent self-catheterization, external catheterization, or incontinence pads or diapers, if habitual voiding or bladder retraining fails.
• Assess the client for acute causes of incontinence before applying diapers.

Home care
• Assess the client for functional disabilities.
• Assess the client's home toilet facilities.

• Instruct the client or caregiver on maintaining accurate bladder records.
• Teach the client and caregiver habitual voiding techniques, relaxation methods, and Kegel exercises.
• Discourage the use of indwelling catheters.
• Remove indwelling catheters whenever possible, and institute a bladder retraining program.

SELECTED REFERENCES

Baigis-Smith, J., et al. "Managing Urinary Incontinence in Community-Residing Elderly Persons," *Gerontologist* 29(2):229-33, April 1989.

Burgio, K.L., et al. "Urinary Incontinence in the Elderly," *Annals of Internal Medicine* 104:507-75, October 1985.

Greengold, B., and Ouslander, J. "Bladder Retraining," *Journal of Gerontologic Nursing* 12(6):31-35, June 1985.

Halker, S. "Disposable vs. Reusable Incontinence Products," *Geriatric Nursing* 6(6)1:345-47, November/December 1985.

Kniep-Hardy, M.J., et al. "Managing Indwelling Catheters in the Home," *Geriatric Nursing* 6(5):280-85, September/October 1985.

Morishita, L. "Nursing Evaluation and Treatment of Geriatric Outpatients with Urinary Incontinence," *Nursing Clinics of North America* 23(1):189-206, March 1988.

Newman, D.K. "The Treatment of Urinary Incontinence in Adults," *Nurse Practitioner* 14(6):21-23, June 1989.

Newman, D.K., and Smith, D.A. "Incontinence: The Problem Patients Won't Talk About," *RN* 52(3):42-45, March 1989.

Ouslander, J.G. "Urinary Incontinence: Geriatric Challenge," *Diagnosis* 42-52, July 1986.

Simons, J. "Does Incontinence Affect Your Client's Self Concept?" *Journal of Gerontological Nursing* 11(6):37, June 1985.

Smith, D.A. "Continence Restoration in the Homebound Patient," *Nursing Clinics of North America* 23(1):207-18, March 1988.

GENITOURINARY SYSTEM

Benign Prostatic Hypertrophy and Prostate Cancer

The prostate gland, a walnut-shaped structure located at the base of the bladder surrounding the first urethral segment, is a major source of worry and discomfort for many elderly men. Palpable only during a rectal examination because of its anatomic position, the prostate gland is clinically significant largely because of its affinity for inflammation, hyperplasia, and cancerous growth.

Benign prostatic hypertrophy (also known as prostatitis or enlargement of the prostate gland) is the most common cause of bladder outlet obstruction in men over age 50. An age-related condition whose onset typically occurs between ages 60 and 70, prostatic hypertrophy affects about one half of all elderly males, 75% of whom are symptomatic after age 70.

Prostate cancer, the second leading form of cancer in men over age 80 and the third leading cause of cancer-related death in men of all ages, is an insidious adenocarcinoma that, even in its later stages, commonly leaves the client asymptomatic. Its rate of growth varies according to the individual. In some clients, prostate cancer grows slowly over an extended period; in others, it grows aggressively within a short period. Regardless of its rate of growth, however, this cancer typically spreads by one of three routes: by direct extension (beginning locally, then spreading to other, outlying tissue), through the bloodstream, or through the lymphatic system. Staging is normally based on the extent of growth.

ETIOLOGY
Prostatic hypertrophy results from an increase in the number of cells, particularly the prostatic stromal, epithelial, and muscular cells. Although its exact etiology is still unknown, the condition is related directly to advancing age and possibly to hormonal (androgen) imbalances, high zinc levels in the prostate gland and recurrent urinary tract infections (UTIs). Race may also be a contributing factor, as the incidence of prostatic hypertrophy is significantly higher among white males.

Although theorists have hypothesized about the cause of prostate cancer, no single theory provides a satisfactory explanation. Suggested causes include advancing age (prostate cancer rarely affects men under age 50); genetic predisposition (the cancer tends to occur in families); race (prostate cancer has a higher incidence among blacks); hormonal imbalance (most prostate cancers depend to some degree on androgen production); exposure to chemical carcinogens, including those in the diet; and industrial or environmental exposure to cadmium.

HEALTH HISTORY FINDINGS
In a health history interview, the client may report or the nurse may detect many of these findings:
• urinary hesitancy or difficulty in initiating voiding
• loss of urinary stream force and caliber (especially in the morning and during the night)
• double-streamed urination
• post-voided dribbling
• increasing nocturia
• weakened or delayed urge to void
• interrupted urine stream while voiding
• burning or pain on urination
• dark amber or blood-tinged urine
• urinary frequency and urgency
• hematuria
• weight loss
• anorexia (may indicate prostate cancer)
• gradual onset of back pain
• history of diabetes mellitus
• history of UTIs or prostate surgery
• use of anticholinergic or sympathomimetic agents
• use of antidepressant, diuretic, or antiparkinsonian medications
• heavy caffeine or alcohol consumption

PHYSICAL FINDINGS
In a physical examination, the nurse may detect many of these findings:

Genitourinary
• palpable and percussable bladder
• suprapubic tenderness
• smoothly surfaced prostate—either firmer than usual (fibromuscular) or soft and boggy (adenomatotic)
• enlarged prostate—either symmetrically or asymmetrically

DIAGNOSTIC STUDIES
The following studies may be performed to evaluate the client's health status:
• serum acid phosphatase studies—to detect cancer; levels are usually elevated in prostate cancer; normal levels, however, do not accurately reflect the absence of disease, especially in the early stages; false-positive results may occur if a specimen is drawn within 48 hours of either a prostate examination or a prostatic massage
• complete blood count (CBC)—to detect anemia, which is common in chronic renal failure and metastatic prostatic adenocarcinoma

• urinalysis and urine culture—to detect infection and altered renal function; red blood cells in the urine may indicate benign prostatic hypertrophy
• urethral catheterization—to obtain an assessment of post-voided residual urine (a residual volume greater than 100 ml indicates urine retention); inability to insert a catheter may indicate prostate enlargement
• uroflow urodynamic testing—to assess the extent of urethral outlet obstruction
• cystoscopy—to visualize the urethra, prostate, and bladder and to determine the size of the prostate and degree of obstruction; indicated if obstructive symptoms are severe
• radiographic studies (including abdominal and pelvic ultrasonography and intravenous pyelography)—to detect prostate enlargement, upper urinary tract obstruction, trigonal involvement, ureteric obstruction, and bladder calculi

• magnetic resonance imaging (MRI)—to aid in differentiating benign tissue from cancerous tissue
• needle biopsy of the prostate gland—to confirm a carcinoma; positive confirmation should be followed with staging the cancer

POTENTIAL COMPLICATIONS
• symptoms of chronic urinary obstruction, including urinary incontinence, urine dribbling, bladder fullness or distention, and recurrent UTIs.
• urinary tract infection
• renal dysfunction (long-standing obstruction)
• anxiety and fear
• urinary incontinence
• sexual dysfunction
• infection
• pain
• depression
• multiple-organ metastasis

Nursing diagnosis: *Potential for infection related to acute prostatitis*

NURSING GOAL: To prevent bacterial overgrowth and subsequent UTI

Signs and symptoms
• foul-smelling, cloudy urine
• elevated temperature
• dysuria
• abdominal discomfort
• urinary frequency
• chills and fever
• positive urine culture (more than 100,000 white blood cells/ml of urine)

Interventions

1. Assess the client for signs and symptoms of prostatitis, including burning, urinary frequency, hematuria, and foul-smelling or cloudy urine.

2. Obtain a urine specimen for urinalysis and urine culture; report positive findings to the physician.

3. Instruct the client to drink at least eight 8-ounce glasses (2,000 ml) of fluid each day.

4. Instruct the client to consume foods and fluids that form acid ash, including cranberry and prune juices, meats, eggs, and fish. Also instruct him to limit his intake of milk and dairy products.

5. Assess the client for signs of urethral obstruction, including urine dribbling, abdominal pressure and pain, and decreased urine output. Insert a suprapubic catheter, as ordered.

6. Encourage the client to engage in frequent sexual intercourse or masturbation, if appropriate.

Rationales

1. Prostatitis can present either as a systemic febrile illness or as a localized inflammation.

2. Because acute prostatitis typically results from a bacterial infection, such tests are necessary to identify specific pathogens and to determine the appropriate course of treatment.

3. Adequate fluid intake helps dilute the urine, thereby decreasing the bacterial count and degree of infection.

4. Foods that form acid ash acidify the urine, thereby inhibiting bacterial growth. Milk and dairy products alkalinize the urine and should therefore be limited.

5. If the assessment reveals a urinary obstruction, suprapubic catheterization, rather than urethral catheterization, may be ordered to bypass the inflamed prostate and urethra.

6. Frequent sexual intercourse reduces prostatic congestion.

OUTCOME CRITERION
• The client will be free of infection related to acute prostatitis.

Nursing diagnosis: *Potential for injury related to postoperative infection and hemorrhage*

NURSING GOALS: To prevent incisional infection and minimize postoperative bleeding

Signs and symptoms
• excessive bloody drainage
• elevated temperature
• incisional pain
• erythema
• anemia

Interventions

1. Assess the client's incision for signs and symptoms of infection, including malodorous, purulent drainage; induration; and erythema. Obtain a wound culture, if indicated.

2. Change the client's wound dressings while maintaining sterile technique, and wash the skin around the incision site. Note and record the color, odor, and amount of drainage.

3. Take measures to prevent coughing, sneezing, or straining during defecation. Ask the physician to order a stool softener or to prescribe a cough medication or antihistamine, if necessary.

4. Instruct the client on proper perineal care after bowel movements.

5. Assess the incisional drain and suprapubic catheter for patency.

6. Obtain an order for sitz baths.

7. Avoid performing rectal examinations on the client or administering enemas to him for at least 1 week.

8. Use an oral thermometer when taking the client's temperature.

9. Consult the physician about removing the catheter as soon as the urine clears and becomes clot-free.

10. Advise the client to avoid strenuous activity for 6 to 8 weeks postoperatively.

Rationales

1. Because skin is the first line of defense against infection, wound cultures are essential to identifying the causative bacteria.

2. Dressings collect urinary drainage, which can cause bacterial overgrowth, and therefore require frequent changing. Washing the skin around the incision site removes urine, which can cause irritation and infection.

3. Increased intra-abdominal pressure could cause the wound to hemorrhage.

4. Perineal care prevents wound infection caused by fecal cross-contamination.

5. Blood may collect at the catheter tip, causing obstruction, urine retention, stasis, and infection.

6. Sitz baths clean the wound and promote healing.

7. Rectal examinations and enemas may increase bleeding because of referred irritation to the prostate.

8. Rectal thermometers may irritate or traumatize the surgical area.

9. Removing the catheter promptly helps to prevent the risk of UTI.

10. Avoiding strain promotes optimal healing and prevents complications.

OUTCOME CRITERIA
• The client will have minimal bleeding.
• The client's wound will be free from infection.

Nursing diagnosis: *Potential for injury related to radiation and estrogen replacement therapy*

NURSING GOAL: To identify and prevent injury from radiation and estrogen replacement therapy

Signs and symptoms
• nausea and vomiting
• impotence
• gynecomastia
• thrombophlebitis
• fluid retention

Interventions

1. Administer estrogen, as ordered.

2. Advise the client that estrogen therapy causes impotence and gynecomastia. Discuss the implications of these changes.

3. Instruct the client to report signs of thrombophlebitis, including calf tenderness, swelling, and redness.

4. Instruct the client to take estrogen after meals to control its resultant nausea and vomiting. If nausea and vomiting persist, consult the physician about the possible use of medications to relieve side effects.

5. Discuss with the client the use of radiation therapy. Explain that radiation therapy may involve treatment with an external beam (which is reserved for the client who is not considered a good surgical candidate) or interstitial seed implantation (which is associated with fewer complications in comparison to external radiation or radical prostatectomy).

Rationales

1. Orally administered estrogen helps to slow tumor growth and maintain normal acid phosphatase levels by suppressing the release of luteinizing hormone, which indirectly decreases the amount of testosterone in the blood. Estrogen replacement causes fluid retention that can lead to heart failure and is therefore contraindicated in clients with cardiac disease.

2. Impotence occurs in all male clients on estrogen therapy. Gynecomastia may cause physical discomfort, from breast tenderness and enlargement, and alter the client's body image.

3. Estrogen therapy is contraindicated for those with or at high risk for developing thrombophlebitis.

4. Most side effects, including nausea and vomiting, can be managed with medication.

5. Radiation may be used before or after surgery to reduce the size of the tumor or to cure the cancer.

OUTCOME CRITERION
• The client will experience no harmful side effects or discomfort from estrogen therapy.

Nursing diagnosis: *Altered patterns of urinary elimination related to prostate enlargement and chronic prostatitis*

NURSING GOALS: To alleviate urinary symptoms and complications of urine retention and to maintain optimal bladder functioning

Signs and symptoms
• urinary hesitancy
• decreased force and caliber of urinary stream
• intermittent or double-streamed urination
• nocturia
• post-voided dribbling
• perineal discomfort

Interventions

1. Assess the client for suprapubic distention and discomfort.

2. Instruct the client to void every 2 to 3 hours and to perform Credé's maneuver (manually squeezing the bladder to empty the urine) when voiding. Also instruct him on intermittent self-catheterization, if indicated.

3. Caution the client to avoid using antihistamine, bronchodilator, and anticholinergic medications.

4. Catheterize the client to obtain a post-voided residual urine volume.

5. Encourage the client to decrease his fluid intake after 6 p.m., preferably eliminating his intake 2 to 3 hours before bedtime.

6. Advise the client to avoid drinking caffeinated and alcoholic beverages.

7. Consult the client's physician about the possible use of prostatic massage and sitz baths to reduce discomfort.

Rationales

1. Increased distention and discomfort may signal urine retention.

2. Regular voiding, bladder emptying, and intermittent self-catheterization help to prevent urine retention, thereby reducing the risk of infection.

3. Such medications can contribute to urine retention, which can lead to infection.

4. In clients with benign prostatic hypertrophy, nodules grow and compress the urethra, which obstructs urine flow. Catheterization helps to determine the presence or recurrence of urine retention and the need for further intervention.

5. Limiting fluids in the evening decreases nocturia.

6. Caffeine and alcohol cause diuresis and urinary frequency.

7. The combination of prostatic massage (digital stroking of the prostate via the rectum) and sitz baths helps to decrease the amount of prostatic secretions and edema.

OUTCOME CRITERIA
- The client will regain bladder control as evidenced by a decrease in urinary frequency and nocturia.
- The client will have improved bladder emptying.

Nursing diagnosis: *Stress incontinence related to prostate surgery*

NURSING GOAL: To help the client remain continent

Signs and symptoms
- urinary dribbling
- urinary frequency and urgency
- urine leakage upon exertion

Interventions

1. Explain to the client that urinary incontinence is common postoperatively and that it typically subsides within 6 months.

2. Teach the client pelvic muscle-strengthening (Kegel) exercises (see "Urinary Incontinence," pages 128 to 137).

Rationales

1. Because internal and external bladder sphincter muscles lie close to the prostate gland, they may be injured during surgery, particularly when a perineal prostatectomy is performed. Such injury can cause temporary incontinence. Also, use of an indwelling catheter can cause a temporary loss in bladder tone, resulting in incontinence.

2. Kegel exercises actively strengthen the pelvic floor muscle, which increases the client's ability to remain continent when intra-abdominal pressure increases.

3. Advise the client and caregiver on the temporary use of condom catheters or disposable pads during periods of incontinence.

3. Using condom catheters or disposable pads can help the client to achieve a sense of continence; however, they may foster dependence, thereby promoting incontinence.

4. Advise the client to call the nurse or physician if signs and symptoms of obstruction (such as hesitancy or decreased urine volume or stream force) recurs.

4. Regrowth of prostate tissue is common and can lead to obstruction.

OUTCOME CRITERIA
• The client will practice Kegel exercises several times a day.
• The client will have fewer incontinence episodes.

Nursing diagnosis: *Pain related to the surgical incision and bladder spasms*

NURSING GOALS: To alleviate pain and to prevent complications

Signs and symptoms
• sharp, intermittent bladder spasms
• urgency to void or defecate
• urine leakage around the catheter site
• incisional pain

Interventions

1. Assess the client's pain, noting its location and intensity.

2. Inform the client that bladder spasms typically resolve within 24 to 48 hours. Administer oxybutynin chloride (Ditropan) or belladonna and opium rectal suppositories (B & O Supprettes), as ordered.

3. Maintain catheter patency by gently irrigating the catheter with 80 to 100 ml of normal saline solution while maintaining aseptic technique.

Rationales

1. Postoperative pain may result from the surgical incision or bladder spasms. The client who has undergone transurethral resectioning or suprapubic prostatectomy sometimes has bladder spasms and severe pain caused by the surgical incision into the bladder, whereas the client who has undergone retropubic or perineal prostatectomy typically has minimal spasms and only mild pain because an incision was unnecessary.

2. Such information reassures the client that his discomfort is a normal, self-limiting consequence of surgery. Antispasmodics and rectal suppositories are usually administered to help relax the bladder; however, their use is contraindicated in the client with glaucoma or severe cardiac disease.

3. Bladder distention or irritation caused by the opening of the catheter balloon can cause painful bladder spasms and bleeding. Irrigating the bladder helps to control bleeding and maintain catheter patency.

OUTCOME CRITERION
• The client will have relief from bladder spasms.

Nursing diagnosis: *Knowledge deficit related to prostatectomy*

NURSING GOALS: To educate the client and the client's family about prostatectomy and to reduce their fear and anxiety

Signs and symptoms
• expression of concerns regarding the possible outcome of surgery (such as impotence and incontinence)

Interventions

1. Explain to the client and the client's family the surgical methods involved in prostatectomy, including transurethral resectioning (TURP) and the suprapubic transvesical, retropubic, and perineal methods. Explain that the TURP procedure, which offers the fastest recovery, involves removal of obstructing tissue through the urethra; the suprapubic transvesical method, removal through a low midline incision into the bladder; the retropubic method, removal through a low abdominal incision; and the perineal method, removal through the scrotum and rectum.

2. Inform the client and caregiver about the client's expected postoperative condition. For example, prepare them for the sight of an indwelling catheter connected to an irrigation solution, hematuria, and a large amount of bloody drainage from the wound.

3. Inform the client that his presurgical symptoms of urinary frequency and urgency may continue after the surgery.

Rationales

1. The client and family need to know the details about the surgical method involved to anticipate the client's physical appearance and expected recovery.

2. Explaining to the client and family about the client's expected condition helps to allay their fears of the unknown.

3. These symptoms may persist because of poor bladder muscle tone resulting from surgical trauma and catheterization.

> **OUTCOME CRITERIA**
> • The client and caregiver will understand the techniques used in prostate surgery.
> • The client and caregiver will be prepared for the client's postoperative condition.

Nursing diagnosis: *Sexual dysfunction related to prostatectomy*

NURSING GOAL: To educate the client about changes in sexual function

Signs and symptoms
• verbalization of sexual inadequacy
• antisocial behavior
• impotence
• retrograde ejaculation
• difficulty maintaining intimate relationships

Interventions

1. Encourage the client to express his concerns about his sexual functioning.

2. Inform the client about the possibility of postoperative retrograde ejaculation.

3. Refer the client for sexual counseling if sexual dysfunction persists 6 months after surgery.

Rationales

1. The client who has undergone perineal prostatectomy and radical dissection may experience sexual dysfunction because of swelling, bleeding, pain, impotence, or inability to maintain an erection. However, except for a lack of seminal fluid, sexual capacity and enjoyment should return to presurgery levels within 2 months.

2. After prostatectomy, the bladder neck remains open, causing ejaculated semen to pass retrogradely from the proximal urethra into the bladder via the distal urethra and meatus, thereby giving the ejaculate a milky appearance. Retrograde ejaculation, although a permanent condition, does not interfere with sexual activity.

3. The client may have preexisting psychological problems that are causing his sexual dysfunction.

4. Advise the client to avoid sexual intercourse for at least 3 weeks after surgery.

4. This allows adequate time for tissue healing.

5. Advise the client to avoid using tranquilizers and certain antihypertensive agents such as methyldopa (Aldomel).

5. These drugs may decrease libido.

OUTCOME CRITERIA
• The client will feel sexually adequate.
• The client will learn to cope with a temporary change in sexual performance.

Nursing diagnosis: *Body image disturbance related to orchiectomy*

NURSING GOAL: To help the client adapt to his altered body image

Signs and symptoms
• sadness
• anger
• grief
• depression
• refusal to touch or look at the surgical area
• withdrawal

Interventions

1. Discuss with the client and the client's family the indications for orchiectomy and the potential side effects, including impotence, gynecomastia, nausea, and vomiting.

Rationales

1. Orchiectomy, the surgical removal of one or both testes, depresses androgen production, thereby eliminating the source of male hormones and possibly depressing cancer growth. It also is thought to reduce the pain associated with prostatic cancer. Bilateral orchiectomy is the treatment of choice for clients who have cardiovascular disease or who have not complied with drug therapy.

2. Encourage the client to discuss his feelings about his orchiectomy and its impact on his life.

2. Such discussions enable the nurse to assess the client's body image and self-esteem and to offer appropriate counseling or treatment, if indicated.

3. Allow the client to grieve.

3. Grieving is essential with any loss if the client is to move toward acceptance.

OUTCOME CRITERION
• The client will achieve a more positive body image.

NURSING ACTIONS IN VARIOUS SETTINGS
Nursing actions for a client with benign prostatic hypertrophy or prostate cancer depend on the setting in which care is provided. This section identifies which actions are appropriate in all settings and which pertain to acute care, extended care, or home care situations.

All settings
• Educate the client and the client's family about possible voiding pattern changes characteristic of benign prostatic hypertrophy. Emphasize which changes, such as obstruction, require immediate medical attention.

• Teach all male clients the importance of a yearly rectal examination after age 40, as early detection makes cancer more treatable.
• Advise the client to seek regular follow-up evaluations and to report any postoperative or other problems, such as urinary incontinence that persists 6 months after surgery, to the physician.
• Help the client and the client's family to cope with the psychosocial impact of the diagnosis of a cancer with a high mortality.
• Assess the home of the client with urinary frequency to determine whether he will have safe access to a

bathroom. If the client is prone to falls, provide an alternate toilet device, such as a urinal, bedside commode, or bedpan.

Acute care
• Inform the client about each of the recommended surgical procedures, and prepare him for any potential postoperative complications.
• At discharge, teach the client proper incision care (if applicable), correct use of assistive devices for urine dribbling, and how to perform Kegel exercises.
• Assess the client for urinary incontinence, and inform him that incontinence is temporary.

Extended care
• Assess the client for signs and symptoms of acute urinary obstruction and for adverse reactions to the prescribed treatment. Report significant findings to the physician immediately.
• Maintain the client's dignity, and provide support through the grieving process.
• Observe the client for voiding pattern changes, especially oliguria; report any changes to the physician immediately. Catheterize the client for urine retention.
• Inform the client that his urinary signs and symptoms are caused by his enlarged prostate gland. Assess ways to minimize discomfort and embarrassment (see "Urinary Incontinence," pages 128 to 137, for specific behavioral techniques).

Home care
• Assess the client's home for safety; recommend assistive equipment (such as a bedside commode, urinal, or bedpan), if indicated.
• Instruct the client's family to contact the physician immediately if the client has signs of a urinary obstruction or a urinary or incisional infection (such as decreased urine output, inability to initiate urination, fever, foul-smelling urine, hematuria, and incisional drainage), exhibits any significant behavioral changes (such as irritability, delirium, or confusion), or complains of pain.
• Help the client and the client's family to cope with the psychosocial impact of the diagnosis of a cancer with a high mortality.

SELECTED REFERENCES
Bachers, E.S. "Sexual Dysfunction after Treatment for Genitourinary Cancers," *Seminars in Oncology Nursing* 1(1):18-24, February 1985.
Badalament, R.A., et al. "New Diagnostic Techniques in Prostate Cancer," *Journal of Urological Nursing* 6(4):252-58, October/November/December 1987.
Barker, S., et al. *Principles of Ambulatory Medicine.* Baltimore: Williams & Wilkins Co., 1986.
Crawford, E.D., and Dawkins, C. "Diagnosis and Management of Prostate Cancer," *Hospital Practice* 21(3):159-62, March 1986.
Diseases, 2nd ed. Nurse's Reference Library. Springhouse, Pa.: Springhouse Corp., 1987.
Huben, R., and Murphy, G. "Prostate Cancer: An Update," *CA—A Cancer Journal For Clinicians* 36(5):274-92, September/October 1986.
Joseph, A.C., and Chang, M.K. "A Bladder Behavior Clinic for Post-Prostatectomy Patients," *Urologic Nursing* 9(3):15-19, January/March 1989.
Loughlin, K., and Whitmore, W. "Managing Prostate Disorders In Middle Age and Beyond," *Geriatrics* 42(7):45-56, July 1987.
Sawyer, P.F. "Prostatectomy: Nursing Care, Radical Prostatectomy for Cancer of the Prostate—Nursing Diagnosis and Interventions," *Journal of Urological Nursing* 6(4):266-75, October/November/December 1987.

Urinary Tract Infection

A bacterial invasion of the genitourinary tract that results in at least 100,000 colonies of organisms/ml of urine, urinary tract infection (UTI) is the second leading cause of febrile illness in elderly clients and a major cause of death among nursing home residents. Because elderly clients commonly present with atypical signs and symptoms (such as delirium, confusion, or general malaise) rather than typical signs and symptoms (such as urinary incontinence, burning upon urination, or cloudy and foul-smelling urine), diagnosing UTI is frequently difficult.

About 25% of all women develop a UTI at least once in their lifetime, the risk increasing with age. Men are less prone to this type of infection under age 50, probably because of their anatomic makeup: The male urethra is 7″ to 8″ (17.8 to 20.3 cm) long, whereas the female urethra is only 1″ to 2″ (2.5 to 5.1 cm) long; also, prostatic fluid serves as an antibacterial shield. However, after age 50, the incidence of UTI in men increases sharply: 50% of all men in this age-group develop benign prostatic hypertrophy (enlargement of the prostate gland), which leads to urine retention and decreased bactericidal activity of urine and prostatic secretions.

Asymptomatic bacteriuria, which primarily affects elderly clients, occurs in about 50% of all elderly clients who undergo long-term indwelling urinary catheterization and about 5% of those who are catheterized intermittently. In this type of infection, bacteria ascend between the urethral mucosa and catheter or within the catheter lumen, thereby colonizing in the bladder.

Treatment for persistent asymptomatic bacteriuria is controversial. Because the infection is difficult to eradicate (treatment carries the risk of some clients developing antibiotic-resistant strains of bacteria) and has a high incidence of recurrence, physicians typically have withheld treatment in elderly clients. However, recent studies suggest that elderly clients with untreated asymptomatic bacteriuria may develop renal insufficiency, possibly resulting in death.

ETIOLOGY

Although most UTIs result from a single type of gram-negative enteric bacteria that enters the urinary meatus and travels up the urethra, some result from a systemic infection that descends into the urinary tract. Common pathogens include *Escherichia coli*, which causes up to 85% of all uncomplicated UTIs; *Proteus*, which is especially common in elderly men, frequently resulting in chronic prostatitis; *Citrobacter* and *Providencia*, which frequently affect chronically catheterized clients; *Klebsiella*; *Enterobacter*; *Serratia*; and *Pseudomonas aeruginosa*.

Certain factors predispose elderly clients to urinary infections and sepsis. These include:
• immobility and neuropathy, which result in poor emptying of the bladder
• bladder outlet obstruction from prostatic hypertrophy or upper urinary tract obstructions
• atrophic vaginitis
• ischemia of the bladder wall secondary to distention
• fecal or urinary incontinence
• diminished bactericidal activity of urine and prostatic secretions
• instrumentation of the urinary tract
• indwelling or intermittent catheterization.

HEALTH HISTORY FINDINGS

In a health history interview, the client may report or the nurse may detect many of these findings:
• nocturia
• incontinence or worsening of existing incontinence
• urinary frequency and urgency
• bladder spasms or pain
• urinary dribbling
• burning upon urination
• nausea or vomiting
• constipation or diarrhea
• anorexia
• marked confusion
• history of urologic disorders (such as cystitis, prostatitis, chronic UTI, renal failure, or urinary calculi)
• history of cerebrovascular disease, cardiovascular disease, diabetes, or cancer
• history of pelvic trauma or radiation
• recent prostate surgery
• recent cystoscopy or catheterization
• use of anticholinergic or immunosuppressant medications

PHYSICAL FINDINGS

In a physical examination, the nurse may detect many of these findings:

Genitourinary
• foul-smelling, cloudy urine
• hematuria
• cystocele or prolapsed uterus
• urethrocele
• atrophic changes (such as vaginal atrophy or a pale, dry perineum)

Respiratory
• increased respiratory rate

Cardiovascular
- increased heart rate
- decreased blood pressure
- ischemic electrocardiogram (ECG) changes

Gastrointestinal
- abdominal distension
- suprapubic fullness and pain unrelieved by voiding
- possible fecal impaction
- enlarged prostate

Musculoskeletal
- joint pain
- flank or back pain (possibly signifying pyelonephritis)

Neurologic
- change in mental status (such as confusion or irritability)
- lethargy
- delirium

Other
- fever

DIAGNOSTIC STUDIES
The following studies may be performed to evaluate the client's health status:
- complete blood count (CBC) with differential—to detect sepsis
- serum electrolyte, blood urea nitrogen (BUN), and creatinine studies—to determine altered renal function secondary to UTI
- blood culture—to detect urosepsis or septicemia
- urinalysis with Gram stain—to immediately detect bacteria in the urine; usually positive for white blood cells, bacteria, microscopic hematuria, and gram-negative organisms
- urine culture and sensitivity test—to detect multiple causative agents and bacteria; usually obtained by a clean-catch specimen (or catheterization when the clean-catch specimen is contaminated)
- renal ultrasonography—to determine bladder emptying and urine reflux and to detect bladder tumors
- urodynamic studies (uroflowmetry and cystometrography)—to detect urinary obstructions or bladder-emptying difficulties
- prostatic massage and culture of secretions—to help detect prostatitis; indicated for elderly male clients with recurrent UTIs

POTENTIAL COMPLICATIONS
- pyelonephritis
- renal failure
- disseminated intravascular coagulation
- septicemia

Nursing diagnosis: *Altered renal tissue perfusion related to shock from urosepsis and septicemia*

NURSING GOALS: To stabilize vital signs and support the client during septic episodes

Signs and symptoms
- hypotension
- fever
- delirium
- increased respiratory rate
- hypoxia

Interventions

1. Assess the client's vital signs and mental status hourly during acute septic episodes.

2. Administer I.V. fluids, such as isotonic (normal) saline solution, as ordered.

3. Consult the physician about obtaining blood studies and blood cultures before antibiotic therapy begins.

Rationales

1. Widespread vasodilation in septic shock causes hypovolemia, resulting in hypotension and an increased heart rate. Hypotension impairs cerebral perfusion, resulting in a deterioration in mental status.

2. Clients in septic shock require large quantities of I.V. fluids to replace intravascular fluid losses. Because such clients have impaired lactate metabolism, lactated solutions are contraindicated. Isotonic solutions, such as normal saline solution, are preferred.

3. Obtaining blood for studies and cultures after antibiotic treatment begins renders inaccurate results.

4. Assess the client with recurrent UTIs for possible causes of urosepsis, including urinary retention and prostatitis.

4. Identifying and treating the cause can help prevent recurrence of the infection.

5. Initiate I.V. antibiotic therapy as ordered.

5. Antibiotics fight infectious organisms.

6. Teach the client the early symptoms of UTI, including changes in the color and consistency of urine, urinary frequency, and burning upon urination. Also teach him ways to prevent infection.

6. Recognizing the early symptoms of UTI can lead to prompt treatment. Teaching the client ways to prevent infection helps decrease the risk of recurrent infections.

OUTCOME CRITERION
• The client will not develop additional metabolic problems from sepsis.

Nursing diagnosis: *Potential for infection related to poor hygiene and long-term catheterization*

NURSING GOALS: To treat and eradicate UTIs and to prevent urosepsis

Signs and symptoms
• urinary frequency
• burning upon urination
• cloudy or foul-smelling urine
• dark amber urine
• hematuria
• change in mental status (such as confusion, irritability, or restlessness)
• lethargy
• malaise

Interventions

1. Obtain a urine specimen for urinalysis and culture if the client has symptoms of urinary frequency, burning upon urination, or hematuria

2. Encourage the client to drink eight to ten 8-oz glasses (2,000 to 2,500 ml) of fluid per day.

3. Teach the client and caregiver early signs and symptoms of UTI, including cloudy, odiferous urine; confusion; lethargy; and fever.

4. Teach the female client to clean the perineum from front to back and to wear clean cotton-crotched underwear or pantyhose. Also teach her to avoid laundry bleach, bubble bath, and perfumed vaginal deodorants and douches.

5. Teach the client to urinate after intercourse.

6. Instruct the client on the importance of taking vitamin C and eating foods that acidify the urine, including meats, nuts, prunes, plums, and cranberries.

Rationales

1. A urinalysis is necessary to identify whether the client has an infection and to determine the proper course of treatment.

2. A fluid intake of 2,000 ml or more lowers the urine osmolarity, thereby reducing the nutrients available to sustain bacterial growth.

3. Recognizing these symptoms aids in early detection and prevention of septicemia, one of the most serious complications of UTI.

4. Proper hygiene prevents the spread and colonization of rectal organisms. Wearing cotton-crotched underwear or pantyhose provides ventilation and absorbs any vaginal discharge that can lead to infection. Bath and feminine hygiene products can change the pH of the perineum and reduce tissue integrity.

5. Urinating after intercourse clears pathogens from the urethra.

6. An acid environment inhibits bacterial growth.

7. Take necessary measures to prevent constipation and fecal impaction, such as implementing a bowel regimen (see "Constipation and Fecal Incontinence," pages 97 to 104).

7. Bowel distention causes urine retention, which can lead to infection.

8. Assess the client for urine retention by performing an abdominal examination and a post-voided catheterization.

8. Organisms multiply in residual urine. Residual urine can cause bladder distention, resulting in ischemia of the bladder wall and the inability to resist infection.

9. Administer antibiotics, as ordered. Warn the client to expect a change in the color of his urine.

9. Antibiotics kill bacteria and eliminate symptoms. Some antibiotics, such as sulfisoxazole (Gantrisin), can discolor the urine orange.

10. Teach the client with an indwelling catheter to maintain a closed sterile system. Maintain the client's catheter by observing the following procedures:
• Wash hands before and after manipulating the catheter site or apparatus.

10. Maintaining a closed sterile system prevents bacterial infection.

• Good hand-washing technique is essential to preventing organisms from entering the bladder during catheter insertion. Major portals for bacterial invasion during catheter insertion include the urethral meatus, the junction between the catheter and the collection tube, and the open end of the collection bag.

• Insert the catheter using aseptic technique.

• Aseptic technique, which includes wearing sterile gloves and washing the meatal area with sterile swabs and solution, maintains a closed system.

• Avoid disconnecting the bag from the catheter.

• Opening the junction between the catheter and the collecting tube can introduce bacteria into the catheter.

• Use a sterile needle and syringe to aspirate any necessary urine specimens from the self-sealing plug or by catheter puncture.

• This ensures that the system remains closed and sterile.

• Wash the meatus and surrounding area with soap and water daily.

• Proper cleaning prevents bacteria in urethral secretions from ascending to the bladder.

• Change the catheter every 30 days using the smallest catheter possible and only a 5-cc balloon.

• Smaller catheters minimize urethral trauma and prevent blockage of the paraurethral glands. Using a small balloon helps prevent bladder irritation that can lead to necrosis of the bladder neck and infection.

• Anchor the catheter to the client's upper thigh with a hook and loop fastener (Velcro) strap.
• Empty the collection bag every 4 hours.

• Anchoring the catheter to the thigh prevents urethral trauma and injury.
• Frequent emptying of the collection bag prevents urine stasis and bacterial contamination.

• Keep the collection bag below the client's bladder level and off the floor; avoid kinking the tubing.

• An unobstructed downhill flow prevents urine reflux and the retrograde spread of air bubbles that carry bacteria.

• Discourage the staff from instilling antibacterial agents into the collection bag.

• The instillation of antibacterial agents in a closed catheter system is unnecessary and may promote infection with organisms resistant to the agents.

• Discourage periodic catheter irrigation. Change the catheter if it becomes obstructed by encrustation or debris.

• Irrigation bathes only a small portion of the bladder mucosa and does not reduce overall bacteriuria. It can cause mucosal damage, facilitating bacterial invasion into deeper submucosal layers. Interrupting the closed drainage system allows organisms to enter the drainage system.

11. Discuss with the physician the need for antibiotics in the catheterized client with a positive urine culture who is symptomatic for bacteriuria. Be sure to change the catheter and the entire system after instituting antibiotic therapy.

11. Antibiotic therapy is the treatment of choice for the client who is symptomatic for bacteriuria. Changing the catheter and entire system is necessary to prevent cross-contamination.

12. Assess the client's need for catheterization weekly, and remove the catheter as soon as possible.

12. Few clients require long-term indwelling catheterization. Removing the catheter as soon as possible minimizes the development of complications, including infection.

13. Instruct the client or the client's caregiver on alternative urine collection systems, such as clean intermittent self-catheterization, if indicated. Be sure to demonstrate how to perform self-catheterization and to explain the importance of using minimal lubrication and reliance on touch, not a mirror, for insertion. Also explain the importance of washing the catheter in soapy water, drying the catheter, then storing it in a small container sealed in a plastic bag when not in use.

13. Straight intermittent catheterization rarely causes UTIs because the urine collection does not disrupt the body's normal structures or overwhelm the immune system. The client should receive proper instructions and demonstrations to ensure compliance with the technique. Washing and storing the catheter when not in use helps prevent contamination and reduce the risk of infection.

OUTCOME CRITERION
• The client will remain free of infection by using alternate drainage systems, incorporating measures to prevent infection from catheter use, and using proper hygienic measures.

NURSING ACTIONS IN VARIOUS SETTINGS
Nursing actions for a client with a UTI depend on the setting in which care is provided. This section identifies which actions are appropriate in all settings and which pertain to acute care, extended care, or home care situations.

All settings
• Teach all clients at risk for bacteriuria and the caregivers of chronically ill elderly clients how to prevent UTIs.
• Teach clients and caregivers the early symptoms of UTI, emphasizing that symptoms may be atypical.

Acute care
• Treat sepsis with I.V. medication, as ordered, for 24 to 48 hours after fever resolves.
• Manage shock with supportive therapy.
• Identify which clients require follow-up oral antibiotics after discharge. Assess for toxic reactions to the medications.
• Identify which clients are too weak to perform activities of daily living; suggest home health services upon discharge.

Extended care
• Discourage the use of indwelling catheters.
• Teach nursing assistants proper perineal cleaning techniques, especially for those clients with frequent fecal incontinence.
• Suspect UTI in any client with mild mental status changes, such as confusion or irritability.
gait disturbances.
• Discourage the use of antibiotic prophylaxis, to prevent the development of resistant bacteria.

Home care
• Discourage the use of indwelling catheterization, and suggest the use of intermittent self-catheterization.
• Document the client's mental status at the initial visit. Look for improvement with treatment, and teach the client's family that increasing lethargy and confusion may be early signs of recurrence.
• Teach all clients who require indwelling catheterization how to prevent bacterial contamination. Consult the physician about the use of a low-dose antibiotic during catheter changes in clients, especially males, who are frail or have recurrent sepsis.

SELECTED REFERENCES
Gienjuch, D. "Managing UTIs in Elderly Patients," *Drug Therapy* 68-79, September 1987.
Gluckman, R. "Community-Acquired Bacterial Urosepsis in Elderly Women," *Geriatric Medicine Today* 5(5):73-80, May 1986.
Newman, D.K., and Smith, D.A. "Helping Geriatric Patients Master Self-Catheterization," *RN* 51(5):86, May 1988.
Pritchard, V. "Watch Out! Urinary Tract Infections Must Not Spread," *Journal of Gerontological Nursing* 11(5):16-19, September/October 1985.
Pritchard, V. "Geriatric Infections: The Urinary Tract," *RN* 51(5):36-38, May 1988.
Roe, B. "Catheter Care: An Overview," *International Journal of Nursing Studies* 22(1):45-56, 1985.
Ross, D. "Urinary Tract Infections in Elderly Men," *Drug Therapy* 76-91, April 1987.
Wilde, M.H. "Living with a Foley," *American Journal of Nursing* 86(10):1121-23, October 1986.
Zweig, S. "Urinary Tract Infections in the Elderly," *American Family Practice* 35(5):123-30, May 1987.

GENITOURINARY SYSTEM

Sexual Dysfunction

Although little research has been done on normal sexual activity and aging, certain generalities have emerged: Older adults tend to continue the same sexual patterns they enjoyed while younger, but they tend to have sex less frequently. The sharpest drop in frequency of sexual activity seems to occur after age 65 in women and after age 75 in men. Men, however, tend to maintain a greater interest in sex, even to advanced age.

ETIOLOGY

Sexual dysfunction in older adults can result from any of a number of causes. For example, normal age-related physiologic changes can affect an elderly client's degree of sexual arousal and tension. Chronic health problems, such as diabetes mellitus, chronic pulmonary obstructive disease, or prostate cancer, can alter normal sexual functioning. Certain medications, such as methyldopa, amitriptyline hydrochloride, and imipramine hydrochloride, can also have an effect on sexual function.

Among women, the most significant obstacle to remaining sexually active is the death or lack of a partner. Statistically, married women typically outlive their spouses by a few years, widows outnumbering widowers three to one. Also, most elderly women believe that sex outside of marriage is inappropriate; their families and peers tend to reinforce that belief.

HEALTH HISTORY FINDINGS

In a health history interview, the client may report or the nurse may detect many of these findings:

Male and female clients
• use of antihypertensive, antidepressant, or antihistamine medications
• use of alcohol, barbiturates, or sedatives
• use of narcotics, psychoactive drugs, levodopa, amyl nitrite, caffeine, or vitamin E
• diminished nipple reactions during sexual stimulation
• diminished sexual desire

Male clients
• decreased ejaculatory force
• reduced volume and force of seminal fluid
• decreased pressure to ejaculate
• single-stage expulsion of seminal fluid
• early morning ejaculation
• delayed erection

• inability to attain full erection until immediately before orgasm
• incomplete testicular elevation during an erection
• reduced sperm count
• penile flaccidity immediately after orgasm
• long refractory phase after orgasm
• slow arousal

Female clients
• decreased vaginal lubrication
• vaginal pain during penile penetration
• delayed orgasm
• painful uterine contractions with orgasm

PHYSICAL FINDINGS

In a physical examination, the nurse may detect many of these findings:

Genitourinary
• small, atrophied breasts
• flaccid penis and testes
• loss of fatty genital tissue
• smaller uterus and ovaries
• smaller clitoris
• decreased vaginal expansion, length, and lubrication
• decreased activity of Bartholin's glands
• thin vaginal mucosa and labia
• atrophic changes of the vagina and perineum, including redness
• smaller labia
• atrophic vaginitis

DIAGNOSTIC STUDIES

The following studies may be performed to evaluate the client's health status:
• hormone studies (such as estrogen, testosterone, follicle-stimulating hormone, and prolactin levels)—to identify hormonal imbalances
• psychological, neurologic, endocrine, and metabolic evaluations—to determine the causes of impotence
• noninvasive doppler ultrasonography—to objectively record arterial blood pressures in the penile arteries
• sleep center evaluation—to determine the number of nocturnal penile erections; normal rate is one erection every 90 minutes

POTENTIAL COMPLICATIONS
• impotence
• depression
• altered sexual patterns

Nursing diagnosis: *Altered patterns of sexuality related to aging*

NURSING GOALS: To determine age-related sexual problems and to help the client maintain sexual identity

Signs and symptoms
• widows and widowers syndrome (permanent decline in sexual function after period of inactivity)
• depression
• irritability
• social withdrawal
• impotence

Interventions

1. Assess the client's need to maintain regular sexual activity.

2. Suggest the use of a water-soluble lubricant to female clients, if indicated.

3. Instruct the client to void immediately after sex.

4. Instruct the male client who has trouble achieving an erection on the appropriate technique for inserting a flaccid penis into the vagina.

5. Suggest the use of a penile sheath if the male client cannot achieve a full erection.

6. Discuss the possibility of a penile implant if the client cannot achieve even a slight erection.

7. Discuss alternate methods of achieving sexual stimulation, such as maturbation or oral stimulation, if indicated.

8. Ensure the client's privacy for sexual activity in an institutional setting.

9. Teach female clients the importance of having an annual physical examination and Papanicolaou (Pap) test. Also instruct female clients how to perform a breast self-examination.

10. Discuss the possibility of estrogen and progesterone therapy with female clients.

11. Encourage clients to maintain an attractive, fit appearance.

12. Encourage the client to maintain social activities, such as dating and dancing.

Rationales

1. Regular sexual activity can help maintain sexual response.

2. Water-soluble lubricants help keep the vagina lubricated during sexual intercourse.

3. Voiding after sex prevents urinary tract infections and related problems, such as penile irritation.

4. This technique can help the client to achieve an erection after penetration.

5. A penile sheath allows a penis to become erect.

6. A penile implant is a hydraulic device that is manually manipulated by a subcutaneous pump to release fluid into an implanted cylinder in the penile shaft, thereby forcing an erection.

7. These methods can help the client to maintain sexual function, release tension, and stimulate his sexual desire.

8. Privacy is the right of every individual.

9. Regular health screenings help to detect disease and enable early treatment. Examinations also provide an opportunity for discussion about sexual function.

10. Estrogen and progesterone therapy may help to decrease the incidence of hot flashes.

11. Maintaining appearance enhances sexual self-esteem.

12. Social stimulation helps to maintain sexual self-esteem.

OUTCOME CRITERION
• The client will maintain desired level of sexual activity.

Nursing diagnosis: *Impaired social interaction related to death of a spouse*

NURSING GOALS: To support the client through the grieving process and to encourage the resumption of social and sexual interaction

Signs and symptoms
• depression
• social withdrawal
• somatic complaints, such as generalized malaise, headaches, and fatigue
• impotence

Interventions

1. Help the client through the grieving process.

2. Encourage the client to reminisce about his spouse.

3. Encourage the client's family and friends to maintain contact with the client after the funeral.

4. Encourage the client to maintain his personal appearance.

5. Encourage the client to gradually begin engaging in new or familiar social activities.

6. Provide information about widow and widower support groups.

7. At the appropriate time, discuss with the client the need to maintain sexual functioning.

Rationales

1. Until the grieving process is completed, the client will have difficulty resuming social activity.

2. Reminiscing encourages the client to sanctify his spouse and is a natural part of permanent separation.

3. Many friends and family members withdraw from a person who has experienced the death of a spouse.

4. By maintaining his appearance, the client can retain or improve his sexual self-esteem.

5. Social activities, such as dances, bingo games, or senior citizen meetings, can provide needed socialization.

6. Sharing a common experience, such as the death of a spouse, helps to reduce the pain of separation.

7. Abstaining from sex can sometimes lead to the total loss of sexual functioning.

OUTCOME CRITERION
• The client will maintain an acceptable level of social interaction.

Nursing diagnosis: *Sexual dysfunction related to diabetes mellitus*

NURSING GOAL: To identify the extent of sexual dysfunction related to diabetes mellitus

Signs and symptoms
• decreased rigidity of erection
• difficulty ejaculating
• verbalization of sexual inadequacy
• difficulty maintaining intimate relationships
• decreased genital sensation
• poor self-esteem

Interventions

1. Take a detailed sexual history, noting the client's physical and psychological status, use of medications, availability of a sexual partner, usual sexual activity (including the frequency and duration of sexual encounters), sex-related problems, and feelings about sex-related problems.

Rationales

1. A detailed sexual history provides a baseline for future comparison, particularly as medical conditions contributing to the problem improve.

2. Instruct the client about normal age-related physiologic changes and how such changes relate to impotency. Be sure to discuss problems common to those with diabetes, such as erectile impotence and retrograde ejaculation.

2. Such instruction helps to educate the client and allay his fears. The client should be aware that diabetes can cause certain physiologic reactions that can interfere with sexual functioning. For example, atherosclerosis can reduce penile blood flow during sexual excitement, interfering with the ability to achieve an erection. Retrograde ejaculation, which may result from incomplete closure of the bladder sphincter, can cause the semen to take on a milky appearance.

3. Monitor the client's blood glucose levels.

3. Unregulated blood glucose levels and acute metabolic decompensation can cause erectile impotence within days or weeks.

4. Discuss possible solutions to the male client's sexual dysfunction, including eliminating such drugs as reserpine, cimetidine, antidepressants, lithium, methyldopa, and phenothiazines from the medication regimen; avoiding alcoholic beverages; joining an appropriate support group to reduce psychological stress; and improving overall physical health.

4. Eliminating certain drugs and alcohol from the client's regimen may help to cure his impotence. Encouraging the client to join a support group and to take measures to improve his health can foster feelings of sexual adequacy.

5. Refer the male client to the physician for further evaluation, if necessary.

5. The physician may identify other measures to aid the client, such as a surgical penile implant.

OUTCOME CRITERIA
• The client will feel sexually acceptable and adequate.

Nursing diagnosis: *Altered patterns of sexuality related to chronic obstructive pulmonary disease*

NURSING GOAL: To teach the client safe and comfortable sexual practices

Signs and symptoms
• dyspnea during sexual intercourse
• fear of suffocating during intercourse
• avoidance of physical contact

Interventions

1. Assess the degree of dyspnea the client typically experiences upon exertion.

Rationales

1. Such assessment provides the nurse with clues as to the client's tolerance for sexual intercourse.

2. Inform the client that the energy expended during sexual intercourse is equivalent to the energy expended while walking briskly on a level terrain for 4 to 6 minutes or while walking up or down two flights of stairs.

2. This helps to reassure the client that sexual intercourse is not stressful to the heart or lungs.

3. If the client has trouble breathing, encourage him to try different positions, such as standing or lying on one side, during sexual intercourse.

3. Such positions minimize chest pressure and allow the client to remain relatively passive during intercourse.

4. Explain to the client that shortness of breath during sexual activity is normal and tolerable within limits.

4. Fear of dyspnea can make sexual activity stressful rather than enjoyable.

5. Advise the client to use oxygen delivered by nasal prongs during sexual activity or to use a metered-dose bronchodilator aerosol before sexual activity.

5. These measures help to reduce hypoxia.

6. Teach the client to stop sexual activity at the first sign of anxiety and to resume the activity after the feeling disappears. In the interim, suggest that he try to relax but to contiue touching and talking to his partner.

6. Temporarily stopping sexual activity during periods of anxiety can help the client to overcome the fear of suffocation during intercourse.

7. Suggest that the client avoid sexual activity during the evening and night, when fatigue is the greatest.

7. Avoiding sex when fatigued lessens the chance of respiratory distress and failure.

OUTCOME CRITERIA
- The client will be more relaxed and less anxious when having sexual intercourse.
- The client will continue to enjoy his usual sexual habits despite his illness.

Nursing diagnosis: *Altered patterns of sexuality related to myocardial infarction (MI)*

NURSING GOAL: To promote safe sexual activity

Signs and symptoms
- reduced or absent libido
- fear of sudden death during sexual intercourse
- depression
- isolation
- chest pain or dyspnea during sexual intercourse

Interventions

1. Recommend that the client masturbate initially after returning home from the hospital.

2. Discuss with the client the possibility of participating in manual manipulation or mutual masturbation with his partner before participating in sexual intercourse.

3. Encourage sexual foreplay.

4. Recommend that the client take a shower or bath before sexual activity.

5. Caution the client to avoid excessive amounts of alcohol or food before sexual activity.

6. Caution the client to avoid sexual activity when he is feeling angry, stressed, or tired.

7. Encourage the male client to use a position that is most comfortable and least stressful to the heart, such as a side-to-side, rear-entry vaginal, or female superior position.

8. Instruct the client to avoid extreme water and room temperatures during sexual activity.

9. Advise the client to consider taking prophylactic nitroglycerin or long-acting nitrates before sexual activity if he typically experiences anginal pain during other activities, such as climbing stairs and walking.

Rationales

1. Masturbation allows the client to experiment with achieving an orgasm without the stress of full sexual activity.

2. Manual manipulation allows both partners to feel comfortable with each other again after the MI and hospitalization.

3. Sexual foreplay gradually elevates the heart rate and blood pressure.

4. A bath or shower may help to relax the client.

5. Heavy alcohol and food intake may impair sexual activity and increase the strain on the cardiovascular system.

6. Such emotions increase the heart rate and strain the cardiovascular system.

7. Avoiding the traditional male superior position minimizes the myocardial work load associated with sexual intercourse.

8. Extreme water and environmental temperatures can increase the pulse and blood pressure.

9. Nitroglycerin taken before stressful activity can help prevent angina through vasodilation.

10. Instruct the client to cease sexual activity, then to take his nitroglycerin and rest if he experiences chest pain during sexual activity.

10. Vasodilators and rest help to reduce pain.

11. Consult the physician about substituting medications or readjusting dosages if the client develops sexual dysfunction after his MI.

11. Various medications, such as beta blockers, diuretics, and antihypertensives, may produce sexual dysfunction in some clients.

12. Instruct the client on the normal physiologic changes that occur during sexual activity, such as an altered breathing pattern and increased heart rate.

12. Learning the phases of sexual activity should help the client to feel less anxious about his ability to engage in sexual intercourse.

OUTCOME CRITERIA
• The client will resume his previous pattern of sexual activity.
• The client will be free of chest pain during sexual activity.

Nursing diagnosis: *Sexual dysfunction related to rheumatoid arthritis*

NURSING GOAL: To encourage the client to participate in sexual activity using the most comfortable, safe position

Signs and symptoms
• joint pain
• genital lesions
• inability to perform or engage in usual sexual activity
• loss of self-esteem
• physical deformities
• perceived unattractiveness
• corticosteroid use
• decreased libido

Interventions

1. Assess the importance of sexual activity to the client.

2. Instruct the client on ways to maintain attractiveness, such as by using cosmetics.

3. Instruct the client to apply moist heat to painful joints 10 to 15 minutes before sexual activity.

4. Instruct the client to take pain medication before sexual intercourse.

5. Teach the client to perform nonweight-bearing flexibility and stretching exercises, such as passive range-of-motion exercises, before sexual intercourse.

6. Discuss the possibility of the client using alternative positions for sexual activity, such as lying supine or sitting in a chair, if he has arthritis of the hip.

7. Encourage the client to join an arthritis support group.

Rationales

1. Understanding the client's sexual needs serves as a basis on which to establish goals and appropriate interventions.

2. Maintaining attractiveness helps the client maintain a positive self-image.

3. Moist heat reduces pain.

4. Pain medications, which can reduce discomfort during sexual intercourse, are especially helpful for the female client who customarily uses a frontal (male superior) approach for sexual intercourse, as this involves abduction of thighs and external rotation of the hips.

5. Such exercises help to increase flexibility, thereby reducing pain.

6. Arthritic involvement in the hips impedes abduction and external rotation movements; alternate positioning reduces abduction and allows for flexion.

7. A support group enables the client to discuss his arthritis-related problems with others who have similar problems.

OUTCOME CRITERIA
- The client will be able to describe the methods used to maintain sexual functioning.
- The client will have little or no discomfort during sexual activity.

Nursing diagnosis: *Altered patterns of sexuality related to cerebrovascular accident*

NURSING GOAL: To teach the client and the client's partner measures to overcome sexual disabilities caused by cerebrovascular accident (CVA)

Signs and symptoms
- impotence
- decreased interest in sexual activity

Interventions

1. Assess the client's interest in sexual activity.

2. Assess the impotent male client for nocturnal penile erections, and refer him to a psychotherapist if necessary.

3. Advise the client that he may need to alter his sexual positioning, and encourage him to discuss with his partner which positions are pleasurable or painful.

4. Include the client's partner during all teaching sessions.

5. Suggest that the client with hemiparesis lie on his affected side, leaving the unaffected arm and hand free to caress his partner. Advise him to wedge a pillow behind his back and to attempt a rear vaginal entry.

6. Instruct the client to avoid pulling his penis toward his abdomen while masturbating; suggest that he use firm, downward pressure instead.

7. Instruct the female client to use a water-soluble lubricant if she has little or no vaginal secretions.

8. If the male client remains impotent after recovery, discuss the need for a penile implant.

9. Encourage intimacy, such as kissing, hugging, and caressing, throughout the day.

10. Instruct the client to empty his bowel and bladder before sexual intercourse.

11. If the client suffers from fecal incontinence, advise him to use an enema before intercourse, especially if defecation has occurred during previous sexual encounters.

Rationales

1. Assessing the client's interest in sexual activity helps to determine the direction of therapy and teaching.

2. Erections that occur during sleep or in the morning may indicate that impotence is nonorganic.

3. Communication between sexual partners is important, especially for a client who has had a CVA, as a CVA decreases sexual spontaneity, flexibility, and the range of sexual behaviors.

4. Including the client's partner enables the partner to articulate feelings and needs, which is essential for effective sexual functioning.

5. Stimulating the client's unaffected side enhances sexual pleasure. Wedging a pillow behind the client's back improves the client's balance.

6. Applying firm, downward pressure to the base of the penis constricts the major blood vessels and contains the blood already in the penis, thereby maintaining an erection.

7. A water-soluble lubricant provides lubrication and prevents injury to the vagina.

8. A penile implant will enable the client to achieve an erection.

9. Sexual intimacy is not synonymous with sexual intercourse but can be sexually fulfilling.

10. Emptying the bowel and bladder decreases the risk of voiding during intercourse.

11. An enema reduces the risk of defecation. However, caution the client to avoid overusing enemas, as this can lead to bowel distention and decreased defecation sensation.

12. Advise the female client with an indwelling catheter to tape the catheter to her thigh or abdomen before sexual intercourse; the male client, to run the catheter along the penis, apply a condom, then tape the tubing loosely to the abdomen. Then have the client clamp the catheter and detach it from the tubing and bag.

12. Taping stabilizes the catheter and prevents urethral trauma during sexual intercourse. Applying a condom over the catheter prevents urethral trauma and prevents leakage. Clamping and detaching the catheter prevent a backflow of urine into the bladder.

13. Suggest that the client incorporate positioning of the catheter into sexual foreplay. For example, recommend that the client and his partner discuss how to position the tube to increase stimulation.

13. Incorporating the positioning of the catheter into sexual foreplay helps to alleviate embarrassment and minimizes the "technical" aspect of the sexual intercourse.

14. Instruct the client to wash the catheter and perineum after intercourse.

14. Washing the catheter and perineum reduces the risk of a urinary tract infection.

OUTCOME CRITERIA
- The client will achieve a desired level of sexual functioning.
- The client will incorporate his physical limitations into sexual activity.

Nursing diagnosis: *Altered patterns of sexuality related to Alzheimer's disease*

NURSING GOALS: To help the client's partner understand the changes in sexuality that accompany dementia and to decrease the client's inappropriate sexual behavior

Signs and symptoms
- spouse's expressed loss of the client's mental faculties and availability of a sexual partner
- inappropriate sexual activity
- confusion about inappropriate behavior and sexual exposure

Interventions

1. Inform the client's family that the sex drive typically diminishes early in dementia but that the client may return kisses and hugs for awhile.

Rationales

1. Educating the family can help them learn to interpret the client's sexual behavior.

2. If the client makes inappropriate advances during care or treatment, casually refuse his overtures, then try to distract him. Be sure to avoid negative overreactions.

2. The client with Alzheimer's disease typically loses his capacity to understand social rules. The nurse should avoid overreacting to his advances to prevent violent or verbally abusive episodes.

3. If the client undresses in public, suggest that the family replace his clothing or fasteners. For example, if a male client unzips his trousers, provide him with pants with an elasticized waist and no zipper; if a female client unbuttons and removes her clothing, provide her with dresses and blouses with no buttons or buttons on the back.

3. The client with Alzheimer's disease is unaware of where he is or of the impact of what he is doing. Altering clothing style decreases the risk of inappropriate exposure.

4. If the client masturbates in public, advise the family to distract him and then remove him from the scene.

4. Distraction, which diverts the client's attention, is a useful strategy, especially in public settings.

5. Explain to the client's family that inappropriate sexual exposure may result from the client's feeling hot, needing to urinate, or wearing uncomfortable clothing.

5. Inappropriate sexual exposure often embarrasses families. Explaining to them why the client may be behaving inappropriately should help to ease their embarrassment.

OUTCOME CRITERIA
• The client's family will implement measures to prevent or reduce the incidence of inappropriate sexual behavior.
• The client's family will cope effectively with the client's sexual behavior.
• The client will have an outlet for sexual feelings and needs.

NURSING ACTIONS IN VARIOUS SETTINGS

Nursing actions for a client with sexual dysfunction depend on the setting in which care is provided. This section identifies which actions are appropriate in all settings and which pertain to acute care, extended care, or home care situations.

All settings
• Provide information to the client and the client's family about the effects of aging on sexuality.
• Ensure the client's comfort when discussing intimacy and sexual concerns.

Acute care
• Perform a limited, focused sexual history on the client.
• Listen attentively to the client's complaints or concerns that relate to sexual functioning.
• Provide opportunities for the client to be intimate with his partner.
• Include any health-related sexual changes in the client's teaching plan.

Extended care
• Provide opportunities for conjugal visits, ensuring that such visits meet federal and state regulations concerning residents' rights.
• Provide "dating" rooms for elderly clients.
• Discuss with the nursing staff ways of managing confused, sexually aggressive clients.
• Promote feelings of intimacy and enhanced self-esteem by providing pet therapy, dances, hair dresser appointments, family outings, and visits by children and grandchildren.
• Establish an institutional philosophy that allows for the sexual privacy of all clients; communicate this philosophy to all staff members.

Home care
• Listen attentively to the client's questions and concerns about sexual functioning.
• Assess the client's home environment for barriers to sexual functioning.
• Provide the client and the client's family with appropriate information on community resources and support groups.

SELECTED REFERENCES
Bonner, E., et al. "Sexual Counseling for the Elderly Patient after Myocardial Infarction," *Medical Aspects of Human Sexuality* 21(3):100-08, March 1987.

Burgener, S., and Kogan, G. "Sexuality Concerns of the Post-Stroke Patient," *Rehabilitation Nursing* 14(4):178-81, July/August 1989.

Burnside, I.M. *Nursing and the Aged,* 3rd ed. New York: McGraw-Hill Book Co., 1988.

Carnevali, D., et al. *Nursing Management for the Elderly.* Philadelphia: J.B. Lippincott Co, 1986.

Cooper, A.J. "Sexual Dysfunction and Cardiovascular Disease," *Stress Medicine* 4:273-81, August 1988.

Hahn, K. "Sexuality and COPD," *Rehabilitation Nursing* 14(4):191-95, July/August 1989.

Heckheimer, E.F. *Health Promotion of the Elderly.* Philadelphia: W.B. Saunders Co., 1989.

Jain, H. "Sexual Disorders in the Elderly," *Medical Aspects of Human Sexuality* 21(3):14-25, March 1987.

McCraken, A.L. "Sexual Practice by Elders: The Forgotten Aspect of Functional Health," *Journal of Gerontological Nursing* 14(10):13-18, October, 1988.

Mulligan, T. "Erectile Failure in the Aged," *Journal of the American Geriatric Society* 36:54-62, 1988.

Menopause

Menopause, the last day of a woman's menses characterized by spontaneous amenorrhea, is a useful clinical indicator of female climacteric, the phase during which ovarian function declines and reproductive potential ceases. This phase, also called perimenopause, encompasses certain endocrine, biological, and clinical changes that typically begin years before menopause (premenopause) and continue for at least 1 year after menopause (postmenopause). Natural menopause usually occurs at about age 50, although this date varies according to the individual. Surgical menopause occurs whenever the ovaries are removed.

During the perimenopausal phase, which typically begins at about age 40, many women experience psychological, mood, and somatic changes caused by hormonal and biochemical imbalances. As ovarian function and estrogen production gradually begin to decrease, various clinical manifestations can occur, including menstrual irregularities, increased luteal phase dysfunction, anovulation, oligomenorrhea, atrophy of the vulva and vagina, and dysfunctional bleeding. Lowered estrogen levels can cause hot flashes and sweats, excessive perspiration (especially at night), and hot flushes of the head, neck, and thorax. Estrogen deficiency can also cause other symptoms that may manifest years after the climacteric, including decreased skin elasticity, atrophy of the breasts and genitalia, osteoporosis, hypothyroidism, arthralgia, atherosclerotic vascular disease, and easy weight gain.

Although up to 85% of women exhibit symptoms during their climacteric, only about 20% consider these symptoms serious enough to consult a physician.

ETIOLOGY

Menopause is caused by insufficient production of estradiol, which is necessary to induce endometrial proliferation and subsequent withdrawal bleeding. Although clinical signs of impending menopause vary among individuals, many women experience a shortened menstrual cycle, increased incidence of luteal phase dysfunction or anovulation, oligomenorrhea, and dysfunctional bleeding.

HEALTH HISTORY FINDINGS

In a health history interview, the client may report or the nurse may detect many of these findings:
• shortened menstrual cycle
• hot flashes
• excessive perspiration, especially at night
• frequent urinary tract infections
• depression

• lack of self-esteem
• fatigue
• palpitations
• dysuria or urinary frequency
• stress incontinence
• decreased libido
• dyspareunia
• recurrent vaginal infections or pruritus
• vaginal discharge or pain
• oligomenorrhea or amenorrhea followed by menorrhagia or polymenorrhea
• hip or spinal compression fracture secondary to osteoporosis
• low back pain
• headaches
• insomnia
• nervousness and irritability
• emotional instability

PHYSICAL FINDINGS

In a physical examination, the nurse may detect many of these findings:

Genitourinary
• fewer alveoli and mammary ducts
• breast atrophy
• reduced subcutaneous fat and elastic tissue of the vulva, vagina, and urethra
• decreased vaginal lubrication
• narrowing and shortening of the vaginal vault
• thin, delicate, pale or erythematous vaginal epithelium, with fine petechial hemorrhages
• vaginal ulcerations
• prolapsed uterus, cystocele, rectocele, or enterocele
• shrunken cervix
• rigid and inelastic distal urethra with thin, easily traumatized epithelium

DIAGNOSTIC STUDIES

The following studies may be performed to evaluate the client's health status:
• estrogen index of vaginal mucosa—to show decreased maturation manifested by a lack of superficial cells; wet smear shows atrophic basal cells

POTENTIAL COMPLICATIONS
• atrophic vaginitis
• osteoporosis
• atherosclerosis
• depression
• altered sexual patterns

Nursing diagnosis: *Potential for injury and infection related to atrophic changes in the genitalia*

NURSING GOALS: To prevent vaginal injury and infection and to teach the postmenopausal client proper hygiene

Signs and symptoms
- vaginal itching, burning, pain, dryness, and odiferous discharge
- urinary frequency, dysuria, incontinence, or recurrent infections
- cystocele, urethrocele, and relaxed pelvic floor

Interventions

1. Assess the client for atrophic vaginal changes, including dryness, itching, burning, and pain. If any changes are noted, suggest that the client apply a water-soluble lubricant to her perineum; wear cotton underpants; avoid wearing nylon panty girdles or pantyhose; keep her perineum clean and dry, washing from front to back with a nondrying soap; avoid douching or using vaginal deodorant sprays; and use sitz baths.

2. Perform a pelvic examination, and collect secretions for culture if the client complains of vaginal discharge or odor.

3. Discuss with the physician the need for systemic estrogen replacement therapy or a vaginal estrogen cream. Advise the client to obtain an annual Papanicolaou (Pap) smear while taking estrogen supplements.

4. Assess the client for stress incontinence, and consult the physician about possible treatments.

5. Instruct the client to perform pelvic muscle-strengthening (Kegel) exercises. If the client complains of pelvic heaviness or pressure, discuss with the physician the possibility of a vaginal pessary.

Rationales

1. Applying a lubricant to the perineal area relieves dryness and decreases pain on intercourse. Wearing cotton underpants prevents the accumulation of moisture that can lead to infection. Avoiding nylon garments allows the skin to breathe. Keeping clean and dry prevents infection, dryness, and irritation. Avoiding douches and vaginal sprays maintains the pH of the vaginal flora, preventing the proliferation of bacteria that can lead to infection. Taking sitz baths relieves pain and irritation.

2. Changes in the vaginal pH cause the proliferation of organisms. Culturing of such organisms can help identify bacterial or fungal infections.

3. Systemic estrogen therapy prevents endometrial hyperplasia; estrogen cream helps treat atrophic vaginitis. Estrogen replacement, however, may cause endometrial cancer and therefore necessitates an annual Pap examination.

4. Stress incontinence can result from weakened supporting tissues surrounding the bladder outlet and urethra due to a lack of estrogen.

5. Prolapse of the bladder, uterus, or urethra may occur after menopause as a result of a cystocele or urethrocele. Kegel exercises provide support for the bladder and the urethra. A vaginal pessary device lifts internal pelvic organs and provides support.

OUTCOME CRITERION
- The client will be free from vaginal injury and infection.

Nursing diagnosis: *Altered patterns of sexuality related to menopausal changes and atrophic vaginitis*

NURSING GOAL: To help the client to return to her desired level of sexual functioning

Signs and symptoms
- dyspareunia
- aversion to sexual intercourse
- vaginal dryness and irritation
- pruritus

Interventions

1. Assess the client for menopause-related changes in sexual activity.

2. Explain to the client the normal changes in sexual function that occur with aging.

3. Encourage the client with dyspareunia to use a water-soluble lubricant.

4. Consult the physician about the possibility of estrogen replacement therapy if the client complains of a decline in libido or sexual activity.

5. Refer the client to a sex therapist or counselor if indicated.

Rationales

1. Such assessment is necessary to determine whether the client's changes are related to menopause, the normal aging process, or some other health problem.

2. By understanding the normal changes in sexual activity that occur with aging, the client will feel less isolated and can begin thinking of herself as a sexual being again.

3. Decreased estrogen production and atrophic changes in the vaginal wall cause a decrease in or a lack of vaginal lubrication. Water-soluble lubricants can help relieve dyspareunia.

4. Lowered estrogen levels may be the primary cause of the client's decreased libido. Estrogen replacement therapy can help to increase the libido and may relieve sexual dysfunction caused by genitourinary atrophy.

5. Menopause, for many women, is a significant indicator of age and maturation. Some clients require counseling or therapy to ease the psychological transition between phases of adulthood.

OUTCOME CRITERIA
- The client will return to her desired level of sexual activity.
- The client will experience no pain during sexual intercourse.

Nursing diagnosis: *Body image disturbance related to a change in role performance and personal identity*

NURSING GOAL: To help the client identify changes in mood and body image as relating to climacteric hormonal changes

Signs and symptoms
- depression
- feeling of uselessness
- mood swings
- insomnia
- "empty nest" syndrome

Interventions

1. Encourage the client to verbalize her feelings and to join a self-help group.

2. Allow the depressed client to discuss her interpersonal relationships and changes in her family home environment.

3. Reassure the client that her feelings may be caused by a decrease in estrogen production.

4. If the client's depression persists, consider referring the client to a geropsychiatrist.

Rationales

1. Verbalization and self-help groups provide ongoing support.

2. Depression over interpersonal relationships and changes in family dynamics can complicate the client's losses, such as the loss of reproductive capacity, and make dealing with the primary problem (menopause) difficult.

3. Identifying the cause of her feelings may help the client to understand that her feelings are a normal part of menopause, thereby helping her to accept her altered body image.

4. Prolonged depression is atypical of menopause and may be caused by an underlying psychiatric disorder or medication use.

OUTCOME CRITERION
• The client will express her feelings about personal changes that have occurred since menopause.

NURSING ACTIONS FOR VARIOUS SETTINGS
Nursing actions for a client with menopause depend on the setting in which care is provided. This section identifies which actions are appropriate in all settings and which pertain to acute care, extended care, or home care situations.

All settings
• Assess the client's menopausal history, and identify any knowledge deficits.
• Assess the client for atrophic vaginitis.
• Assess the client for signs and symptoms of urinary incontinence (see "Urinary Incontinence," pages 128 to 137).

Acute care
• Allay the fears and concerns of the client experiencing surgical menopause, and consult the physician about the possibility of estrogen replacement therapy.

Extended care
• Assess the client for signs and symptoms of urinary incontinence.

Home care
• Identify any environmental stressors that may predispose client to psychological problems.
• Assess the client's family for stress imposed by the client's menopausal symptoms.
• If the client agrees, include her spouse in discussions.

SELECTED REFERENCES
Beard, M.K., and Curtis, L.R. "Libido, Menopause, and Estrogen Replacement Therapy," *Postgraduate Medicine* 86(1):225-28, July 1989.
Frazer, J. "The Dilemma of the Perimenopausal Female: A Sexual/Physical Health Issue," *Holistic Nursing Practice* 67-75, August 1987.
McKeon, V.A. "Dispelling Menopause Myths," *Journal of Gerontological Nursing* 14(8):26-29, August 1988.
Nolan, J.W. "Developmental Concerns and the Health of Midlife Women," *Nursing Clinics of North America* 21(1):151-59, March 1986.
Stenchever, M. "Management of Vaginitis in the Older Woman," *Geriatric Medicine Today* 6(10):17-20, October 1987.

Falls

A leading cause of serious injury and death among older adults, falls account for two thirds of all accidents involving elderly clients. Only about 50% of those hospitalized for a fall survive 1 year.

Several factors place older adults at high risk for falls, including age-related physiologic changes, chronic disease, hospitalization, and habitual behavior (such as routinely visiting the bathroom in the middle of the night) or environmental hazards. Elderly women statistically experience more falls than elderly men because they are more likely to live alone, live longer, and have osteoporosis.

About 50% of falls involving older adults result from habitual behaviors or environmental hazards; however, environmental hazards seem to have a lesser impact with advancing age. Most falls are preventable with a few simple precautions or changes in daily routine. Falls in the home are most likely to occur during the daytime, typically in the client's living room or bedroom or on the stairs. Falls that occur outdoors typically occur on the sidewalk or on the front or back steps of the client's home.

For the first week after admission to a hospital or nursing home, elderly clients are at increased risk for falls. Most falls occur at night, usually during a trip to the bathroom. More falls occur when fewer staff members are on duty and when nurses are changing shifts.

Because many older adults do not report falls unless they have been injured, nurses who perform health screenings should always question elderly clients about any recent falls; investigating all falls can help prevent future injuries.

ETIOLOGY

The most common cause of all falls is tripping. Many accidental falls result from a combination of environmental factors (such as poorly lit stairs, loose rugs, low tables, pets, and ice) and normal age-related physiologic changes (such as decreased visual acuity, muscle weakness, and decreased coordination).

Drop attacks—falls that occur for no apparent reason and that leave the client's legs feeling paralyzed—may result from temporary muscle paralysis or stiffness. They may also be related to changes in the vertebral arteries, arthritis, or spondylosis of the spine. Sometimes, movement of the head or neck precipitates an attack. Drop attacks are not considered syncopal episodes because no loss of consciousness occurs.

Vertigo, which may result from acute vasovascular insufficiency, can cause a fall. Typically, vertigo occurs as a single episode and causes the client to experience a rotating or spinning sensation involving himself or his surroundings. It may result in abrupt hearing loss and horizontal nystagmus.

Postural hypotension, resulting from orthostatic blood pressure changes when a client rises too fast from a sitting or lying position, can cause a fall. Use of antihypertensives, diuretics, or certain nonprescription medications may aggravate the condition.

Central nervous system lesions, such as those resulting from a cerebrovascular accident, can cause falls. Vertebrobasilar attacks, resulting from vertebrobasilary insufficiency, and transient ischemic attacks can also cause falls.

Other common causes of falls in elderly clients include boredom, depression, loss of confidence, advanced dementia, medication use, and alcoholism.

HEALTH HISTORY FINDINGS

In a health history interview, the client may report or the nurse may detect many of these findings:
• history of a recent fall with or without a loss of consciousness
• sensation of paralysis in the legs after the fall
• aura preceding the fall
• history of falling in the morning upon rising
• history of falling while urinating or defecating
• generalized weakness
• obesity
• slurred speech
• dyspnea
• chest pain or palpitations
• nausea
• diarrhea
• urinary frequency with incontinence
• syncope
• seizures
• vertigo
• confusion
• history of acute congestive heart failure, chronic pulmonary disease, or diabetes mellitus
• history of a neurologic disease, such as Parkinson's disease, cerebrovascular accident, transient ischemic attack, or epilepsy
• history of a fractured hip
• use of multiple sedative, hypnotic, and analgesic medications
• history of long-term alcohol use

PHYSICAL FINDINGS

In a physical examination, the nurse may detect many of these findings:

Musculoskeletal
• pain in the hip or knee, with the affected leg appearing to be externally rotated, abducted, and shorter than the unaffected leg
• decreased leg mobility

• instability
• pain upon palpation of distal radius, neck of femur, or ulna and humerus
• loss of balance when walking a few steps with arms raised horizontally

Integumentary
• dry skin with poor turgor
• multiple bruises
• hematomas

Respiratory
• crackles

Cardiovascular
• dysrhythmias
• orthostatic hypotension
• carotid bruits and distention

Neurologic
• tremors
• cogwheel rigidity
• poor balance and unsteady gait
• decreased reaction time

Other
• loss of visual field
• nystagmus

DIAGNOSTIC STUDIES
The following studies may be performed to evaluate the client's health status:
• complete blood count (CBC)—to assess for anemia and infection

• serum electrolytes—to assess for hypoglycemia, hyperglycemia, or dehydration; an imbalance may be related to medication use
• thyroid studies—to rule out hypoactive or hyperactive thyroid disease
• electrocardiogram (ECG)—to assess for dysrhythmias or cardiac irregularities
• Holter ECG monitoring—to assess for cardiac irregularities over a 24-hour period
• chest X-ray—to assess for congestive heart failure and pneumonia, which may cause decreased cerebral oxygenation and precipitate a fall
• skull or bone X-rays—to identify fractures or hemorrhages
• neurologic testing, such as computed tomography (CT) scan, EEG, or arteriogram—to evaluate strokes or seizures

POTENTIAL COMPLICATIONS
• fractures
• exacerbation of arthritis
• bruising
• hematomas
• loss of confidence
• social isolation
• depression
• dependence on caregivers or family member
• confusion
• institutionalization

Nursing diagnosis: *Potential for injury related to poor balance, frequent falls, and hazardous environment*

NURSING GOALS: To reduce the client's risk for falling and to help the client and caregiver to identify environmental hazards

Signs and symptoms
• postural instability
• gait changes (proneness to stumbling)
• impaired muscle control

Interventions

1. Assess the client's home for pets, small children, and toys or other small objects.

2. Encourage the client to exercise regularly or to perform other activities that improve balance, such as walking.

Rationales

1. An elderly client with poor vision may not be able to see small objects that might cause him to trip and fall.

2. Exercise improves agility, response time, muscle tone, and confidence.

3. Advise the mobile client to wear properly fitting, comfortable shoes with low heels and nonskid soles; to watch for curbs, ramps, rough ground, and icy or wet pavement; to avoid crossing busy streets; and to be especially careful during twilight, when lighting is poor.

3. Wearing appropriate shoes provides stability and helps prevent falls. Watching for hazardous terrain can prevent falls caused by altered depth perception. Avoiding busy streets is advisable because the elderly client may require more time to receive, process, and respond to information. Being careful during twilight is especially important because the elderly client typically has decreased night vision and a decreased ability to adjust from light to dark.

4. Advise the client to remove all hazards from stairs and hallways. Recommend the following: installing baseboard lights, maintaining adequate lighting (using 100-watt bulbs) near doorsteps and in walkways, positioning light switches so they can be reached easily from doorways and stairs, replacing handrails with ones that are easy to grasp from both sides of the stairs, and painting the top and bottom steps a bright color

4. Because stairs are the most common site of falls, all stairways and hallways should be well lit. Switches should be accessible, and handrails should be positioned for easy grasping and support. Painting the top and bottom steps a bright color alerts the elderly client to the stairs' location and decreases the risk of falling.

5. Teach the client the hazards of standing on chairs, stools, and ladders when changing light bulbs or reaching for objects.

5. Tilting the head backward may cause an imbalance in posture and may also cause vertigo or dizziness because of a reduction in cerebral bloodflow.

6. Assess the client's home for environmental hazards. Suggest appropriate changes, including running exposed extension cords along walls; using thick, shock-absorbent carpeting or padding; checking for proper maintenance and functioning of assistive devices, such as wheelchairs, walkers, and canes; rearranging furniture so that the client can use it for support when walking around, especially if he cannot use a cane or walker in his home; avoiding highly polished or wet floors; maintaining nonskid floor surfaces; removing elevated thresholds; keeping carpets firmly tacked down; avoiding the use of throw rugs that slide; avoiding carpets with busy patterns, especially on stairways; avoiding sharp-cornered, low-lying furniture; and using sturdy chairs with arms.

6. Assessing the client's home is necessary to ensure that environmental hazards are eliminated to prevent tripping and injury from falls.

7. Advise the client at high risk for falls to avoid drinking alcohol.

7. Alcohol alters the client's spatial perception and may contribute to a fall.

8. Teach the client to avoid working on objects, such as ceiling lights or curtain rods, that require him to work with his arms raised above his head.

8. Vascular changes may result in dizziness and drop attacks.

9. Instruct the client to rise slowly from a sitting or lying position and to avoid abrupt movements and head turns.

9. The risk of postural hypotension increases with age, especially in the client who takes diuretic and antihypertensive medications. Aging also causes degenerative changes in the vestibular system of the inner ear, which can cause a loss of balance upon sudden movement.

10. Suggest the installation of a personal emergency call system especially if the client lives alone.

10. An emergency call system allows the client to call for help if he should fall.

11. Reassess the need for certain medications in the client who falls frequently. The medications requiring review are those that induce somnolence (hypnotics), postural hypotension (diuretics, nitrates, antihypertensive agents, and tricyclic antidepressants), and confusion (cimetidine and digitalis).

11. The inappropriate use of drugs is the most frequent antecedent to falls. The dosages of these drugs may require adjustment to minimize side effects.

12. Caution the client who has new bifocals or tinted glasses or who has had recent eye surgery to be alert to the chance of a fall.

12. New supplementary lenses may cause spatial disorientation and dizziness.

OUTCOME CRITERION
• The client will remain free from fall-related injuries.

Nursing diagnosis: *Impaired physical mobility related to trauma from frequent falls*

NURSING GOALS: To evaluate and help improve the client's ability to function independently and to prevent recurring falls

Signs and symptoms
• dizziness
• transient ischemic attacks
• orthostatic hypotension
• vision and hearing impairments
• impaired memory
• pain
• confinement to bed

Interventions

1. Assess the client for perceptual or cognitive impairments.

2. Assess the client's resting pulse and respiratory rates, blood pressure, and muscle strength and mass before beginning an exercise regimen.

3. Instruct the client and family on performing range-of-motion (ROM) exercises. Teach them to move each extremity in a gentle, circular motion and not a jerky, rapid motion; to mobilize the scapulae before exercising the arms; and to mobilize the hips before exercising the legs. Explain the importance of performing the exercises twice daily, performing three repetitions for each joint.

4. Prevent prolonged immobility in the bedridden client.

5. Encourage the client to perform activities of daily living, such as hair combing, dressing, and using a bedside commode or ambulating to the bathroom.

Rationales

1. Such impairments can interfere with the client's drive to move or can generate a fear of movement, either of which can precipitate a fall.

2. These measures serve as a guide for establishing realistic goals and a time schedule. Checking the client's blood pressure is important because prolonged confinement to bed or immobility can lead to orthostatic hypotension, a common cause of falls.

3. General strengthening and conditioning exercises, such as ROM exercises, help prevent the loss of joint mobility and, in some cases, restore lost mobility. Moving the extremities in a gentle, circular motion effectively reduces the degree of muscle spasticity. Mobilizing the scapulae and hips before working on the distal extremities helps to relax all of the joints, thereby facilitating the performance of exercises. Adhering to a strict exercise regimen helps to prevent muscle, tendon, and ligament contractures, which can precipitate falls.

4. Prolonged immobility can affect the normal functioning of muscles and joints, which can precipitate falls. Nurses should keep in mind that it takes an average of 7 days to regain the function lost during 1 day of bed rest.

5. Performing activities of daily living allows the client to remain active and mobile, helping to prevent falls. Hair combing enhances shoulder flexibility and range of motion in the arms. Dressing stimulates fine motor coordination and helps preserve joint mobility. Using a bedside commode or ambulating to the bathroom helps to strengthen the quadriceps.

6. Instruct the client who is immobilized by a cast or traction to perform isometric exercises.

6. Isometric exercises help to maintain muscle tone and strengthen the immobilized body part.

7. Institute "stir-up" movements in the client with orthostatic hypotension by using a tilt table or having the client dangle his legs at the bedside several times a day.

7. These movements promote blood return and are considered a form of light exercise, which is necessary before the client attempts more strenuous exercises.

8. Encourage the client to get out of bed, stand, and ambulate as soon as his condition allows.

8. Standing and bearing weight through the long bones retards bone resorption, prevents contractures, and promotes the return of blood from the extremities to the heart.

9. Evaluate the client's need for bed rails, an overhead trapeze, a rope ladder, or a braided bedpull attached to the foot of the bed.

9. Such devices help the client to transfer in and out of bed, thereby promoting mobility and preventing falls.

10. Consider the use of a motor-driven or spring armchair for the client with arthritis, Parkinson's disease, or any other mobility impairment.

10. These devices can help the client to stand without falling.

11. Assess the client's need for a cane, crutches, a walker, or a wheelchair.

11. A cane transfers up to 25% of the client's body weight away from the legs; crutches and walkers improve balance by reducing weight bearing on both legs by 50%. Each of these devices helps the client to ambulate and, when used properly, helps prevent falls. A wheelchair, which may be necessary for the client who can no longer ambulate, allows for independence and mobility.

12. Assess the client's need for supportive devices, such as a splint or brace.

12. Splints and braces are designed to stabilize joints, relieve pain, and improve function so that the client can ambulate safely.

13. Place high-top sneakers or foam boots on the bedridden client.

13. These foot coverings help to prevent footdrop.

14. Avoid using physical restraints or keeping the bed side rails up unless necessary.

14. Restraints impair mobility considerably and increase the client's risk of falling. Keeping the side rails raised increases the height of a fall, should it occur, as well as the extent of injury.

OUTCOME CRITERIA
• The client will not fall.
• The client will ambulate progressively to achieve optimal mobility and independence.

Nursing diagnosis: *Bathing, toileting, and dressing self-care deficit related to postural hypotension, vertigo, and environmental hazards*

NURSING GOALS: To observe the client's function during bathing, toileting, and dressing and to modify the hazards or obstacles that interfere with the client's ability to complete these tasks

Signs and symptoms
• frequent falls
• visual deterioration
• loss of short-term memory

Interventions

1. Help the client prevent falls when toileting or bathing by ensuring the toilet seat is 18″ (45.7 cm high; placing grab rails on the walls near the toilet and tub; positioning night lights between the bedroom and bathroom; placing a commode at the client's bedside; installing nonskid mats in the tub or using a nonskid shower chair; placing toilet paper within easy reach; and installing an alarm system, such as a handbell.

2. Arrange the client's room to prevent falls while dressing. Consider arranging furniture so that pathways are clear; avoiding furniture with rollers; removing wobbly tables and chairs; instructing the client to not wear long robes or clothing while walking; providing a bedside phone or alarm and instructing the client to request help whenever necessary; providing the client with a flashlight to keep at the bedside or installing a bedside remote-control light switch; clearing objects that might interfere with the client's use of a walker or cane; and placing frequently used items in more accessible locations.

3. Teach the client the correct way to fall: Have him protect his head and face while falling, then have him summon help and keep warm if he cannot get up. If he can get up, instruct him to roll onto his stomach and crawl to a nearby piece of furniture to pull himself up, or to shuffle sideways on his buttocks to a piece of furniture.

Rationales

1. Proper positioning of equipment and fixtures helps prevent falls.

2. All furniture should be safe and properly arranged to prevent accidental stumbling and to provide support. Long clothing increases the risk for tripping and falling and should be avoided. A phone or alarm system enables the client to call for help in case of a fall. A flashlight or remote control light switch provides the client with adequate lighting at all times and enables him to light the room without getting up from bed. Placing items that are frequently used in more accessible locations prevents excessive reaching or bending that can lead to loss of balance and falls.

3. Mobilization will help the client get up or obtain assistance. Staying warm prevents hypothermia.

OUTCOME CRITERIA
• The client will reduce environmental or health hazards that predispose him to falls.
• The client will remain free from injury.

NURSING ACTIONS IN VARIOUS SETTINGS

Nursing actions for a client who suffers falls depend on the setting in which care is provided. This section identifies which actions are appropriate in all settings and which pertain to acute care, extended care, or home care situations.

All settings

• Orient the client to his environment to prevent relocation syndrome.
• Provide adequate nonglare lighting, especially during the evening, to reduce the risk of "sundown syndrome" or confusion.
• Monitor the client who has recently started a new medication for an increased risk of falling.
• Assess the need for side rails, since side rails increase the height of a fall, thereby worsening the injury.
• Avoid using restraints whenever possible because the client may fall if he attempts to get out of bed.
• Teach the client the proper use of medications and the complications associated with alcohol use.
• Encourage the client who fallen to resume normal activities.

• Help the client perform exercises, including walking on different types of surfaces and climbing stairs, to help him regain confidence and mobility.

Acute care

• Inform the nursing staff about the high incidence of falls that occur during the first week of an elderly client's hospitalization, and monitor the client closely.
• Assess all clients, especially those waiting in the emergency room, for falls.
• Educate the night shift staff about falls, as most falls occur at night.
• Keep a call light at the client's bedside, and teach him to use it to call for help.

Extended care

• Provide activities and recreational programs to prevent depression.
• Place the client at high risk for falls close to the nurses' station.
• Attach the call bell cord to the client's gown. Doing so ensures that the client will inadvertently pull the light out of the wall, causing the light go on, if he should attempt to get out of bed.

• Keep the intercom system open to the client's room during the night shift so that moaning or movement can be heard.

Home care
• Complete a comprehensive home environment safety assessment.
• Consider instituting a physical therapy referral for gait training and therapeutic exercises to increase muscle strength, if appropriate.
• Refer the client to social services for assistance in arranging community services.
• Determine the availability of community organizations that perform minor home repairs to improve safety for the low-income elderly client.
• Assess the availability of church groups to provide community services.
• Refer the client to Meals On Wheels, which may help to improve the client's nutritional status and reduce the possibility of falls.
• Institute a buddy system for the client who lives alone. Under a buddy system, friends call each other two to three times per day at specified times. If the phone is not answered, the caller telephones a neighbor, the police, or some other designated person to check on the client.
• Suggest that the caregiver write to the U.S. Consumer Product Safety Commission, Washington, DC 20207, for a copy of "Safety for Older Customers: Home Safety Checklist."

SELECTED REFERENCES

Andrew, R., et al. *Principles of Geriatric Medicine.* New York: McGraw-Hill Book Co., 1985.

Dornbrand, L., ed. *Manual of Clinical Problems in Adult Ambulatory Care.* Boston: Little, Brown & Co., 1985.

Heckheimer, E.F. *Health Promotion of the Elderly in the Community.* Philadelphia: W.B. Saunders Co., 1989.

Mendelsohn, S., et al. "Assessment Protocols for Acute Medical Conditions," *Journal of Gerontological Nursing* 12(7):17, July 1986.

Schulman, B., and Acquabiva, T. "Falls in the Elderly," *Nurse Practitioner* 12(11):33-37, November 1987.

Tack, K.A., et al. "Patient Falls: Profile for Prevention," *Journal of Neuroscience Nursing* 19(2):83-89, April 1987.

Tiderksar, R. "Geriatric Falls: Assessing the Cause, Preventing Recurrence," *Geriatrics* 44(7):57-61, July 1989.

Osteoarthritis and Rheumatoid Arthritis

Osteoarthritis and rheumatoid arthritis are two of the most common musculoskeletal conditions affecting elderly clients. Osteoarthritis, the most common musculoskeletal disorder among older adults, is considered a normal part of aging. Rheumatoid arthritis, a chronic, insidious disease that frequently begins in middle age, most commonly strikes after age 60.

A noninflammatory disorder of moveable joints, osteoarthritis is characterized by the breakdown of articular joint cartilage and subsequent ulceration and by the formation of new bone. As the disease progresses, bony spurs develop adjacent to joints, pinching nerves and commonly resulting in shooting pain, limited movement, and decreased dexterity. Over 90% of those over age 40 show some evidence of osteoarthritis on X-ray, especially in weight-bearing joints. Nearly 16 million Americans are affected severely enough to seek treatment annually.

Rheumatoid arthritis, a chronic systemic disease marked by exacerbations and remissions, is characterized by joint inflammation, anemia, periarticular osteoporosis, and muscle atrophy caused by inflammation (myositis) and disuse. Most prevalent in the early spring, rheumatoid arthritis begins with an inflammation of the synovial membrane, which thickens and adheres to the adjacent articular cartilage. It frequently affects the organ systems, including the skin, eyes, lungs, and heart, as well as the vascular system. Rheumatoid arthritis is three times more common in women than men and has a tendency to run in families. Nearly 6.5 million Americans seek medical care for rheumatoid arthritis annually. Prognosis usually depends on the disease course and treatment.

ETIOLOGY

Although the exact cause of osteoarthritis is unknown, the following factors may contribute to its development: congenital abnormalities, such as congenital dysplasia of the hip or knock-knees; hormonal influences, such as decreased estrogen; genetic factors, particularly factors that involve the terminal interphalangeal joints; joint injury or excessive joint use; local joint stress, such as bow-leggedness; sex and age, as osteoarthritis is more prevalent in men under age 45 and women over age 55; environmental influences, such as a damp, moist climate; and obesity.

Rheumatoid arthritis is thought to develop as a result of an autoimmune reaction characterized by inflammation of the synovial membranes lining the joints, ultimately leading to the weakening and destruction of underlying cartilage. Genetic factors may also play a role: The genetic marker HLA-DW4 is measurable in about half of all those with rheumatoid arthritis. However, this marker also appears in individuals who do not have the disease.

HEALTH HISTORY FINDINGS

In a health history interview, the client may report or the nurse may detect many of these findings:

Osteoarthritis
• dull, aching pain with intermittent sharpness
• localized stiffness that is relieved by passive activity
• pain at rest, upon awakening, and during the night
• asymmetrical pain
• pain occurring over several years, primarily in weight-bearing joints

Rheumatoid arthritis
• severe symmetrical, polyarticular pain
• stiffness ("gelling" phenomenon) after periods of inactivity
• multiple inflamed joints developing over several months
• symmetrical pain and swelling in the hands and feet
• fatigue, anorexia, or myalgia
• family history of arthritis
• fatigue
• malaise
• weight loss
• shortness of breath
• dyspnea on exertion
• cough
• constipation
• joint deformities
• intolerance to extreme heat or cold

PHYSICAL FINDINGS

In a physical examination of a client with *osteoarthritis*, the nurse may detect many of these findings:

Musculoskeletal
• local joint tenderness
• decreased joint motion
• crepitus in finger joints
• synovitis
• joint enlargement and deformity
• muscle spasms

Integumentary
• bony protuberances at the distal interphalangeal joints (Heberden's nodes) that are achy, red, and tender and produce a clumsy, tight feeling
• bony protuberances at the proximal interphalangeal joints (Bouchard's nodes)

Other
• obesity

In a physical examination of a client with *rheumatoid arthritis,* the nurse may detect many of these findings:

Musculoskeletal
• symmetrically warm, swollen, and tender joints
• guarded movements
• decreased range of motion
• decreased muscle strength
• decreased medial arch
• "fallen" metatarsal heads

Integumentary
• red palms, with an enlarged vein on the dorsum of the hand
• firm, movable, flesh-colored rheumatoid nodules over pressure points
• swollen interphalangeal joints ("spindle fingers")
• shiny, stretched skin over the affected joint
• synovial cysts on the knees, wrists, or elbows
• leg ulcers

Gastrointestinal
• splenomegaly

Neurologic
• carpal tunnel syndrome
• peripheral neuropathies

Other
• slight fever
• tissue inflammation over the sclera
• decreased salivary, lacrimal, and vaginal secretions (Sjögren's syndrome)

DIAGNOSTIC STUDIES
The following studies may be performed to evaluate the client's health status:

Osteoarthritis
• aspiration of synovial fluid from the affected joint—to rule out other inflammatory problems
• complete blood count (CBC)—to identify infection, anemia, or blood dyscrasins; findings include a normal white blood cell count, anemia from aspirin and nonsteroidal anti-inflammatory medications, and occult blood loss
• erythrocyte sedimentation rate (ESR)—to identify inflammation; may be elevated with acute inflammation
• X-rays of the affected joint—to assess bony destruction or to rule out other diseases, such as metastatic disease; findings include osteophytes and cystic change in the bone beneath the area of denudation

Rheumatoid arthritis
• ESR and gamma globulin levels—to detect inflammation; elevated in 60% of clients with rheumatoid arthritis
• serum rheumatoid factor—to help diagnose the disease; factor is found in 76% of clients with rheumatoid arthritis
• X-rays of the affected joint—to reveal periarticular soft tissue swelling and periarticular osteoporosis
• chest X-ray—to reveal pulmonary fibrosis and nodules
• aspiration of synovial fluid—to assess the degree of inflammation; fluid is typically thin and watery with an increased white blood cell count

POTENTIAL COMPLICATIONS
• pain and joint tenderness
• contractures
• immobility
• limited life-style
• joint swelling (rheumatoid arthritis)
• fatigue
• body image disturbance
• depression
• isolation
• loss of self-esteem

Nursing diagnosis: *Chronic pain related to inflamed, stiff joints*

NURSING GOAL: To provide relief from arthritic pain and discomfort

Signs and symptoms
• local joint pain
• joint tenderness and swelling
• immobility
• weakness and fatigue

Interventions

1. Assess the client's pain, noting its severity, location, and duration.

2. Apply ice packs to hot, inflamed, and acutely painful joints.

Rationales

1. Such assessment is necessary to determine the appropriate treatment to relieve the pain.

2. Cold effectively reduces acute pain associated with hot, inflamed joints.

3. Apply heat to recently developed contractures while performing range-of-motion exercises over the affected site.

4. Assess the client's respiratory rate and auscultate his lungs before implementing heat therapy. If the client cannot tolerate heat, consider using cold therapy.

5. Teach the client and caregiver about superficial heat therapies—such as hot moist packs, heat lamps, electric pads, paraffin wax baths, and blown hot air—and deep heat therapies, such as diathermy.

6. If the client has acute inflammation, avoid using superficial or deep heat therapy. Apply cool compresses instead.

7. Evaluate the need for ultrasound therapy, especially in clients with periarticular and capsular tightening. ·

8. Evaluate the need for hydrotherapy, in which all or part of the client's body is immersed in water. If appropriate, monitor the client's pulse and blood pressure during immersion.

9. Administer acetaminophen (Tylenol), as ordered, to the arthritic client who has pain but no inflammation.

10. Administer aspirin or nonsteroidal anti-inflammatory agents, such as indomethacin (Indocin), as ordered.

3. Heat applied during exercise increases collagen extendibility, thereby helping to resolve contractures.

4. The elderly client has a decreased tolerance for heat, especially when submerged in warm water. Heat intolerance may be evidenced by a decrease in respiratory and pulmonary functions. Although heat therapy is usually effective for subacute or chronic rheumatoid arthritic joints, cold therapy may be necessary for the client who cannot tolerate heat.

5. Superficial heat therapy is usually recommended for the client with subacute or chronic rheumatoid arthritis. Moist heat is usually preferred over dry heat when used at the same temperature, as moist heat penetrates the joints deeper. However, when dry heat is recommended, it is best tolerated at higher temperatures. Deep heat, such as diathermy (heat produced by electromagnetic waves) is contraindicated in the client with acutely inflamed joints, as increased temperature accelerates cartilage destruction. Although diathermy and superficial heat are equally effective, diathermy is typically used on the client who does not benefit from superficial heat.

6. Heat can damage an acutely inflamed joint by increasing proteolytic enzyme activity.

7. Ultrasound effectively combines with exercise to increase range of motion after periarticular and capsular tightening has occurred.

8. Warm, submersive heat loosens joints and muscles for therapeutic water exercise. Immersion of large body portions increases the pulse rate and decreases blood pressure.

9. Acetaminophen, which is inexpensive and has few side effects, is the treatment of choice to control mild to moderate pain, especially if the pain is recent and not caused by inflammation or a prostaglandin-mediated process.

10. Physicians start treatment with the least toxic medications and progress if necessary. These medications decrease inflammation by blocking the arachidonic acid pathway, which produces prostaglandins. Aspirin may be the only drug needed; however, the elderly client should not take more than 8 to 10 g/day to avoid GI irritation and central nervous system side effects.

11. Monitor the client receiving aspirin and anti-inflammatory agents for the following signs and symptoms: tinnitus, drowsiness, headaches, or insomnia; skin rash; upper GI problems, such as gastritis, nausea, vomiting, or peptic ulcer disease; and renal dysfunction, such as a decreased sodium clearance.

11. Tinnitus is the primary symptom of aspirin toxicity. Skin rashes, such as urticaria, maculopapular eruptions, or photosensitivity, are a common side effect of aspirin use. Upper GI symptoms are a common side effect of aspirin use and can be avoided by administering aspirin with meals. However, because aspirin can increase GI bleeding and decrease platelet adhesiveness, periodic monitoring of the client's blood count and guaiac testing are necessary. Aspirin and anti-inflammatory medications block prostaglandin E2 at the kidneys, which decreases renal blood flow and creatinine clearance and can lead to renal failure. Although most clients recover their previous level of renal function after the drugs are discontinued, those with previously impaired renal function, dehydration, or depleted intravascular volume should be monitored carefully.

12. Monitor the client receiving indomethacin (Indocin) for sodium retention.

12. Sodium retention can lead to congestive heart failure in the elderly client.

13. Administer corticosteroids (Prednisone), aurothioglucose (Solganal), gold sodium thiomalate (Myochrysine), D-penicillamine (Cuprimine), or hydroxychloroquine (Plaquenil), as ordered.

13. These agents are useful in a small percentage of clients with persistent, active, inflammatory disease. Corticosteroids suppress inflammation and acute pain but do not prevent joint destruction and deformities. Dosages should be as small as possible for as short a time as possible to prevent side effects. Gold salts (such as aurothioglucose and gold sodium thiomalate), one of the most effective treatments for rheumatoid arthritis, interfere with the function of mononuclear cells, thereby reducing inflammation. Hydroxychloroquine, an easily administered antimalarial, has a low incidence of toxicity. Its usual side effects include GI distress, rash, retinopathy, and CNS disturbances.

14. Discuss the possibility of orthopedic surgery (such as synovectomy of the involved joint, osteotomy, or total joint arthroplasty) with the client who, despite medical management, has joint destruction from inflammation.

14. Synovectomy protects large joints for up to 5 years, but results in a significant loss of range of motion. Osteotomy corrects misalignment and eliminates abnormal joint stress, which slows the disease's progress. Total joint replacement, usually performed on the hips, knees, and shoulders, can help the client with severe destructive arthritis to remain ambulatory and functional rather than bedridden.

OUTCOME CRITERIA
- The client will verbalize temporary pain relief.
- The client will have fewer muscle spasms.
- The client will have increased range of motion.

Nursing diagnosis: *Impaired skin integrity related to immobility, the use of a splint, and decreased function*

NURSING GOAL: To prevent dermatologic complications caused by decreased physical function

Signs and symptoms
- skin breakdown around nodules and functional splints
- reddened, inflamed skin over joints

Interventions	Rationales
1. Assess the client's skin for redness and irritation, especially over nodules.	1. Nodules increase the client's risk for skin breakdown.
2. Assess the client's skin under the splint.	2. Splints increase pressure points, especially when first used.
3. Turn the client, or encourage client to turn, at least every 2 hours while in bed.	3. The client may require bed rest during episodes of acute inflammation. Frequent turning prevents skin breakdown.
4. Use minimal amounts of soap and avoid deodorant soaps when bathing the client.	4. Soap dries the skin.
5. Apply lotion to the client's skin, and massage bony prominences.	5. Lotion moisturizes the skin, and massage increases circulation over pressure points.
6. Apply wool or sheepskin protectors to the client's affected joints.	6. These keep the joints warm and protect the skin during immobilization.

OUTCOME CRITERION
• The client will be free from skin breakdown during acute episodes of rheumatoid arthritis.

Nursing diagnosis: *Impaired physical mobility related to stiffness, inflammation, pain, or loss of locomotor ability.*

NURSING GOALS: To teach the client proper joint mechanics and to assist him in planning activities that require movement

Signs and symptoms
• localized stiffness
• red, inflamed leg joints
• pain
• myalgia
• obesity
• fatigue

Interventions	Rationales
1. Encourage the client with rheumatoid arthritis to rest frequently and to elevate or splint the affected limb during episodes of acute inflammation.	1. Inflammation is a destructive process that is treated by decreasing stress through rest and elevation. Rest and immobilization of the joint also enhance the effect of nonsteroidal anti-inflammatory medications. Splinting an inflamed joint limits movement during episodes of acute inflammation but does not cause a permanent loss of joint mobility.
2. Promote frequent rest periods, and avoid disturbing the client during rounds.	2. The client with active arthritis may complain of fatigue. Rest reduces pain, retards the degenerative process, and decreases the stress of weight bearing and the effect of gravity on the bones.
3. Provide emotional rest by encouraging the client to meditate, join support groups, or participate in diversional activities.	3. Emotional stress can exacerbate arthritic symptoms.

4. Encourage the obese client to lose weight, especially if he has arthritis of the spine and lower extremities.

4. Although obesity does not cause osteoarthritis, extra weight stresses weight-bearing joints, such as the hips, knees, back, and feet. This extra stress can cause joint pain and damage.

5. Recommend that the client use a cane, walker, or crutches.

5. Assistive devices provide stability, relieve strain on weight-bearing joints, and increase mobility.

6. Teach the client to maintain good posture by encouraging him to avoid flexing painful joints, bend at the knees when lifting, and stand straight.

6. Flexed positions lead to stiffness, loss of joint motion, and deformity. Good body mechanics reduce joint stress by using large muscles to work against gravity. Standing straight helps to relieve back pain.

7. Encourage the client with rheumatoid arthritis to practice slow, progressive isometric exercises.

7. Isometric exercises increase muscle power and strength and decrease joint stress. They are particularly suitable for the client with swollen and painfully inflamed or severely damaged joints.

8. Teach the client with osteoarthritis to practice passive, nonstressful range-of-motion (ROM) exercises.

8. Passive ROM exercises maintain joint mobility and function.

9. Recommend that the client bicycle, swim, or perform water aerobic exercises.

9. Bicycling exercises the knees and ankles and improves leg strength; swimming and water exercises improve muscle tone and exercise joints while reducing stress on weight-bearing joints.

10. Teach the client to wear properly fitting footwear, such as shoes that provide medial lateral stability, arch support, and good shock absorption. Assess whether the client needs rocker bottom shoes.

10. Improper footwear increases joint stress. Because clients with osteoarthritis lift their feet rather than roll over painful joints, they lose propulsion, which increases instability and pain.

11. Encourage the client with osteoarthritis to avoid walking down stairs.

11. Walking down stairs increases stress on weight-bearing joints.

12. Teach the client with rheumatoid arthritis how to splint joints. Explain that he should use a functional splint for such activities as washing clothes and making beds; tell him to wear the splint initially for 1 hour at a time, gradually increasing the time to 6 to 8 hours. Explain that he should use a resting splint at night. Tell him to check the skin around the splint for redness or soreness after each use and to use alcohol, not hot water, to clean the splint. Advise him to avoid leaving the splint in hot areas.

12. A functional splint stabilizes the joint during use; gradually increasing its use reduces the risk of skin breakdown. A resting splint stabilizes and immobilizes a joint, such as the wrist, in a desired position; however, this type of splint interferes with normal joint functioning, so it should only be used when joint movement is unnecessary. Checking the skin after each use helps in the early detection of pressure areas, thereby helping to prevent pressure sores. Heat changes the shape of adjustable splints and should be avoided.

OUTCOME CRITERIA
• The client will move all joints within their normal range of motion.
• The client will function at an acceptable level.

Nursing diagnosis: *Body image disturbance related to deformed arthritic joints*

NURSING GOAL: To encourage the client to express his feelings about his body changes

Signs and symptoms
• lethargy
• lack of interest in activity
• prolonged immobility
• disheveled appearance
• depression
• frequent sleeping

Interventions

1. Encourage the client to express his concerns about the disease and its long-term effects on his body.

2. Provide emotional support for the client.

3. Provide opportunities for the client to enhance his appearance, such as with the use of make-up or different clothing.

4. Dress the client in warm, comfortable, easily donned clothing, and help him to maintain a stylish appearance.

5. Encourage the client to participate in a local arthritis support group and to contact the Arthritis Foundation.

Rationales

1. Encouraging verbalization allows the nurse to provide support and counseling.

2. The client who has had rheumatoid arthritis for years may be experiencing despair and depression related to the pain and chronicity of the disease.

3. Enhancing one's appearance helps to boost morale.

4. Clothes should be both functional and attractive to maintain morale.

5. Support groups encourage the verbalization of feelings and concerns, which lessens the internal stress associated with the disease.

OUTCOME CRITERION
• The client will verbalize increased confidence in his ability to deal with his illness as well as the changes in his appearance and life-style.

Nursing diagnosis: *Impaired home maintenance management related to decreased mobility, loss of dexterity, and decreased strength*

NURSING GOAL: To help the arthritic client manage at home by modifying his environment

Signs and symptoms
• localized or generalized pain
• joint swelling and tenderness
• muscle atrophy
• pain
• limited movement

Interventions

1. Evaluate the client's preference for either hot or cold therapies. Also evaluate the ease of use and cost associated with each therapy.

2. Provide the client with multiple choices of hot and cold therapies.

3. Evaluate the advantage of using assistive devices, such as long-handled combs, hooks for opening car doors, extension mirrors, button hooks, wide-gripped eating utensils, or canes or walkers.

4. Have the client demonstrate how to use hot and cold therapy and assistive devices.

5. Teach the client and caregiver to organize ADLs to minimize repetitive, wasteful motion.

Rationales

1. Identifying the client's preference will help ensure compliance.

2. If one treatment is unavailable, the client can substitute another therapy and still avoid pain.

3. Assistive devices help to decrease stress on the affected joints. Canes and walkers improve stability and safety while allowing the client to perform activities of daily living (ADLs).

4. Demonstrations ensure that the client understands how to use the treatments, thereby preventing injuries, falls, or other problems.

5. Simplifying work conserves energy.

6. Teach the client to avoid tightening his grip when turning doorknobs, opening jars, or using scissors. Also instruct him to avoid prolonged holding or pressures that misalign joints.

6. These activities increase joint pressure and pain.

7. Provide the client with raised car and toilet seats.

7. Conventional car and toilet seats are typically too low and increase knee pain.

OUTCOME CRITERIA
• The client will have improved joint function.
• The client will maximize functional capacity to perform ADLs independently and safely.

NURSING ACTIONS IN VARIOUS SETTINGS

Nursing actions for a client with osteoarthritis or rheumatoid arthritis depend on the setting in which care is provided. This section identifies which actions are appropriate in all settings and which pertain to acute care, extended care, or home care situations.

All settings

• Emphasize the importance of reporting to the physician any signs of disease progression, such as increased stiffness or deformity.
• Administer nonsteroidal anti-inflammatory agents with meals.
• Reevaluate the effectiveness of adaptive devices, self-help aides, and assistive devices as the client's disease progresses. Also, evaluate the need for additional devices.
• Reevaluate the client's need for physical or occupational therapy throughout the disease's progression.

Acute care

• Discontinue the client's aspirin use at least 7 days before any surgery because of the risk of reduced platelet adhesiveness.
• Ensure that the client's environment remains safe to decrease the risk of injury from instability.
• Assist the client with early postoperative mobilization to prevent contractures and increased stiffness.

Extended care

• Provide clients with necessary self-help aids and assistive devices.
• Institute support groups for clients with signs of arthritic disease.
• Administer tub baths as a method of therapeutic hydrotherapy.
• Provide daily recreational and activity programs to maintain mobility and joint function.
• Provide diversional activities for clients with chronic pain.
• Provide ongoing cosmetic services to help maintain the client's self-esteem.

Home care

• Assess the client's home environment to identify any obstacles or potential hazards.
• Assess the client's use of prescription and nonprescription medications.
• Refer the client to the local chapter of the Arthritis Foundation, and encourage him to join a local arthritis support group.
• Initiate a support group if none is available in the community.
• Identify organizations that can modify the client's home, at a minimal cost, to promote safety and conserve energy.
• Discuss ineffective nonmedical therapies and treatments with the client and the client's family to prevent their wasting money for potentially harmful products and services.

SELECTED REFERENCES

Andres, R., et al. *Principles of Geriatric Medicine.* New York: McGraw-Hill Book Co., 1985.

Bell, C.L. "Rheumatoid Arthritis: Current Practices and Rehabilitation," *Topics in Geriatric Rehabilitation* 4(3):10-22, April 1989.

Dornbrand, L., ed. *Manual of Clinical Problems in Adult Ambulatory Care.* Boston: Little Brown & Co., 1985.

Heckheimer, E.F. *Health Promotion of the Elderly in the Community.* Philadelphia: W.B. Saunders Co., 1989.

Joseph, N. "Arthritis Medications from A to Z," *Caring* 8(1):14-17, January 1989.

Panush, R.S. "Exercise and Arthritis," *Topics in Geriatric Rehabilitation* 4(3):23-31, April 1989.

Portnow, J., and Helfgott, S. "Rehabilitation of the Elderly Arthritic Patient," *Geriatric Medicine Today* 6(9):63-69, September 1987.

Osteoporosis

Osteoporosis is an age-related disorder characterized by decreased bone mass, which results in skeletal fragility and proneness to fractures that can occur spontaneously or after minimal trauma. Initially, the disease affects trabecular bone, the spinal vertebrae, the femur head, and the distal end of the radius. Because trabecular bone has a faster rate of remodeling than does cortical bone, it is the site of most bone resorption.

Osteoporosis can be categorized according to two main types: postmenopausal and senile. Postmenopausal osteoporosis typically occurs during the early postmenopausal years and affects the trabecular bone of the vertebral column, causing vertebral fractures. Senile osteoporosis occurs in all elderly clients and affects both the trabecular and cortical bone of the vertebrae and the articulating bones of the hip, causing fractures mainly in the vertebrae and hips.

Approximately 25% to 50% of all women over age 60 suffer from osteoporosis. The condition is the most common form of metabolic bone disease and the cause of nearly half of all adult fractures. Although new treatment regimens are available to slow bone loss, early diagnosis—and, therefore, early treatment—is difficult to establish.

ETIOLOGY
Osteoporosis occurs when bone resorption exceeds bone formation. Bone loss from aging occurs in everyone, although it proceeds more rapidly in women than in men because of an accelerated bone loss in the perimenopausal years. Although the cause of osteoporosis is unknown, the condition is strongly related to estrogen deficiency.

Clients who are at risk for osteoporosis include women, Caucasians and Asians, those with a positive family history for osteoporosis, those who have undergone early menopause, and those with low body weights, sedentary life-styles, calcium deficiencies, high-protein diets, or histories of smoking. Those on prolonged heparin or steroid therapy are also at risk.

Osteoporosis often accompanies stress diseases, such as diabetes, metastatic disease, hyperthyroidism, rheumatoid arthritis, chronic hepatic disease, malnutrition, chronic obstructive pulmonary disease, malabsorption, hyperparathyroidism, and Cushing's disease. However, in these instances the etiology is unclear.

HEALTH HISTORY FINDINGS
In a health history interview, the client may report or the nurse may detect many of these findings:
• loss of 2″ (5.1 cm) in total body height
• acute or chronic mid- to low-back pain
• marked joint discomfort when sitting or standing
• decreased mobility
• paralysis (lower motor neuron disease)
• loss of appetite
• history of Cushing's disease, hyperthyroidism, or hyperparathyroidism
• history of bone marrow tumors or fractures
• history of chronic hepatic disease, diabetes mellitus (type 1), or renal tubular acidosis
• history of idiopathic hypercalcemia
• history of prolonged use of heparin, steroids, or analgesics
• use of supplemental vitamins and minerals
• use of long-acting psychotropic drugs
• history of deficiencies in calcium and vitamin C
• history of smoking and alcohol use
• family history of osteoporosis or multiple fractures
• history of living alone and relying on community support
• inability to perform activities of daily living (ADLs)
• history of early menopause (or oophorectomy)

PHYSICAL FINDINGS
In a physical examination, the nurse may detect many of these findings:

Musculoskeletal
• muscular weakness
• aching pain with position changes
• increasing loss of stature
• kyphotic deformity
• mid- to low-back pain

Gastrointestinal
• acute abdominal pain, radiating from the back
• abdominal distention

Other
• thinness (females)
• periodontal disease

DIAGNOSTIC STUDIES
The following studies may be performed to evaluate the client's health status:
• X-rays—to show decreased bone density; only apparent after a loss of more than 40% of total bone mass
• single and dual photon absorptiometry—to determine the risk of fracture to the distal and midshaft radius
• computed tomography (CT) scan—to detect vertebral trabecular bone loss

POTENTIAL COMPLICATIONS
• pain
• self-care deficit
• accidental injury
• knowledge deficit

Nursing diagnosis: *Pain related to fractures*

NURSING GOAL: To provide relief of pain associated with bone fractures

Signs and symptoms
• aching pain over fracture area
• restricted mobility secondary to pain
• frequent requests for analgesics

Interventions

1. Assess the client's pain for location, duration, and severity.

2. Maintain the client with vertebral fractures who has acute pain on complete bed rest for 2 to 4 weeks, and administer analgesics every 4 to 6 hours, as needed or as ordered.

3. Apply heat packs and administer gentle massage.

4. Administer stool softeners to help the client with back pain avoid constipation.

5. Administer pain medications before any scheduled activity.

6. Teach the client passive range-of-motion and isometric exercises.

7. Begin ambulation as soon as possible, using assistive devices, such as walkers and canes, as needed.

8. Provide diversional activities.

Rationales

1. An assessment will determine the degree of pain and the precipitating factors.

2. Rest and analgesics are the treatment of choice for vertebral fractures.

3. Heat and massage relax muscles and increase circulation.

4. Constipation commonly results in straining on defecation, which can lead to increased back pain.

5. Providing an analgesic approximately ½ hour before an activity decreases pain and the fear of pain.

6. Exercise will prevent contractures and functional decline.

7. Ambulation decreases complications associated with immobility and osteoporosis, such as fractures, pain, and discomfort.

8. Diversional activities decrease the client's focus on pain.

OUTCOME CRITERIA
• The client will be free from pain after undergoing the appropriate therapy.

Nursing diagnosis: *Potential for injury related to limited mobility and frequent falls*

NURSING GOALS: To provide a hazard-free environment and to promote safety

Signs and symptoms
• diagnosed osteoporosis
• history of fractures
• lack of social support
• safety hazards in the home or room
• decreased visual acuity
• repeated falls

Interventions

1. Assess the client's gait; obtain a physical therapy evaluation, if necessary, for gait training and assistive devices.

Rationales

1. A steady gait and the appropriate use of assistive devices can prevent falls.

2. Advise the client to wear shoes with low rubber heels and cushioned soles.

2. Appropriate shoes reduce back trauma during walking.

3. Instruct the client to avoid flexion exercises of the spine, including sit-ups and waist-bending exercises.

3. Flexion exercises increase vertical compression forces on the vertebrae.

4. Teach the client proper body mechanics, and caution her to avoid lifting heavy objects.

4. Using improper body mechanics and lifting heavy items may cause spontaneous fractures.

5. Advise the client to avoid participating in jarring activities, such as jogging.

5. This type of motion could cause a compression fracture.

6. Administer estrogens, as ordered. Recommended treatment includes oral conjugated estrogen or transdermal estrogen and progesterone.

6. Estrogens prevent postmenopausal bone loss, even if some bone loss has already occurred. Transdermal estrogen avoids first-pass liver metabolism and, therefore, minimizes liver side effects. Adding progesterone to estrogen therapy removes the risk of estrogen-induced endometrial and breast cancer and promotes new bone formation.

7. Assess the client's home for safety hazards, such as steps, throw rugs, and inappropriately placed furniture. Suggest modifications as needed.

7. Modifying the client's home enviornment can help prevent falls.

8. Consult a social worker to assess the client's community support system.

8. Many communities have organizations that provide housekeeping and shopping services. Such services can help decrease physical stress and the risk of a spontaneous fracture.

OUTCOME CRITERIA
• The client will sustain no further fractures.
• The client will suffer no injuries.

Nursing diagnosis: *Bathing and dressing self-care deficit related to decreased functional ability*

NURSING GOAL: To return the client to a prefracture level of independence in performing ADLs and to prevent learned helplessness

Signs and symptoms
• recent loss of ability to perform ADLs
• immobility
• fear of pain

Interventions

1. Assess the client's ability to perform ADLs.

2. Provide adequate time for the client to perform self-care activities.

3. Schedule the administration of the client's pain medications for ½ hour before self-care activities.

Rationales

1. Such assessment can help the nurse to determine the client's degree of functional disability.

2. Allowing adequate time promotes a feeling of accomplishment and decreases feelings of helplessness. Allowing client to perform self-care prevents learned helplessness.

3. Oral pain medication requires approximately ½ hour for absorption. Administering pain medication before the client performs self-care activities should decrease the severity of the client's pain as well as her fear of pain.

4. Periodically evaluate the client's progress in his ability to perform ADLs.

4. Monitoring the client's progress will enable the nurse to identify areas that need further rehabilitation and will reveal factors that may be contributing to the client's disability.

5. Positively reinforce the client's accomplishment of self-care tasks.

5. Positive reinforcement should increase the client's self-confidence and encourage her to perform more tasks.

6. Identify support systems that can help the client to perform ADLs. Consider consulting a visiting nurse agency and a physical or occupational therapist.

6. Support systems can help meet the client's basic care needs. Other health care disciplines can contribute to holistic health care.

OUTCOME CRITERION
• The client will bathe and dress herself.

Nursing diagnosis: *Knowledge deficit related to the disease and its treatment*

NURSING GOAL: To enhance the client's knowledge of the disease's progression and usual treatments

Signs and symptoms
• inadequate calcium intake
• sedentary life-style
• high protein intake
• excessive alcohol intake
• smoking
• early menopause
• family history of osteoporosis

Interventions

1. Assess the client's knowledge of the disease. Incorporate the client's family or caregiver in the learning process.

2. Review with the client and caregiver the importance of a diet high in calcium. Suggest adding foods with a high calcium content, including milk and other dairy products (such as American and Swiss cheeses, yogurt, ice cream, and cottage cheese), fish (such as sardines and salmon), and vegetables (such as tofu, spinach, and beet, turnip, mustard, and dandelion greens). Consider recommending calcium carbonate supplements.

3. Help the client to develop an exercise program to discourage immobility. Suggest walking or bicycling.

4. Devise realistic goals to help the client quit smoking. Provide positive reinforcement.

Rationales

1. Such assessment will help the nurse determine appropriate interventions. Involving the client's family or caregiver in teaching enhances compliance and decreases confusion.

2. The client may be deficient in dietary calcium. Postmenopausal women usually need 1,500 mg of calcium a day to normalize calcium balance. Calcium carbonate tablets contain 40% calcium, which is the highest content in any type of calcium salt.

3. Weight-bearing exercise stimulates bone formation, while inactivity leads to excess bone resorption.

4. Smoking accelerates bone loss. Setting realistic goals helps the client to feel that her goals are attainable. Positive reinforcement enhances feelings of accomplishment.

OUTCOME CRITERIA
• The client will increase her calcium intake through diet or supplements.
• The client will eliminate behaviors that predispose her to further bone resorption.

NURSING ACTIONS FOR VARIOUS SETTINGS

Nursing actions for a client with osteoporosis depend on the setting in which care is provided. This section identifies which actions are appropriate in all settings and which pertain to acute care, extended care, or home care situations.

All settings
• Inform the client and caregiver that, although osteoporosis is incurable, the progression of disease can be halted.
• Assist the client and caregiver in identifying reversible risk factors of osteoporosis.

Acute care
• Assess the client for pain.
• Consult social services for home care coordination; if necessary, refer the client to a home health agency for a homemaker or visiting nurse.

Extended care
• Monitor the client's dietary intake of calcium, protein, vitamin C, and alcohol.
• Schedule exercise and rest periods.
• Monitor the client for indications of pain, and intervene appropriately.
• Consult a physical therapist.

Home care
• Monitor the client's functional status.
• Reinforce health care practices that help to decrease the risk of osteoporosis.

SELECTED REFERENCES

Coralli, C.H., et al. "Osteoporosis: Significance, Risk Factors and Treatment," *Nurse Practitioner* 11(9):16-20, 25-35, September 1986.

Hallal, J.C. "Osteoporotic Fractures Exact a Toll," *Journal of Gerontological Nursing* 11(8):13-19, August 1985.

Liddel, D. "An In-Depth Look at Osteoporosis," *Orthopaedic Nursing* 4(3):23-28, March 1985.

Lindsay, R. "Managing Osteoporosis: Current Trends, Future Possibilities," *Geriatrics* 42(3):35-40, March 1987.

Lindsay, R. "Osteoporosis: An Updated Approach to Prevention and Management," *Geriatrics* 44(1):45-54, January 1989.

Miller, G. "Osteoporosis—Is It an Inevitable?" *Journal of Gerontological Nursing* 11(3)5:10-15, March 1985.

Mines, A. "Osteoporosis: A Detailed Look at the Clinical Manifestations and Goals for Nursing Care," *The Canadian Nurse* 45-48, January 1985.

Pogrund, H., et al. "Preventing Osteoporosis: Current Practices and Problems," *Geriatrics* 41(5):55-58, 61-71, May 1986.

Reed, A.T., and Birge, S.J., "Screening for Osteoporosis," *Journal of Gerontological Nursing* 14(7):18-20, July 1988.

Talbot, J., et al. "Drug Therapy for Prevention and Treatment of Osteoporosis," *Topics in Geriatric Rehabilitation* 4(2):37-57, February 1989.

MUSCULOSKELETAL SYSTEM

Gout

Gout, or gouty arthritis, is a form of chronic arthritis characterized by recurrent episodes of sudden, severe joint pain, typically in the big toe. Such pain is caused by inflammation from accumulated sodium urate crystals within the joint. Each episode typically resolves after several days or weeks, even if untreated; it usually is followed by an interval without symptoms.

Most clients with gout are men who suffered their first attack between ages 40 and 50. Women, who are rarely affected, typically suffer their first attack only after menopause. The condition is most prevalent among those who are obese, drink large amounts of alcohol, have diabetes mellitus, and are hypertensive. More than half of all clients suffer a second attack within 2 years.

ETIOLOGY
Normally, the kidneys excrete uric acid, a waste product of purine metabolism. In some clients, the uric acid crystalizes and settles in joints and surrounding tissue. These crystals then begin irritating and inflaming the joint lining, causing the pain characteristic of an acute gout attack. The reason why uric acid crystals settle in joints is still unclear.

Although no positive connection can be made between gout and hyperuricemia, which is typically caused by an overproduction of uric acid or from failure of the kidneys to excrete uric acid, most clients with gout also have hyperuricemia. Some individuals, however, have hyperuricemia without gout. Both conditions, which can be inherited, are commonly precipitated by diuretic use, excessive food and alcohol consumption, surgery, and crash diets. Decreased renal function that occurs with advancing age does not seem to be a precipitating factor.

HEALTH HISTORY FINDINGS
In a health history interview, the client may report or the nurse may detect these findings:
• extreme pain in the joints of the big toe, finger, foot, ankle, elbow, wrist, or knees
• increased pain with slight pressure
• pain typically occuring between 4:00 a.m. and 5:00 a.m.
• malaise
• history of renal disease, diabetes mellitus, coronary artery disease, hypertension, or congestive heart failure
• recent surgery
• recent trauma
• family history of gout

• use of thiazides or low doses of aspirin
• use of cytotoxic agents, fructose, nicotinic acid, or vitamin B_2
• long-term consumption of alcohol
• recent increase in exercise
• history of crash dieting

PHYSICAL FINDINGS
In a physical examination, the nurse may detect many of these findings:

Musculoskeletal
• extreme joint tenderness
• inflamed, hot joint
• tophi (chalky urate crystal deposits) around cartilaginous areas, such as the ear
• pain limited to two or three joints, primarily in the legs or feet

Integumentary
• shiny, red or purple skin over the inflamed joint
• desquamation over the joint

Other
• obesity
• moderately elevated temperature

DIAGNOSTIC STUDIES
The following studies may be performed to evaluate the client's health status:
• serum uric acid studies—to determine excessive levels; levels are usually more than 8 mg/dl, but may be normal
• erythrocyte sedimentation rate (ESR)—to help in diagnosis; usually elevated during attacks
• calcium pyrophosphate dehydrate (CPPD) levels—to identify abnormal levels; usually elevated in pseudogout (inflammation of a joint that mimicks gout but results from other causes, such as sepsis)
• white blood cell count—to help in diagnosis; sometimes elevated in an acute gout attack
• X-rays of the affected joint—to diagnose various types of arthritis and gouty arthritis; findings are normal early in the disease
• aspiration of synovial fluid—to confirm the diagnosis; performed only on large joints
• Gram stain and culture—to rule out septic gout; performed if synovial fluid is especially cloudy

POTENTIAL COMPLICATIONS
• pain
• decreased mobility

Nursing diagnosis: *Pain related to acute inflammation*

NURSING GOAL: To relieve and prevent the recurrence of pain associated with acute gout attacks

Signs and symptoms
• severe joint pain, typically in the big toe
• pain in the elbow, finger, ankle, foot, wrist, or knee
• inflamed, warm, and tender joint
• skin desquamation after the attack

Interventions

1. Administer colchicine, indomethacin, or phenylbutazone, as ordered. Monitor the client receiving oral colchicine for diarrhea, nausea, or abdominal cramps.

2. Administer probenecid, sulfinpyrazone, or allopurinol, as ordered, to prevent recurrence of acute gout pain. Inform the client taking allopurinol about the possibility of an acute gout attack during the first 6 months of therapy.

3. Assess the client receiving allopurinol for a skin rash. If a rash is noted, notify the physician and discontinue the medication.

4. Review the client's medication record for possible drug interactions, such as from captopril, azathioprine, mercaptopurine, and warfarin sodium.

5. Monitor the client for increased pain during administration of uricosuric agents. Administer anti-inflammatory medications, as ordered.

6. Avoid administering aspirin to clients receiving uricosuric agents.

7. Place a foot cradle over the client's bed.

8. Apply cool, moist soaks to affected joints.

9. Encourage the client to drink six to eight 8-oz glasses (1,500 to 2,000 ml) of fluid each day.

Rationales

1. Colchicine, an antigout agent, provides immediate pain relief and may be used as a diagnostic tool; when given orally, this agent can cause severe GI upset. Other nonspecific anti-inflammatory medications, such as indomethacin and phenylbutazone, may be given to help reduce pain and inflammation.

2. These drugs help prevent the recurrence of acute gout attacks by blocking the reabsorption of uric acid by the proximal renal tubule. Uricosuric agents (probenecid and sulfinpyrazone) may be ordered to help increase uric acid secretion, thereby lowering the serum acid level. These agents are contraindicated in acute gout attacks, and may, in fact, exacerbate acute pain. Allopurinol, which blocks uric acid production to decrease serum uric acid levels, is typically ordered for clients with abnormal kidney function or those prone to kidney stone development. Like probenecid and sulfinpyrazone, allopurinol is contraindicated for acute gout. During the first 6 months of allopurinol therapy, serum uric acid levels drop rapidly, possibly leading to increased joint inflammation and pain. Informing the client of this possibility promotes medication compliance.

3. A rash may signal hypersensitivity to the drug and may occur before more severe reactions, such as vasculitis.

4. Allopurinol enhances the activity of these drugs. A client taking these medications should not be given allopurinol.

5. At the start of uricosuric therapy, the crystals in the joints begin to dissolve, increasing inflammation and the frequency of attacks. Anti-inflammatory agents are usually effective in relieving pain.

6. Aspirin blocks the effect of uricosuric agents, causing uric acid levels to rise.

7. Even slight pressure on the joint produces pain.

8. Cool, moist soaks can reduce inflammation and decrease pain.

9. Adequate hydration minimizes the risk of kidney stone formation.

10. Provide other comfort measures, such as back massages and turning and positioning, as often as possible and as tolerated.

10. These measures promote comfort and distract the client from his pain.

11. Teach the client to avoid high-purine foods, such as anchovies and sardines, especially if he has renal impairment.

11. The kidneys excrete uric acid. Uricosuria may increase in the client who has a diet high in purine and impaired renal function.

12. Weigh the client weekly, and encourage him to lose weight slowly.

12. Crash diets may increase the client's uric acid formation, increasing his risk of a gout attack.

OUTCOME CRITERIA
• The client will verbalize relief of pain.
• The client will comply with the medication regimen.
• The client will remain free from adverse reactions to the drugs.

NURSING ACTIONS IN VARIOUS SETTINGS
Nursing actions for a client with gout depend on the setting in which care is provided. This section identifies which actions are appropriate in all settings and which pertain to acute care, extended care, or home care situations.

All settings
• Explain to the client the importance of taking all medications as prescribed. Emphasize that, even though a gout attack may subside, the underlying arthritic problem remains.
• Instruct the client to limit his consumption of beer, wine, and champagne to one 4-oz glass per day and to restrict his intake of hard liquor to 2 oz per day.
• Instruct the client to drink four 8-oz glasses (950 ml) of nonalcoholic fluid each day.

Acute care
• Promptly assess the client who may be experiencing a gout attack, as such attacks are considered medical emergencies. Notify the physician immediately.
• Teach the night nursing staff to be particularly alert to the signs and symptoms of gout attacks, as attacks often occur during the night.

Extended care
• Keep oral and I.V. colchicine available for clients who have a history of gout.
• Conduct a staff inservice on the procedure for handling a client with an acute gout attack.

Home care
• Instruct the client on medication use and on diet and alcohol restrictions.
• Provide the client and the client's family with information about the Arthritis Foundation.
• Instruct the client's caregiver to take the client to an emergency room if an acute gout attack occurs.

SELECTED REFERENCES
Calkins, E., et al. *The Practice of Geriatrics.* Philadelphia: W.B. Saunders Co., 1986.
Dornbrand, L., et al. *Manual of Clinical Problems in Adult Ambulatory Care.* Boston: Little, Brown & Co., 1985.
Fox, I.H., et al. "Gout and Pseudogout in Primary Care," *Patient Care* 84-126, July 15, 1989.
Hoole, A.J., et al. *Patient Care for Nurse Practitioners,* 3rd ed. Boston: Little, Brown & Co., 1988.
McGill, P.E. "Gouty Arthritis in the Geriatric Patient," *Geriatric Medicine Today* 5(71):59-73, July 1987.
Reichel, W. *Clinical Aspects of Aging.* Baltimore: Williams & Wilkins Co., 1989.

Dementia and Alzheimer's Disease

Dementia is an organic mental disorder characterized by intellectual deterioration, marked personality changes, and progressive inability to carry out activites of daily living (ADLs). Typically, the loss of cognitive abilities becomes severe enough to interfere with the client's capacity to live independently.

Frequently, dementia begins insidiously; its diagnosis is made by a process of exclusion. Alzheimer's disease, the most common form of dementia in elderly clients, can be categorized according to three stages of progressively deteriorating mental capacity (see *Staging Alzheimer's Disease,* page 198). Other forms of dementia include reversible dementia and multi-infarct dementia.

A multifaceted disorder that affects the client, the client's family, and society, dementia is a leading cause of death among older adults. Between 2 and 3 million people, mostly older adults, suffer from some form of dementia. The disorder affects 1 in 10 American families. Because families typically provide ongoing care for demented clients for years without much support or assistance, nursing care is directed toward enhancing knowledge and providing support.

ETIOLOGY
About 15% of all demented clients have reversible dementia, or pseudodementia, which can result from sepsis, drug toxicity, benign hydrocephalus, brain tumor, subdural hematoma, or depression. About 25% to 30% have a multi-infarct form of dementia that is closely linked with cardiovascular disease. In this form, which results from a series of minor cerebrovascular accidents that destroy tissue throughout the brain, the disorder follows a pattern in which the client's level of functioning drops step by step over the course of about 15 years, with a maintenance period following each step.

About 50% to 60% of all demented clients have dementia of the Alzheimer's type. In this disease, which is characterized by the destruction of brain cells, the client typically survives 5 years. A brain biopsy of a client with Alzheimer's disease shows the classic appearance of neurofibrillary tangles and plaques. Although the exact cause of this disease is unknown, researchers have learned that the brain cells of those with Alzheimer's disease lack certain neurotransmitters, such as acetylcholine and norepinephrine, which may cause the cognitive changes characteristic of the disease. No evidence indicates that Alzheimer's disease results from a virus or an accumulation of toxic substances, such as aluminum.

A small percentage of clients with dementia obtain the disorder by viral transmission. This rare form of dementia typically results from an infection that was acquired 10 to 20 years before the onset of the disease. The most common of the viral dementias is Creutzfeldt-Jakob disease. After the symptoms manifest, the disease progresses rapidly, often producing severe dementia within 6 months to 1 year.

Dementia is considered a terminal illness. If the cause of reversible dementia is not identified and treated, the individual will not improve. The most common cause of death in demented clients is from infection, such as pneumonia. Severely demented clients may be prone to infection because of their generally debilitated state. In Alzheimer's disease, the immune system is usually affected, placing clients at even higher risk for infection.

HEALTH HISTORY FINDINGS
In a health history interview, the client may report or the nurse may detect many of these findings:
- confusion
- decreased functional ability
- mood or personality changes
- vision and hearing deficits
- chronic constipation
- fecal or urinary incontinence
- decreased libido
- impotence
- stilted and slowed gait (middle and late stages)
- depression
- mania
- anxiety
- paranoia
- situational disturbances
- violent outbursts
- uncontrolled crying
- inability to cooperate
- recent memory loss
- adverse reaction to a newly prescribed medication
- recent weight gain or loss
- withdrawal from work or social situations
- reversal of usual sleep patterns (such as sleeping during day and remaining awake at night)
- increased restlessness and confusion in the evening
- history of multiple sclerosis, syphilis, or Parkinson's disease
- history of cerebral atherosclerosis or Huntington's disease
- history of Creutzfeldt-Jakob disease or Pick's disease
- frequent falls
- history of a subdural hematoma
- history of a hip replacement
- misuse of prescribed medications
- use of psychotropic, antidepressant, or antihypertensive medications
- history of overeating
- history of alcohol use
- family history of dementia
- family history of Down's syndrome

PHYSICAL FINDINGS

In a physical examination, the nurse may detect many of these findings:

Neurologic
• slowed reflexes
• visual and spatial deficits

Integumentary
• rashes

Gastrointestinal
• hypoactive bowel sounds
• distention from constipation and gas
• fecal impaction

Musculoskeletal
• gait disturbance
• loss of coordination

Psychological
• global and progressive changes in cognitive function
• loss of memory and sense of time
• altered speech
• difficulties in naming objects and people
• arithmetic miscalculations
• score of less than 22 on the Folstein Mini-Mental State examination (see "Delirium," pages 225 to 229)

DIAGNOSTIC STUDIES

The following studies may be performed to evaluate the client's health status:
• drug studies—to identify drug toxicity as a cause; medications that can cause mental confusion include digoxin, theophylline, and phenytoin
• thyroid function studies—to rule out hypothyroidism, which can mimic early signs of dementia
• complete blood count (CBC) with differential—to rule out septicemia; dementia may be the only presenting symptom in a client with septicemia
• electrolyte studies—to identify potassium and sodium deficits and hypoglycemia, which can cause mental confusion
• computed tomography (CT) scan—to rule out brain tumors, subdural hematomas, and hydrocephalus
• positron emission tomography (PET) scan—to determine the uptake of glucose by the brain; abnormal findings include reduced glucose metabolism in the temporal-parietal cortex
• magnetic resonance imaging (MRI) scan—to reveal detailed structural changes in the brain; used with or instead of the CT scan
• evaluation for depression—to rule out depression as a cause of dementia (see "Depression," pages 264 to 269)

POTENTIAL COMPLICATIONS
• malnutrition
• constipation
• urinary incontinence
• family conflict and stress
• infection
• depression (early stages)
• insomnia

Nursing diagnosis: *Altered thought processes related to memory loss, confusion, and disorientation associated with dementia*

NURSING GOALS: To help the caregiver manage the client's behaviors caused by mental deterioration and to implement measures that compensate for dementia

Signs and symptoms
• paranoia
• repetitive behavior
• violent or aggressive outbursts

Interventions

1. Provide the client with a consistent, routine environment.

2. Avoid reorienting clients more than once per encounter

3. If the client tends to repeat questions or gestures during conversations, try to divert his attention by changing the subject.

Rationales

1. A consistent routine helps the client function with his limited capabilities.

2. Reorientation frustrates the demented client because he cannot remember.

3. Diverting the client will interrupt his train of thought.

4. Permit common behaviors, such as hoarding objects or wandering, as long as they are conducted in a safe environment. To prevent hoarding, keep items out of the client's view.

4. The client with Alzheimer's disease commonly exhibits certain behaviors, such as wandering, pacing, hoarding or hiding objects, inappropriate sexual behavior, "sundowning" (exhibiting increased confusion, agitation, pacing, and handwringing in the late afternoon, typically resulting from fatigue), catastrophic reaction (overreacting to minor problems with uncontrolled crying, shouting, or violence), and violence (typically resulting from frustration). In many cases, these behaviors are difficult to prevent; therefore, permitting the nonviolent or unoffensive behaviors in a safe environment is often less agitating to the client.

5. Assess the client for signs of depression, such as a mood disturbance or insomnia.

5. Depression can aggravate dementia and, therefore, requires treatment.

6. To decrease the client's agitation and restlessness, implement the following: maintaining a structured, consistent environment and establishing a routine that is easy for the client and caregiver to follow; creating a picture book of familiar people and places from the client's past; promoting regular physical activity and art therapy, such as finger painting; playing old, familiar music during periods of agitation; and, if feasible, instituting pet therapy.

6. The client typically remains calmer in a familiar environment. A picture book of familiar people and places from the client's past is an effective calming tool, as the client with Alzheimer's disease tends to retain long-term memories. Physical activity and art therapy provide diversion and help to prevent agitation. Music, especially old familiar melodies, can calm the client who has become agitated. A pet can have a calming effect on elderly client.

7. Consult the client's physician on the possible use of lorazepam if other therapies are unsuccessful.

7. Small doses of tranquilizers or antipsychotic medications may help to lessen the client's agitation, anxiety, and unpredictable behavior.

8. Avoid administering benzodiazepines. If prescribed, discuss their discontinuation with the physician.

8. Benzodiazepines tend to increase confusion and cause paradoxical agitation.

9. Recommend that the client's family or caregiver obtain an identification bracelet for the client. Advise them to sew labels with the client's name and address onto the client's clothing.

9. These measures will help identify the client if he should become lost.

10. Place labels or name tags on the objects, rooms, and people with which the client has regular contact.

10. Labels help the client to remember.

11. Provide clues or reminders about the identity of objects and about the client's duties. For example, place a large calendar in the client's room, and mark an "X" through each day so that the client can identify the correct date; make a schedule of the day's activities; compile lists of things the client needs to remember; decorate the client's room to indicate the holidays; make large, simple signs identifying rooms and activities, such as "Brush your teeth" and "This is the bathroom."

11. These measures may reorient the client and help him function more successfully.

12. Instruct the client's family or caregiver to restrict the client's alcohol intake.

12. Alcohol may contribute to confusion.

OUTCOME CRITERIA
• The client will be more functional.
• The caregiver will understand which environmental modifications best facilitate the client's functioning.

Nursing diagnosis: *Impaired verbal communication related to deteriorated cognitive condition*

NURSING GOALS: To establish effective verbal and nonverbal communication with the client and to understand the client's needs as his dementia increases and verbal skills decline

Signs and symptoms
- repetition of words
- mental search for words
- use of nonsensical language
- agitation
- hostility

Interventions

1. Gently approach the client with an open, friendly, and relaxed manner and expression.

2. Speak to the client in a clear, low-pitched tone.

3. Always identify yourself and look directly at the client.

4. Assess the client's hearing and vision; if deficits are noted, refer the client for further evaluation and treatment.

5. Assess the client's nonverbal behaviors, such as facial expressions, body language, posture, grimacing, and increased restlessness.

6. Minimize background noise when talking with the client.

7. Encourage the client to describe stories or situations from his past, prompting him when necessary.

8. Maintain a routine to minimize the need for communication.

9. Use a reminiscence therapy book, including pictures from the client's past.

Rationales

1. Clients with Alzheimer's disease tend to mirror the affect of those around them.

2. High-pitched tones convey anxiety and tension.

3. Identifying yourself and looking at the client captures the client's attention.

4. Hearing and vision deficits contribute to communication problems.

5. Nonverbal cues may be the client's only way of communicating pain or discomfort.

6. Background noise may be a source of distraction.

7. Typically, those with Alzheimer's disease retain long-term memories until the later stages of the disease. Allowing the client to talk about things he remembers is soothing.

8. If a client and caregiver follow a routine, verbal communication is unnecessary.

9. Visual prompts stimulate long-term memory, especially when used repeatedly. A reminiscence book gives the client something specific on which to focus.

OUTCOME CRITERIA
- The caregiver will demonstrate an improved ability to understand the client's needs.
- The caregiver will be less frustrated by a lack of ability to communicate with the client.

Nursing diagnosis: *Potential for aspiration related to dysphagia*

NURSING GOALS: To prevent aspiration and to promote safe eating habits

Signs and symptoms
- difficulty swallowing
- elevated temperature
- acutely increased confusion
- increased chest congestion
- coughing while eating

Interventions

1. Assess the client's ability to chew and swallow.

2. Feed the client in an upright position, and allow him to remain upright for 45 minutes after meals.

3. Frequently offer the client soft foods in small amounts, such as eggs, cottage cheese, and pudding.

4. When feeding the client, place the food on the back of his tongue and encourage him to eat slowly.

5. If the client has difficulty swallowing liquids, provide fruit slush instead. To prepare the fruit slush, blend a 48-oz can of fruit cocktail with 8 oz of orange juice in a blender.

6. If the client has difficulty taking oral medications, try crushing the medications and mixing them into apple-sauce.

7. Teach the caregiver how to perform abdominal thrusts in case the client chokes.

Rationales

1. Such assessment should help identify any eating difficulties and enable the nurse to develop a plan of care.

2. Remaining upright propels food toward the stomach and helps prevent aspiration.

3. Soft foods are easy to swallow. The client can handle small meals easier than large ones.

4. Eating in this way facilitates swallowing.

5. Thick liquids are easier to swallow. A fruit slush mixture equals one day's liquid intake.

6. This should facilitate swallowing and will ensure that the client receives his medication.

7. The caregiver should know this maneuver, as the demented client is at risk for choking.

OUTCOME CRITERIA
- The client's airway will remain clear.
- The client will receive adequate nutrition and hydration.
- The client will remain free from aspiration while eating.

Nursing diagnosis: *Potential for trauma related to inappropriate judgment and wandering*

NURSING GOAL: To ensure the client's safety as he loses his ability to make sound judgments

Signs and symptoms
- forgetfulness
- inability to make sound judgments
- wandering
- gait disturbance
- frequent falls

Interventions

1. Assess the client's home for environmental safety hazards; help the client's family to make necessary changes. For example, advise them to unplug the stove when not in use; place combination or child-proof locks on the outside of all doors; use a nightlight; store all knives, scissors, medications, matches, firearms, and toxic household chemicals safely out of the client's reach; remove small rugs from hallways and heavily trafficked areas; place handrails in hallways and bathrooms; and allow the client to smoke only under supervision.

2. Avoid the use of restraints or bed rails. If necessary, keep the client's mattress on the floor.

Rationales

1. Confusion, faulty judgment, and gait disturbances predispose the client to accidental injury.

2. Restraining the client may promote agitation and paranoia and may contribute to injury.

3. Help the client's family or caregiver to evaluate the client's ability to drive. Suggest the possibility of hiding the car keys or locking the steering wheel, if necessary.

3. Driving may be contraindicated for a demented client because of perceptual difficulties and a loss of sense of direction. Families sometimes have difficulty deciding whether clients are capable of driving and may need assistance.

OUTCOME CRITERIA
• The client's environment will be modified to ensure safety.
• The client will not be a safety hazard to others.

Nursing diagnosis: *Altered patterns of urinary elimination related to loss of memory*

NURSING GOALS: To assess for acute symptoms of incontinence and to institute bladder retraining, if necessary

Signs and symptoms
• urinary or fecal incontinence
• functional deterioration
• decreased mental status
• use of incontinence pads or diapers
• urinary tract infection
• perineal skin breakdown

Interventions

1. Assess the client for acute causes of incontinence, such as infection, urinary retention, or delirium.

2. Assess the client's pattern of incontinence, and use the information to devise a planned toileting schedule.

3. Assist the client with toileting by posting a large, colorful sign or a picture of a commode on the bathroom door; watching for nonverbal cues that signal the need for elimination and reminding the client to go to the bathroom; assisting the client with removing or adjusting his clothing as necessary; helping the client to position himself correctly for elimination; and cueing the client or talking him through each step of the task, if necessary.

4. Assess the client for constipation by keeping an accurate stool record

5. Ensure that the client drinks six to eight 8-oz glasses (1,500 to 2,000 ml) of fluid a day, but restrict his fluid intake after 6 p.m.

6. Suggest that the incontinent client wear disposable incontinence pads or adult diapers.

Rationales

1. An assessment is the first step in evaluating the cause of incontinence and provides the nurse with a basis on which to build interventions.

2. Planned, scheduled voiding (habit training) is more successful if the client has an individualized schedule.

3. The client with Alzheimer's disease sometimes loses the ability to recognize or respond to appropriate voiding signals, such as the need to void, the location of the bathroom, and the normal toileting routine.

4. Constipation or hard stool in the distal colon increases pressure on the bladder, which can lead to urine leakage.

5. Adequate fluids dilute the urine and decrease the risk of bladder irritation and accidents. Restricting fluids after 6 p.m. decreases the load on the bladder during sleep, decreasing the risk of nighttime incontinence.

6. Although incontinence can be reduced, the problem can not always be eliminated. Disposable incontinence pads or adult diapers can help prevent embarrassing bladder accidents and give the client a sense of security.

OUTCOME CRITERIA
• The client will have fewer urinary incontinence episodes.
• The client will have fewer environmental barriers to toileting.

Nursing diagnosis: *Sleep pattern disturbance related to dementia*

NURSING GOAL: To minimize sleep disturbances common in dementia

Signs and symptoms
• increased restlessness and anxiety as nighttime approaches
• frequent awakening
• frequent position changes during sleep
• wandering

Interventions

1. Teach the client's family or caregiver the sleep pattern changes common in dementia, such as frequent awakening, moving about during the night, and remaining awake for prolonged periods.

2. Institute behavioral approaches, such as rising at same time each morning, eliminating afternoon naps, and promoting regular exercise.

3. Establish a bedtime routine for the client, and strive for consistency.

4. Ensure the client's safety for nighttime wandering and restlessness. Make sure the environment has special hard-to-reach locks on the outside doors, an unplugged stove, an easy chair in the client's room to allow him to move from the bed to the chair, a lack of restraints, and a gate at top of the stairways.

5. Avoid administering benzodiazepines for long-term management of insomnia.

6. Reorient the client in a soft, soothing manner if he awakens during the night and becomes confused and agitated.

7. Assess the client for "sundowning" syndrome during the late afternoon or early evening. If necessary, limit the client's evening activities, offer companionship, turn on lamps before evening, and provide soft music or social stimulation in the late afternoon.

Rationales

1. Knowledge of these changes can relieve the caregiver's anxiety and help to establish realistic expectations.

2. In the early and middle stages of dementia, these approaches help to promote sleep at night.

3. A consistent routine is comforting and helps the client prepare for rest.

4. Ensuring the client's safety, rather than attempting to prevent expected nocturnal behaviors, is more practical.

5. Long-term use of benzodiazepines may worsen the client's sleeping problem. Dependence on sedative-hypnotics can create psychological problems for caregivers caught up in the conflict of providing or not providing such medication.

6. A soothing manner reduces the possibility that the client will become agitated and lose control.

7. Sundowning syndrome, which is characterized by increased confusion, agitation, anxiety, pacing, wandering, and hand wringing, typically manifests in late afternoon or early evening. This condition is typically related to fatigue and the inability to handle stress.

OUTCOME CRITERION
• The client and caregiver will take appropriate measures to minimize the client's sleeping problems.

Nursing diagnosis: *Feeding, bathing, hygiene, dressing, grooming, and toileting self-care deficit related to fatigue, weakness, impaired motor control, and memory loss*

NURSING GOAL: To assist the client to perform self-care tasks

Signs and symptoms
- inability to dress, feed, or bathe self
- urinary or fecal incontinence
- foul body odor
- poor hygiene
- unkempt appearance

Interventions

1. Assess the client's physical and cognitive status.

2. Teach the client's family or caregiver to provide the client with necessary care.

3. Provide step-by-step instructions and simplify tasks to allow the client to complete as many tasks as possible on his own.

4. Help the client bathe by following the client's old routine as much as possible; having all supplies at hand and talking him through one task at a time; avoiding discussions about the necessity of the bath; checking the temperature of the water and using safety devices, such as grab bars, nonskid mats, or a bath chair; encouraging the caregiver to shower with the client, if necessary; and removing everything from the bathroom except the items needed for the bath.

5. Help the client to dress by laying out clothes in the order in which they should be put on, using simple garments with hook and loop (Velcro) closures or large zippers, and by allowing ample time.

6. Assist the client with eating by allowing him to feed himself, giving him ample time to eat, and providing straws, training cups, and large utensils with built-up handles.

7. Plan a toileting schedule to manage incontinence (see "Urinary Incontinence," pages 128 to 137).

Rationales

1. Such assessment helps the nurse to evaluate the client's capabilities.

2. The caregiver without formal training may require instruction about basic care.

3. This process allows the client to maintain functional status and increases his feelings of self-worth.

4. Following familiar routines prevents agitation. Targeted step-by-step assistance promotes independence and minimizes falls and injury. Limiting or avoiding discussion about the need for a bath prevents agitation. Checking the water temperature and providing safety devices prevents falls and subsequent injury. Removing extra items prevents the possibility of inappropriate use and injury.

5. Laying out the clothes relieves the client of having to make decisions. Simple garments facilitate independence and prevent frustration. Allowing ample time for dressing eliminates the possibility of frustration and agitation.

6. Encouraging self-feeding promotes independence. Allowing the client enough time for meals prevents frustration and agitation. Providing appropriate utensils and cups facilitates eating.

7. Incontinence in late dementia often results because of the client's inability to perceive the need to void as well as his inability to toilet himself.

OUTCOME CRITERIA
- The client will perform as much self-care as possible.

Nursing diagnosis: *Ineffective family coping: compromised, related to knowledge deficit and increased demands*

NURSING GOAL: To help the client's family learn to cope with the client's dementia

Signs and symptoms
- family's or caregiver's inability to cope effectively in different situations
- family's or caregiver's stated lack of knowledge about dementia

Interventions

1. Assess the family's and caregiver's knowledge level by asking appropriate questions about their understanding of dementia, the common behaviors exhibited by demented clients, appropriate family and caregiver roles, and need for respite from the client.

2. Involve all family members in teaching sessions.

3. Explain and demonstrate necessary nursing care, including how to manage constipation, care for the incontinent client's skin, pad the incontinent client's bed, and handle sleep disturbances.

4. Suggest ways for the client's family to enhance their understanding of the client's problem, such as by joining a support group or local Alzheimer's disease association or by reading appropriate supportive material.

Rationales

1. An assessment of the family's status provides the nurse with a baseline for determining the best approach and needed interventions.

2. Because the client with Alzheimer's disease requires long-term care, all family members must learn to cope effectively with this chronic, progressive disease.

3. The family is apt to be unaware of how to manage nursing problems and may require detailed instruction.

4. Support groups help to enhance the coping abilities of the family and caregiver of the Alzheimer's disease client. Sharing information about similar or common problems helps the family and caregiver to adapt to expected change.

OUTCOME CRITERIA
• The client's family and caregiver will learn more about the disease.
• The client's family and caregiver will learn how to care for the client.
• The client's family and caregiver will identify appropriate coping mechanisms.

Nursing diagnosis: Altered family processes related to the situational crisis of a chronically ill family member, to disruption of family life, and to altered family roles

NURSING GOALS: To reduce family conflict and to increase the capacity for caregiving

Signs and symptoms
• role reversals
• expressed inability of the family or caregiver to cope
• caregiver's or family's lack of respite

Interventions

1. Encourage the family and caregiver to express their feelings, frustrations, and problems to appropriate health care professionals, interested family members, or trusted friends.

2. Offer support, understanding, and reassurance to family members.

3. Help the caregiver to learn about newly assumed responsibilities.

4. Refer the client's family to social services or a discharge planner to assist with home care or nursing home placement.

5. Encourage the caregiver to use respite services, such as adult day care and home health aides.

Rationales

1. Ventilating feelings and problems frequently helps with coping and finding appropriate solutions.

2. Caring for a client with Alzheimer's disease is frequently a frustrating and thankless task that leaves family members drained.

3. The caregiver sometimes needs help with new tasks, such as managing finances.

4. Social services can often link the caregiver with support systems and answer questions about long-term care.

5. Respite provides the caregiver with renewed energy.

OUTCOME CRITERIA
• The client's family will learn to cope with their newly assumed roles.
• The client's family will be aware of available respite resources.

Nursing diagnosis: *Social isolation (client and family) related to anxiety about the client's disability and memory loss and to the inability to leave the client alone*

NURSING GOAL: To prevent social isolation of the client and the client's family

Signs and symptoms
• expressed feelings of isolation by the client or family
• lack of support

Interventions

1. Assess the client's ability to communicate and the family's level of social isolation.

2. Discuss with the client's family the possibility of relying on friends for support and respite.

3. Identify alternative support systems for the family so that caregivers can maintain a social life.

Rationales

1. The client sometimes suffers from isolation because of his inability to communicate effectively. The family is often embarrassed about the problem of dementia and withdraw from social situations.

2. The family often needs help to realize that friends, if informed, can offer support and respite.

3. The demands of caregiving often cause isolation. Formal support groups and friends can provide necessary comfort and support.

OUTCOME CRITERIA
• The client and the client's family will feel less isolated.
• The client's family will learn to identify and use appropriate support systems.

NURSING ACTIONS IN VARIOUS SETTINGS
Nursing actions for a client with dementia or Alzheimer's disease depend on the setting in which care is provided. This section identifies which actions are appropriate in all settings and which pertain to acute care, extended care, or home care situations.

All settings
• Encourage the client's family to have the client evaluated for dementia if such evaluation has not been performed previously.
• Educate the client's family about dementia and its common behaviors and about appropriate support groups, including the Alzheimer's Disease Association, church groups, adult day care, and home health services.
• Emphasize to the client and client's family the importance of planning for the progression of the disease and the client's eventual death.
• Encourage the client to make any decisions about money and legal matters early, while he is still able to function effectively and make sound judgments.

• Suggest that the client and the family consult a lawyer about a durable power of attorney, a will, and a living will.

Acute care
• Educate the client's family about any necessary testing.
• Consider whether the hospitalized client should be placed in a semiprivate room or whether a relative spend the night.
• Prepare the family for the client's discharge by referring them to a home health agency or specific support group.

Extended care
• Plan to prevent such complications as dehydration and constipation.
• Educate the nursing staff about dementia and how to care for the demented client; encourage their participation in care conferences and support groups.
• Strive to provide consistent caregivers and a consistent routine.

STAGING ALZHEIMER'S DISEASE

Alzheimer's disease, whose usual course is smooth and progressive, is staged according to the manifestation of symptoms that mark the client's deteriorating condition. The chart below indicates characteristic symptoms during the early, middle, and late stages of the disease.

	Early stage	Middle stage	Late stage
Memory	• Short-term memory loss • Difficulty remembering names, words, or thoughts • Misplacing familiar items, such as eyeglasses or keys • Forgetting telephone messages • Missing appointments • Getting lost on familiar trips	• Unawareness of all recent events • Ability to recall distant past intact	• Inability to learn new concepts or to formulate memories • Total memory loss of recent and distant events
Language	• Decreased communication • Unaffected speech • Reduced vocabulary • Difficulty in finding appropriate words • Making irrelevancies • Decreased verbal communication	• Continual use of repeated words or phrases • Slowed speech with pauses and interruptions • Inability to complete sentences or continual need to revise speech	• Significantly reduced vocabulary • Increased use of invented terms • Inability to read • Need for repeated instructions • Severely limited vocabulary (use of only one or two words) or inability to speak • Repetition of words or sentences without understanding their meaning • Total loss of comprehension
Mood and behavior	• Mood swings • Withdrawal or depression • Easy distractibility • Need to seek out familiar people and surroundings • Less initiation and spontaneity • Denial of forgetfulness and confusion	• Frequent mood swings • Increased self-absorption and insensitivity to others' feelings • Little display of warmth • Need to pace or wander • Increased agitation, suspicion, hallucinations, and delusions • Sleep disturbances	• Frequent agitation • Obliviousness to others and the environment • Inability to recognize caregiver
Coordination and motor skills	• Good control over coordination and motor skills • Slowed reaction time • Possible inability to drive	• Loss of coordination and balance • Difficulty walking • Difficulty writing (often illegible)	• Total inability to walk, sit, smile, or swallow • Possible stuporous or comatose condition
Cognitive skills	• Difficulty handling finances (such as paying bills, balancing checkbooks, or making change) • Difficulty performing complex but familiar tasks (such as playing bridge or golf) • Inability to work	• Difficulty making decisions • Inability to perform simple arithmetic • Difficulty concentrating • Inability to follow a story • Need for instructions to perform tasks • Poor judgment • Loss of sense of time or place	• Little observable cognitive function
Self-care	• Ability to complete activities of daily living with little or no assistance	• Need for assistance with deciding what to wear, putting on clothing, and bathing • Fear of bathing • Inability to remember the bathroom's location • Urinary and fecal incontinence	• Need for extensive assistance in performing activities of daily living • Possible total reliance on others for care

Home care
• Help the client's family or caregiver to establish a simple, predictable routine that promotes the client's independence.
• Encourage the client's family to evaluate nursing homes before one is necessary.
• Help the family to obtain respite.
• Provide the family with appropriate educational material.
• Assess the client for potential complications, and plan ways to prevent them.
• Assess the client periodically for neglect or physical abuse.
• Encourage the client's family or caregiver to seek help from other family members, friends, and health care professionals.
• If the caregiver plans to be away from home for a long period, plan to have meals delivered to the client.

SELECTED REFERENCES
Caseta, M., et al. "Caregivers to Dementia Patients: The Utilization of Community Services," *Gerontologist* 27(2):209-14, 1987.

Chenoweth, B., and Spencer, B. "Dementia: The Experience of Family Caregivers," *Gerontologist* 26(3): 267-72, 1986.

Gomez, A., and Gomez, E. "Dementia? or Delirium?" *Geriatric Nursing* 10(3):141-43, May/June 1989.

Johnson, L., and Lohr-Keller, K. "Staging Alzheimer's Disease," *Geriatric Nursing* 10(4):196-97, July/August 1989.

Laney, P. "Pharmacological Considerations in the Treatment of Alzheimer's Disease," *Geriatric Medicine Today* 6(9):29-53, September 1987.

Mann, L. "Community Support for Families Caring for Members with Alzheimer's Disease," *Home Health Care Nursing* 3(1):8-10, 1985.

"Losing a Million Minds: Confronting the Tragedy of Alzheimer's Disease and Other Dementias," OTA-BA-323, Washington, D.C.: U.S. Government Printing Office, April 1987.

Read, S., and Cummings, J. "Alzheimer's Disease: Past, Present and Future," *Hospital Medicine* 23(4):63-83, April 1987.

Reisberg, B., et al. "Patient and Caregiver Management," *Drug Therapy* 65-93, October 1986.

Scott, J., et al. "Families of Alzheimer's Victims," *Journal of the American Geriatric Society* 34(3):349-54, May 1986.

Thorton, J., et al. "Alzheimer's Disease Syndrome," *Journal of Psychological Nursing* 24(5): 16-22, May 1986.

Zgola, J. *Doing Things.* Baltimore: The Johns Hopkins University Press, 1987.

Cerebrovascular Accident

Cerebrovascular accident (CVA), or stroke, is a suddenly occurring condition caused by an acute vascular brain lesion typically resulting from a hemorrhage, a ruptured or leaking aneurysm, a thrombus, or an embolus. A leading cause of death among older adults, CVA commonly results in hemiplegia, numbness, aphasia, and arthralgia.

Strokes are generally defined by the area of the brain affected. For example, a left CVA indicates a lesion on the left side of the brain, which typically causes right-sided weakness or paralysis; a right CVA, a lesion on the right side of the brain, which typically causes left-sided weakness or paralysis. Because the left side of the brain controls speech, analytical thinking, and verbal and auditory memory, clients who have suffered a stroke in this area commonly have difficulty communicating. Because the right side of the brain controls spatial and visual perception, creativity, and nonverbal memory, a lesion in this area causes sensory input disturbances.

Furthermore, because the brain's right and left hemispheres each contain four separate lobes that control specific functions, a lesion in any of these areas disrupts those functions. For instance, the frontal lobe controls voluntary muscle movements and houses Broca's area, and the anterior portion of the frontal lobe controls emotional behavior and complex intellectual ability. The parietal lobe receives and transmits sensory information to the skin, muscles, joints, and tendons. These sensations enable a person to distinguish pain, heat, cold, and pressure; to determine the size, shape, and texture of objects; to identify the location and intensity of stimuli; and to locate and feel his body parts. The occipital lobe receives and interprets visual stimuli, and the temporal lobe controls hearing, taste, and smell.

Lesions affecting Wernicke's area in the temporal lobe cause fluent aphasia, a condition in which the client comprehends little and cannot follow directions or understand questions. Although the client speaks at a normal rate and has a normal inflection pattern, he may have any of the following language problems: phonemic or literal paraphasia, which involves placing sounds out of sequence or adding or substituting other sounds for the target word (for example, saying "splorkle'" instead of "fork"); semantic or verbal paraphasia, which entails substituting a related or an unrelated word for the target word (for example, saying "mother" instead of "wife"); neologism, which involves the invention of words (such as "dumbocob" or "a piece of dumbo"); nonsensical sentence construction, which involves placing real words in an order that does not make sense (for example, saying "the thing over there is to do those other things under it").

Lesions in Broca's area, which lies close to the motor speech area, cause nonfluent aphasia. With this type of aphasia, the client understands speech better than he can express it. Since the client has trouble planning all motor movements, speech is a struggle. While the rate of speech and inflection patterns remain unchanged, verbal output only includes content words and omits function words (telegraphic speech). As a result, speech is broken and choppy. Also, the client realizes that his speech does not always make sense.

ETIOLOGY
In nearly 75% of all elderly CVA clients, stroke results from a thrombus that occludes a blood vessel, preventing blood flow to an area of the brain. Another leading cause of CVA in elderly clients include an embolus that originates from a heart thrombus and lodges in a cerebral artery, causing a brain infarction. Finally, CVA may result from a cerebral hemorrhage caused by hypertension or a ruptured aneurysm. Hypertension causes bleeding into the brain tissue, whereas a ruptured aneurysm bleeds into the subarachnoid space.

Older adults with a history of hypertension, diabetes, cerebrovascular or coronary artery disease, obesity, anticoagulant medication therapy, heavy alcohol and nicotine consumption, a sedentary life-style, a history of transient ischemic attacks (TIAs), or a family history of strokes are at high risk.

HEALTH HISTORY FINDINGS
In a health history interview, the client may report or the nurse may detect many of these findings:

Thrombotic stroke
• TIAs lasting hours or months
• TIAs lasting 30 minutes
• return to normal function after a TIA

Embolic stroke
• abrupt onset of hemiplegia or impaired vision during activity
• headache on the affected side

Hemorrhagic stroke
• severe headache
• vomiting
• sudden onset of symptoms during activity
• loss of consciousness
• symptoms lasting from hours to days
• focal neurologic signs and symptoms

General findings
- diplopia
- blindness
- absent or diminished taste
- hoarseness
- difficulty swallowing
- nausea or vomiting
- fecal or urinary incontinence
- headache
- decreased attention span
- memory loss
- behavioral changes
- history of hypertension or cardiac disease
- history of diabetes mellitus, anemia, or migraine headaches
- recent head trauma
- use of anticoagulant, sedative, or diuretic medications
- history of diet high in fat and calories
- history of long-term smoking
- family history of CVA
- recent work or family crisis

PHYSICAL FINDINGS
In a physical examination, the nurse may detect many of these findings:

Neurologic
- weakness or paralysis on opposite side of brain lesion
- poor proprioception
- hemianesthesia
- neglect of affected half of body and its surrounding space
- apraxia
- dyslexia
- impaired facial sensation with pain
- ideomotor apraxia (difficulty performing complex acts)
- ataxia
- quadriplegia
- agnosia (inability to recognize familiar objects)
- decerebrate rigidity
- altered or absent oculovestibular reflexes
- aphasia (fluent, nonfluent, or global)
- dysarthria
- paraphasia
- impaired voluntary movement

Integumentary
- bruises and scrapes on the left side of the body

Respiratory
- hyperventilation or hypoventilation
- labored respirations

Cardiovascular
- decreased or increased blood pressure
- decreased pulse rate
- dysrhythmias
- carotid bruits

Gastrointestinal
- impaired gag reflex

Musculoskeletal
- decreased muscle strength

Psychological
- impulsive behavior (right CVA)
- sensory input disturbances (right CVA)
- spatial or perceptual disorientation (right CVA)
- inability to recognize familiar objects (right CVA)
- cautious and plodding movements (left CVA)
- recent memory loss (left CVA)
- decreased attention span
- loss of higher cognitive function
- fatigue
- emotional lability
- depression
- flat affect
- euphoric indifference
- personality changes
- semiconsciousness
- coma

Other
- fever
- obesity
- homonymous hemianopia
- impaired spatial perception
- inability to see objects on the affected side
- nystagmus
- paralyzed gaze
- blindness or impaired vision
- fixed and dilated pupils
- deafness
- tinnitus
- vertigo

DIAGNOSTIC STUDIES
The following studies may be performed to evaluate the client's health status:
- complete blood count (CBC)—to determine amount of blood lost from a hemorrhage
- blood glucose levels—to identify diabetes or hypoglycemia, which can lead to complications
- prothrombin time (PT) and partial thromboplastin time (PTT)—to determine a baseline value; clients with a CVA resulting from a thrombus may need anticoagulant therapy
- urinalysis—to assess renal function and identify urinary tract infection
- computed tomography (CT) scan of the head—to differentiate an infarction from a hemorrhage and to reveal the extent of bleeding and brain compression; also, to rule out other conditions, such as a brain tumor
- cerebral angiography—to reveal the site of bleeding or blockage
- skull and cervical spine X-rays—to rule out fractures, especially if the client suffered a fall with the CVA

• positron emission tomography (PET) scan—to determine alterations in cerebral blood flow, volume, and metabolism

POTENTIAL COMPLICATIONS
• immobility
• falls
• hyperthermia
• coma
• cardiopulmonary arrest

• constipation or fecal impaction
• contractures
• pneumonia
• urinary and fecal incontinence
• urinary tract infection
• urine retention
• dehydration
• depression
• dependence on caregiver, family members, or nursing staff

Nursing diagnosis: *Ineffective breathing pattern related to acute CVA*

NURSING GOAL: To maintain effective breathing patterns while preventing pulmonary complications

Signs and symptoms
• unresponsiveness
• decreased breath sounds
• hypoventilation

Interventions

1. Assess the client's airway every 15 to 60 minutes.

2. Assess the client's neurologic status, including his level of consciousness, orientation, grip, and pupillary response, every hour.

3. Auscultate the client's lungs, and suction his airway as needed.

4. Assess the client's respirations, including the rate and characteristics of respirations, skin color, and degree of restlessness. Report any abnormalities to the physician.

5. Assess the client's temperature every hour.

6. Assess the bedridden client for signs of a thrombus or pulmonary embolus, including chest pain, shortness of breath, calf pain, or redness and swelling in an extremity.

7. Provide oxygen therapy, as ordered.

8. Humidify the client's room air and supplemental oxygen.

9. Position the hemiplegic client on his affected side only briefly. Avoid positioning the client's hemiplegic arm over his abdomen.

Rationales

1. Secretions can accumulate and obstruct the client's airway or cause atelectasis or pneumonia. Respiratory infection is a primary cause of death in the client with CVA.

2. Neurologic assessments help to identify the early signs of neurologic deficits from decreased blood flow, cerebral edema, or hemorrhage.

3. Abnormal lung sounds, such as crackles or rhonchi, may indicate complications from hypoventilation.

4. Increased respiratory rate, tachypnea, ashen or cyanotic coloring, or increased restlessness signal hypoxemia. Early detection facilitates prompt treatment.

5. A CVA may alter the client's temperature regulator, causing hyperthermia.

6. Immobilization and bedrest increase the risk for thrombus formation, which can lead to an emboli.

7. The brain uses 20% of the oxygen normally available to the body. When a CVA causes cerebral ischemia, supplemental oxygen may help prevent brain tissue death.

8. Humidity helps to thin secretions and maintain airway patency.

9. Positioning the client on his affected side may cause secretions to pool, which cannot be cleared because of the client's hemiplegic condition. The weight of a paralyzed arm over the client's abdomen may reduce thoracic expansion.

10. Avoid administering tranquilizers, sedatives, and narcotics.

10. These medications may depress the client's respirations and mentation.

11. Provide a call button or another means of signaling help within easy reach of the client's unaffected arm.

11. Because of the client's risk for airway obstruction, a call system is essential.

OUTCOME CRITERIA
• The client will have a clear airway and clear lung sounds.
• The client will be free from pulmonary complications related to an acute CVA.

Nursing diagnosis: *Potential for aspiration related to neuromuscular weakness and dysphagia*

NURSING GOALS: To maintain airway patency and to prevent aspiration

Signs and symptoms
• choking
• continual coughing
• absence of gag reflex
• drooling
• increased oral secretions
• coma

Interventions

1. Assess the client's neurologic status. If the client is unconscious, elevate the foot of the bed 6″ to 9″ (15.2 to 22.9 cm) or place the bed in the Trendelenburg position, unless contraindicated; position him on the unaffected side with one pillow between his legs and one pillow against, not beneath, his head; clear his mouth of accumulated secretions; and maintain good oral hygiene.

2. Assess the client's ability to chew and swallow.

3. Have the client sit upright while he eats.

4. Provide foods that are easy to chew and swallow, such as semisolid foods. Place small bites of food on the unaffected side of the client's mouth.

5. Keep emergency suctioning equipment close to the client's bedside.

Rationales

1. Elevating the foot of the bed increases blood flow to the brain, thereby increasing perfusion. Lying on the unaffected side prevents the pooling of secretions, which can occur if the client lies on his affected side. Clearing the mouth of accumulated secretions and maintaining good oral hygiene prevents the risk of airway obstruction and aspiration pneumonia.

2. Hemiplegia and dysphagia predispose the client to aspiration of food.

3. This position facilitates swallowing.

4. The client with CVA can tolerate semisolid foods better than liquids. Placing small bites of food on the unaffected side decreases the risk of aspiration; also, the client is better able to swallow food that he can feel and manipulate with his tongue.

5. Suctioning equipment may be necessary if aspiration should occur.

OUTCOME CRITERIA
• The client will have a decreased risk for aspirating food, fluids, and secretions.
• The client will not develop pulmonary complications related to dysphagia.

Nursing diagnosis: *Impaired physical mobility related to arm weakness or paralysis*

NURSING GOALS: To increase the range of motion (ROM) in the client's arms, to minimize the effects of immobility, and to prevent associated complications

Signs and symptoms
• arm weakness or paralysis
• contractures
• painful affected shoulder
• reflex sympathetic dystrophy syndrome

Interventions

1. Keep the bedridden client positioned flat and properly aligned, provided he has no signs of increased intracranial pressure.

2. Assess the client's affected arm for edema.

3. When obtaining blood specimens or inserting I.V. needles, be careful to use only the client's unaffected side.

4. Elevate the client's edematous affected arm, and measure its circumference daily. Document and report the findings.

5. Support the client's affected arm in a neutral position while he is in bed, and elevate it periodically.

6. Apply resting splints to the client's wrist and fingers.

7. Use a draw sheet to move or lift the client who is confined to bed.

8. Maintain a positioning schedule at the client's bedside.

9. Support the client's arm with a sling or pillow whenever he is out of bed.

10. Periodically place the client's shoulder in an abducted position while he is supine. Avoid using the sling continuously while the client is confined to bed.

11. Provide passive ROM exercises to all of the client's affected joints at least four times a day, beginning 2 days after the CVA. Repeat each exercise three to five times per extremity during the early flaccid stage, and increase the number of repetitions during the spastic stage.

12. Avoid overstretching the client's weakened muscles during ROM exercises or through such activites as arm dangling.

13. Assist the client with transfers, such as from the bed to a chair, by placing your arms under the client's arms and around his trunk. Avoid pulling the client's arms during the transfers.

Rationales

1. Maintaining proper body alignment prevents contractures and deformities. Nurses should keep in mind that the client with increased intracranial pressure should be positioned with the head of the bed elevated to minimize cerebral edema and pressure.

2. Edema and tissue damage result from loss of muscle contractions and decreased venous return.

3. Inserting needles into the client's affected side may further damage tissue or contribute to shoulder-hand syndrome.

4. Elevation prevents tissue damage by reducing edema. Measuring the arm's circumference provides objective data about any improvement or worsening of the condition.

5. A neutral position with periodic elevation prevents contractures and minimizes edema.

6. Splints maintain hand function.

7. Using a draw sheet prevents twisting or injuring the client's shoulder.

8. This record documents the amount of time that the client remains in any one position. The client and his family can help determine the positioning schedule and assist with turning.

9. The force of gravity on paralyzed shoulder muscles can sublux the joint. A sling will keep the humerus in the glenoid space, preventing debilitating pain.

10. A sling abducts and internally rotates the shoulder. The client needs balance between abduction and adduction.

11. Exercise maintains muscle tone, decreases the risk of contractures, and increases the development of new motor pathways to the brain. The number of repetitions is the key to developing new neuronal connectors.

12. Overstretching muscles impedes recovery and may cause injury or pain.

13. Proper transfer maneuvers prevent the risk of injury from traction or twisting of the client's shoulder.

14. Apply heat packs or administer nonsteroidal anti-inflammatory medications, as ordered, before passive ROM exercises.

14. Heat and anti-inflammatory medications reduce pain, especially during exercise.

15. Evaluate the effectiveness of biofeedback on the client's spastic arm.

15. Biofeedback strengthens weak muscles and may relieve spasticity in muscles over which the client has some voluntary control.

16. Consult a physical therapist about planning a rehabilitation schedule with the client and the client's family.

16. A collaborative schedule helps the client set goals, provides a sense of control, and measures progress.

17. Consult an occupational therapist about the client's need for a homemaker or adaptive equipment.

17. An interdisciplinary approach to rehabilitation ensures maximal functioning.

OUTCOME CRITERIA
- The client will be free from arm, shoulder, and hand contractures.
- The client will be free from shoulder pain.
- The client will be free from edema in his affected arm.

Nursing diagnosis: *Impaired physical mobility related to leg weakness or paralysis*

NURSING GOAL: To prevent thrombophlebitis, deformities, and physical deterioration

Signs and symptoms
- weakness or paralysis
- inability to ambulate

Interventions

1. Immobilize the client's affected leg with rolled sheets or sandbags while he is confined to bed.

2. Attach a footboard to the client's bed, or place high-top sneakers on the client's feet. Assess the soles of the feet for skin breakdown, and provide passive ROM exercises.

3. Teach the bedridden client to move by rolling. Have him clasp his hands together and reach upward, bend his knees, turn his head in the direction of the turn, then allow his knees to follow the turn to complete the rolling movement.

4. Have the bedridden client perform gluteal-setting and thigh-strengthening exercises five times daily. To perform the exercises, have the client contract his buttocks for a count of five, then relax the buttocks for count of five. Have him repeat the exercise while pushing his inner thighs into the bed.

5. Avoid applying direct pressure to the client's popliteal area while he is confined to bed.

6. Teach the client to perform quadriceps-setting exercises while sitting in bed by contracting the muscles of his unaffected thigh and raising his heel. Assist the client with the exercises on the affected leg.

Rationales

1. Immobilizing the affected leg prevents outward rotation and joint impairment.

2. These measures help prevent foot drop.

3. Rolling is an excellent activity to develop normal bilateral segmental movement and to develop the trunk rotation required for balance.

4. Gluteal-setting exercises strengthen the muscles required to ambulate; thigh-strengthening exercises reduce the risk of developing knee contractures.

5. Pressure on the popliteal area decreases venous return and increases flexion.

6. These exercises strengthen the muscles necessary for ambulation.

7. Provide antiembolism stockings, as ordered.

7. Antiembolism stockings promote venous return and decrease the risk of thrombus formation caused by immobility.

8. Assess the client's ability to balance before allowing ambulation.

8. Assessing the client's balance helps prevent injury from a fall.

9. Apply a short-leg brace, as ordered.

9. A brace corrects foot drop, provides correct foot placement on the heel strike, and stabilizes the knee.

10. Teach the client to lead with his unaffected side when transferring from the bed to a chair.

10. Effective transfer technique reduces the client's risk of falling.

11. Prevent prolonged plantar flexion when the client is out of bed.

11. Overstretching weakened muscles impedes recovery and may increase pain once the client begins to ambulate.

12. Keep the bedridden client's affected hip in a neutral position by placing pillows, rolled towels, or sandbags against the client's lateral thigh and calf.

12. This technique prevents external rotation of the client's leg and foot or dislocation of the hip.

13. When medically appropriate, help the client to walk, first using parallel bars, then progressing to a mobile walking aid.

13. Rapid ambulation prevents the client from becoming dependent on fixed support and assists with muscle conditioning.

14. Encourage the use of a four-legged hemwalker or quad-cane if the hand of the client's affected arm is functional.

14. These devices provide better balance and stability than a two-handed walker.

15. Evaluate the possibility of using biofeedback if the client has weak ankle dorsiflexion.

15. Biofeedback may strengthen muscles so that an orthosis is unnecessary.

16. Initiate stair climbing once the client can ambulate on a level surface.

16. The client should be able to maintain his balance on stairs once he can walk on a level surface.

17. Instruct the client to grip handrails with his unaffected hand when going down stairs.

17. Grasping with the unaffected hand decreases the risk of falls.

18. Teach client to lead with his unaffected foot when climbing up stairs and to lead with his affected foot when going down stairs.

18. This method provides better balance and decreases the client's risk of falling.

OUTCOME CRITERION
• The client will achieve maximum independence while remaining free from injury.

Nursing diagnosis: *Pain related to shoulder-hand syndrome*

NURSING GOALS: To promote comfort and to decrease pain

Signs and symptoms
• shoulder pain
• hand swelling from vasomotor instability
• hand coolness
• wrist and finger pain with passive ROM exercise
• reflex sympathetic dystrophy syndrome
• tissue atrophy
• contractures
• osteoporosis

Interventions

1. Assess the client's pain, noting its location, duration, and severity.

2. Initiate an active physical therapy program, including ROM exercises to the client's wrist and fingers.

3. Teach the client to exercise his affected side by using his unaffected hand.

4. Initiate more passive exercises if severe shoulder pain and arm paralysis persist.

5. Administer pain medications as ordered, especially before performing passive ROM exercises.

6. Administer oral corticosteroids, as ordered.

Rationales

1. Such assessment helps the nurse to determine the degree of pain and any associated symptoms.

2. Exercise reduces edema and prevents contractures.

3. This technique helps the client to exercise independently.

4. In this situation, the nurse's goal is to help the client maintain bathing and dressing abilities, rather than pursuing aggressive therapy for full ROM recovery. Passive ROM exercises will help the client to perform activities of daily living.

5. Reducing the client's pain allows him to exercise more effectively.

6. Corticosteroids help reduce tissue swelling.

OUTCOME CRITERIA
- The client will have no shoulder pain.
- The client will have no edema in his hand and arm.

Nursing diagnosis: *Impaired verbal communication related to aphasia and dysarthria from right-sided CVA*

NURSING GOALS: To minimize communication deficits and to establish some form of verbal or nonverbal communication

Signs and symptoms
- dysarthria
- aphasia
- isolation
- depression
- sensory deprivation

Interventions

1. Assess the client's communication abilities daily by naming familiar objects around the room and asking the client to point to them, by testing his ability to follow oral commands, and by asking the client to repeat phrases.

2. Ensure consistency in care by maintaining a routine daily schedule and providing the same caregiver.

3. Protect the client from excessive auditory and visual stimulation, such as from noisy sitting areas, televisions, and radios.

Rationales

1. Daily assessments of the client's communication skills provide a baseline for planning daily care and rehabilitation.

2. Consistency decreases the client's uncertainty and confusion and promotes stability.

3. This decreases the risk of sensory overload and allows the client to focus attention on the task at hand.

4. Establish effective verbal communication through the following measures: capture the client's attention before giving him a message; repeat statements if the client appears not to have understood; avoid the use of childlike speech; ask questions during a conversation; allow time for communication; give only one command at a time, increasing the number of commands as appropriate; teach the caregiver to initially ask yes-no questions, then progress to open-ended questions; suggest the use of songs to communicate, if appropriate; accept the client's speech efforts; and use simple gestures while speaking.

4. Capturing the client's attention enhances communication. Repeating a statement ensures that the client received the message. Avoiding childlike speech prevents feelings of inferiority that can contribute to the client's sense of helplessness. Asking questions ensures that the client follows the conversation as the topic changes. Giving only one command at a time breaks down communication into its simplest form for easy comprehension. Asking simple questions, then progressing to more difficult ones, increases the opportunities for the client to speak. Suggesting songs may be appropriate for some clients, as those with aphasia sometimes can communicate better that way. Accepting the client's speech by not correcting his words or sentences should enhance his desire to communicate. Using simple gestures enhances speech and facilitates communication.

5. Establish nonverbal communication by observing the client and interpreting his gestures; talking to the client even if he does not respond; having the client write messages, provided he does not have alexia; and using a communication board with pictures.

5. The CVA client may effectively communicate through gestures. Talking to the client, even if he does not respond, encourages speech. Written messages may be a more effective form of communication for a client who can write better than he can verbalize. However, nurses should keep in mind that a client with a comprehensible aphasia or fluent aphasia may also write incomprehensible messages. A communication board decreases the amount of verbalization needed to communicate.

6. Use simple words, common phrases, and short sentences when giving the client instructions.

6. Complex explanations may cause neurosensory overload and unnecessary frustration.

7. Reassure the client, and redirect his attention to another task or topic when he swears, cries, or has an emotional outburst.

7. The client who has suffered a CVA typically exhibits excessive or inappropriate emotions because of the brain injury. These clients are often unable to control their emotional responses, and an excessive reaction by the family caregivers may add to the client's distress.

8. Nonverbally praise the client for completed tasks, such as by patting him on the back.

8. The client who has suffered a CVA usually can understand nonverbal praise and encouragement.

9. Provide diversional activities when the client becomes extremely frustrated.

9. Diversion decreases the client's frustration.

10. Avoid referring to the client's past superior abilities.

10. Referring to past abilities will only depress the client and slow progress.

11. Have the client plan a task by dividing it into a specific number of steps.

11. By focusing on small, manageable goals, the number of the client's successes will increase.

12. Encourage the client's family to maintain telephone contact.

12. Even if the client cannot respond, a telephone call allows him to maintain contact with the outside world.

13. Refer the client with significant speech deficits to a speech therapist for a comprehensive evaluation and rehabilitation.

13. A speech therapist can identify and treat specific speech problems.

OUTCOME CRITERIA
• The client will demonstrate an increased ability to understand and express himself.
• The client will meet personal and environmental communication needs.

Nursing diagnosis: *Potential for impaired skin integrity related to prolonged immobility*

NURSING GOALS: To prevent skin breakdown and pressure sore formation

Signs and symptoms
• pressure sores
• skin tears
• red, excoriated skin over bony prominences

Interventions	Rationales
1. Assess the client's skin every 8 hours, and report any red or broken skin areas immediately.	1. An elderly client is apt to have delicate skin, particularly if he is debilitated. Prompt intervention helps prevent serious skin problems.
2. Assess the client's occiput, sacrum, greater trochanter, and malleoli for redness, inflammation, or skin tears.	2. These sites are especially prone to skin breakdown.
3. Assess the client for decreased sensation on his affected side.	3. Decreased or absent sensation places the client at greater risk for skin breakdown.
4. Keep all bedding materials clean and dry.	4. Moisture promotes bacterial growth and increases the risk of skin breakdown.
5. Provide special mattresses or foam or sheepskin padding, as necessary.	5. Special mattresses and padding redistribute pressure to prevent skin breakdown.
6. Use a drawsheet to turn the client in bed.	6. Using a drawsheet reduces the risk of shearing the client's skin and prevents twisting the client's affected shoulder, which can cause severe pain.
7. Allow the client to lie on his affected side for only 20 to 30 minutes at a time.	7. Because of decreased tissue perfusion, the skin on the client's affected side is at greater risk for tissue breakdown.
8. Place the client in a prone position for at least 15 minutes every day.	8. A prone position promotes hyperextension, which is necessary for walking, and helps prevent knee and hip flexion contractures.
9. Regularly elevate the client's arm and leg on his affected side.	9. Paralysis decreases or eliminates muscle pumping and slows venous return, which causes edema. Elevating the affected extremities increases venous return and decreases edema.
10. Protect the client's skin from the effects of a hypothermia blanket used during the acute stage of CVA by applying a sheet or bath blanket over the hypothermia blanket, next to the client's skin, and by liberally applying mineral oil to the exposed skin.	10. These measures protect the client's skin and prevent the risk of breakdown.

OUTCOME CRITERION
• The client will maintain intact skin.

Nursing diagnosis: *Altered patterns of urinary elimination related to decreased immobility and incontinence*

NURSING GOALS: To develop and implement a bladder retraining program, to avoid using an indwelling catheter, and to involve the caregiver in the retraining program

Signs and symptoms
• frequent incontinence
• indwelling catheter use

Interventions

1. Assess the client's voiding pattern by using a voiding diary or bladder record.

2. Question the client and caregiver about the client's voiding pattern and number of incontinence episodes before the CVA.

3. Obtain a specimen for a urinalysis and urine culture if the client complains of urinary frequency, dysuria, or hematuria.

4. Prompt the client to void every 2 hours by assisting him to the bathroom or bedside commode or by offering him a bedpan or urinal.

5. Teach the client to use deep-breathing and relaxation techniques to control his urge to void.

6. Teach the client pelvic muscle-strengthening (Kegel) exercises.

7. Avoid the use of an indwelling catheter to treat incontinence.

8. Involve the client's family in all incontinence teaching sessions and explain the rationales for the interventions.

9. Recommend that the client use reusable diapers or bed pads if enuresis occurs.

Rationales

1. A bladder record follows the client's response to treatment and can also identify symptoms of incontinence.

2. Knowing the client's previous voiding pattern establishes a baseline and helps the nurse to determine the degree of change brought on by the CVA. Preexisting incontinence may be attributed to some cause other than the CVA.

3. A urinalysis and culture can rule out a urinary tract infection and help identify bladder retention.

4. Such prompts encourage the client to void habitually, thereby encouraging him to use the toilet independently.

5. Using these techniques should help the client to progressively lengthen the time between voidings, thereby helping him to remain continent.

6. These exercises strengthen the pelvic muscle, which increases outlet resistance around the urethra, thereby helping the client to remain continent.

7. Catheters cause several complications that result in increased morbidity and mortality. Also, indwelling catheters diminish bladder capacity, which decreases the client's chance for successful bladder retraining.

8. Family members need to know that incontinence may not be permanent and that they can help the client become become independently continent.

9. Absorbent pads and diapers help manage incontinence. Reusable products are less expensive than disposable ones.

OUTCOME CRITERIA
• The client will develop a normal voiding pattern, voiding every 3 to 4 hours while awake, within 2 months.
• The caregiver will understand appropriate interventions and will support them.
• The client will not need an indwelling catheter to treat his incontinence.

Nursing diagnosis: *Tactile and auditory sensory-perceptual alteration related to homonymous hemianopia, impaired proprioception, and hearing loss*

NURSING GOALS: To minimize the effects of the client's perception deficits and to help the client maintain and accentuate unaffected sensory functions

Signs and symptoms
- aphasia
- deafness
- homonymous hemianopia
- isolation
- confusion
- withdrawal

Interventions

1. Assess the client for deficits involving hearing, vision, speech, or touch.

2. Position the client so that his unaffected side is closest to the room entrance. Provide music, a television, or a radio, as appropriate.

3. Provide visual stimulation, such as posters, near the area where the client exercises.

4. Decorate the client's environment in bright colors.

5. Avoid exposing the client to sensory overload, such as intercom noises, or performing one-on-one therapy in an area with background noise.

6. Touch and exercise the client's unaffected side.

7. Turn the client's head, and perform passive ROM exercises on his unaffected side.

8. About 1 week after the client's CVA, begin instructing him to turn his head to the unaffected side and to scan with his eyes.

9. Initially approach the client only from his right side. Gradually begin approaching him from the left side, and encourage the client to turn that way. Place prominent visual anchors, such as a picture of the client's spouse, to the extreme left.

10. Teach the client to touch the walls and other boundaries.

11. If the client has diplopia, keep one of his eyes patched, alternating the eye every 4 hours.

12. Rearrange the client's room so that objects are in the client's direct line of vision.

13. Draw the client's attention to visual reference points in the room, such as doorways and furniture.

Rationales

1. Ischemia or infarction can impair sensory perception on the client's affected side.

2. Positioning the client in this way and providing auditory stimulation increases sensory input.

3. These items help capture the client's attention and help him to focus on the task at hand.

4. Bright colors appropriately stimulate the client's senses, especially since elderly clients tend to have reduced sensation.

5. The client may withdraw if the environment is too overwhelming.

6. These nonverbal activities establish contact, decrease anxiety, and increase the client's awareness of his affected side.

7. These activities help establish new neuromuscular pathways to the uninjured portions of the client's brain.

8. This increases the client's awareness of the space on his unaffected side. Waiting 1 week allows the nurse to objectively evaluate the residual effects of the CVA.

9. These actions increase the client's awareness of his left visual field.

10. Touching physical boundaries helps the client compensate for spatial perception deficits.

11. Patching decreases diplopia.

12. The client cannot see objects on his affected side.

13. Drawing attention to reference points helps to increase spatial awareness when the client suffers unilateral neglect.

OUTCOME CRITERIA
- The client will interpret his environment appropriately.
- The client will develop necessary skills to compensate for sensory deficits.

Nursing diagnosis: *Eating, bathing, dressing, and toileting self-care deficit, related to right-sided CVA*

NURSING GOALS: To ensure a safe environment for performing self-care and to assist client with self-care activities

Signs and symptoms
• inability to perform activities of daily living (ADLs)
• spatial-perceptual deficits
• inability to recognize potentially dangerous situations
• one-sided vision (inability to see things on the affected side)

Interventions

1. Assess the client's ability to perform ADLs, such as eating, dressing, toileting, and bathing, independently.

2. Assess the client's hearing by using a tuning fork or ticking watch or by whispering.

3. Provide adequate lighting when the client attempts to eat, dress, or perform personal hygiene.

4. Keep the client's environment free from clutter while he is dressing, bathing, feeding, or toileting.

5. Teach the client how to perform ADLs, limiting the sessions to 10 to 15 minutes.

6. Praise the client for all completed tasks, no matter how small.

7. Place maps or colored dots along the client's regularly travelled pathway, including the way to the bathroom, kitchen, dining area, and the client's room.

8. Instruct the client to dress in front of a full-length mirror.

9. Teach the client to button his clothes from bottom to top.

10. Approach the client initially from his right side, and remember to place all food and objects to his right.

11. Teach the client to move slowly, especially when removing objects from the table.

12. Have the client practice picking up and manipulating small objects, such as coins, combs, and eating utensils.

13. Mark the client's clothing and shoes to indicate the right or left side. Place landmark objects consistently on the same side of the client's body. For example, always place the client's watch on his right wrist.

Rationales

1. Such assessment serves as a baseline of the client's capabilities. Spatial-perceptual deficits may be difficult to recognize.

2. The client may have presbycusis, a common age-related condition, as well as other hearing deficits resulting from his CVA.

3. Adequate lighting enhances the client's vision.

4. Removing clutter decreases the risk of injury.

5. The client has a decreased attention span and cannot benefit from longer teaching sessions.

6. Praise decreases discouragement. The client with right-sided CVA can understand the spoken word.

7. These measures help to orient the client and reduce his difficulty with spatial relationships.

8. The client with unilateral neglect may fail to attend to his left side. A mirror will help the client see his left side.

9. This is typically the easiest method of buttoning for a client with apraxia.

10. The client with a visual field cut can only see objects to his right.

11. Moving slowly compensates for poor proprioception.

12. Picking up small objects enhances proprioception.

13. These measure help the client distinguish left from right.

OUTCOME CRITERIA
• The client will be free from complications.
• The client will compensate for physical and intellectual losses.

Nursing diagnosis: *Knowledge deficit related to medication use, rehabilitation, and long-term care for CVA*

NURSING GOALS: To teach the client and the client's family about necessary medications and rehabilitation, to decrease the client's anxiety, and to ease the caregiver's fears and concerns about caring for the client

Signs and symptoms
• anxiety and frustration
• caregiver's verbalization of feelings of being overwhelmed
• multiple questions from the client and the client's family about the recovery process

Interventions

1. Reassure the client and the client's family that functional recovery is possible with patience and consistent rehabilitation.

2. Teach the client and the client's family about the proper use of prescribed medications, such as anticoagulants (heparin and warfarin sodium), antiplatelet aggregation agents (aspirin and dipyridamole), and antihypertensives.

3. Provide written instructions to the client and caregiver about anticoagulant therapy, including the usual dosage, schedule, and action of the medication; the need for frequent laboratory tests (including PTT and PT) to determine the need for dosage adjustments; the importance of observing for signs of bleeding (such as melena, petechiae, easy bruising, hematuria, black stools, hemoptysis, and epistaxis) and reporting them immediately; the need to avoid aspirin and other over-the-counter medications; the need to protect the client from falls or other injury; and the importance of notifying all of the client's other health care providers, including his dentist, about the client's anticoagulant therapy.

4. Teach the client the importance adjusting his lifestyle to minimize the risk of another CVA. Such changes may include controlling weight, stopping smoking, modifying dietary intake, controlling blood pressure, and reducing stress.

Rationales

1. Maintaining hope is essential for an optimal recovery. Family support and understanding can help boost the client's morale.

2. Anticoagulants inhibit the progression of CVA and may reduce the incidence of recurring thromboembolic events. Heparin inactivates thrombin to prevent fibrin clot formation; warfarin interferes with vitamin K production, thereby decreasing the synthesis of several clotting factors. Antiplatelet aggregation agents inhibit platelet aggregation and embolus formation. Many clients who have had a CVA have preexisting hypertension and therefore require antihypertensive medication.

3. Because anticoagulants can cause life-threatening bleeding, the client and the client's caregiver must be made aware of the importance of strictly adhering to the regimen, the need for follow-up laboratory testing, and the need to inform other health care professionals about the client's condition and medication use.

4. These factors contribute to the risk for CVAs.

OUTCOME CRITERIA
• The client will alter his life-style, as necessary, to decrease the risk for another CVA.
• The client and his caregiver will list the dosage and potential side effects of each of the client's medications.

NURSING ACTIONS IN VARIOUS SETTINGS

Nursing actions for a client with CVA depend on the setting in which care is provided. This section identifies which actions are appropriate in all settings and which pertain to acute care, extended care, or home care situations.

All settings

• Reassure the client and the client's family that functional recovery is possible with patience and consistent rehabilitation.
• Explain to the client's family that emotional lability commonly occurs but that it should decrease over time.
• Discuss the impact of the client's illness and the expected prognosis with the client and caregiver.
• Encourage the client's family to communicate regularly with the client.
• Determine the client's functional ability level before the CVA.
• Assess the client's capacity to learn new material.
• Reassess the client's bowel and bladder continence throughout his recovery.
• Maintain a consistent interdisciplinary approach to the client's rehabilitation.

Acute care

• Provide primary care nursing.
• Use an interpreter to communicate with non-English-speaking clients.
• Provide adaptive aids whenever possible.

Extended care

• Identify family and community resources for non-English-speaking clients.
• Provide adaptive aids whenever possible.
• Provide pet therapy, if appropriate.
• Provide daily diversional activities.
• Assess the client's rehabilitation potential.
• Assess the client's social situation and his options for returning to the community.
• Assess the client's ability to cooperate with the rehabilitation team.
• Determine the client's age, and identify specific health problems that may interfere with rehabilitation efforts.

Home care

• Advise the client's family to reorganize the client's home to aid his memory and prevent injury.
• Evaluate the client's need for continued physical and occupational therapies.
• Identify appropriate support groups in the client's community.
• Refer the client to Meals On Wheels if he lives alone and cannot prepare his own meals.
• Help the client contact volunteer organizations that can adapt his home to his disabilities.

SELECTED REFERENCES

Andres, R., et al. *Principles of Geriatric Medicine.* New York: McGraw-Hill Book Co., 1985.

Dornbrand, L., ed. *Manual of Clinical Problems in Adult Ambulatory Care.* Boston: Little, Brown & Co., 1985.

Gary, R., et al. "Stroke: How to Start the Long Road Back," *RN* 49(6):49-55, June 1986.

Hahn, K. "Left Versus Right: What a Difference a Side Makes in Stroke," *Nursing 87* 17(9):44-47, September 1987.

Loustau, A., and Lee, K. "Dealing with the Dangers of Dysphagia," *Nursing 85* 15(2):47-50, February 1985.

Passarella, P., and Lewis, N. "Nursing Application of Bobath Principles in Stroke Care," *Journal of Neuroscience Nursing* 19(2):106-09, April 1987.

Reedy, D.F. "The Client with Aphasia: The Nurse's Assessment of Language Abilities," *Topics in Clinical Nursing* 8(1):67-73, April 1986.

Roth, E.J. "The Elderly Stroke Patient: Principles and Practices of Rehabilitation Management," *Topics in Geriatric Rehabilitation* 3(4):27-61, July 1988.

Whitney, F.W. "Relationship of Laterality of Stroke to Emotional and Functional Outcome," *Journal of Neuroscience Nursing* 19(3):158-64, June 1987.

Parkinson's Disease

Parkinson's disease, a degenerative neurologic disorder of the brain's basal ganglia, is characterized by a clinical syndrome (parkinsonism) marked by tremors, rigidity, bradykinesia, postural instability, and gait abnormalities. The disease progresses over time, the exact rate varying with each client.

The incidence of Parkinson's disease rises sharply in adults over age 55, affecting about 5% of all whites over age 70. The disease, which is less prevalent among blacks and Orientals, affects men and women equally.

Tremors, one of the hallmark signs of parkinsonism, are usually observed when the client's hands are resting or outstretched but not moving. These movements, which are usually not disabling, sometimes affect the legs, head, and lips or chin.

Rigidity, another classic sign, refers to increased resistance to passive stretching. Such rigidity is most evident when the client actively moves one arm or leg while passively moving the other. In many clients, the rigidity affects only one side of the body and may be designated as cogwheel (muscle rigidity that abates in a series of jerks), lead-pipe (diffuse muscle rigidity), or clasp-knife (increased muscle resistance that suddenly gives way with further pressure) in nature.

Bradykinesia, characterized by slow, deliberate movements, or akinesia, characterized by a lack of spontaneous movments, are two of the more disabling features of parkinsonism. Typically, these signs manifest through diminished expressive facial movements and hand gestures.

Postural instability usually occurs late in the disease. The client typically assumes the characteristic posture of a bowed head, bent trunk, and drooping shoulders, with arms flexed at the elbow and hands positioned in front of the body. Because the client's center of gravity is displaced forward, he has a tendency to fall.

Gait abnormalities, including shuffling (festination) and short-stepping, are typical of clients with parkinsonism. Clients often have difficulty initiating the first step, and, once they do initiate walking, they tend to walk uncontrollably faster and faster (propulsion).

Other changes can occur in those with Parkinson's disease. For example, the client's speech may change because of bradykinesia and rigidity of the tongue and other muscles. Handwriting may become progressively smaller over the course of a single line. Orthostatic hypotension, impotence, and constipation may occur as a result of autonomic insufficiency.

Mental changes, including dementia, occur in about 20% of clients with Parkinson's disease; however, the client's slow responses may give the impression of dementia even when the client is cognitively normal. Some researchers feel that dementia is part of the natural progress of Parkinson's disease. Clients who exhibit mental status changes require evaluation to rule out a treatable cause. The evaluation should include temporarily stopping anti-parkinsonian medications, as they can cause mental status changes.

ETIOLOGY

Although the exact cause of true Parkinson's disease is unknown, studies indicate that the dopamine-containing cells of the substantia nigra degenerate with the disease, and the resultant imbalance in neurotransmitter activity between dopamine and acetylcholine cause parkinsonian symptoms. Recent studies suggest that dopamine deficiencies in other areas of the brain, as well as abnormalities of other neurotransmitters, such as norepinephrine and serotonin, may also contribute to the cause.

Parkinsonian symptoms may also occur with other syndromes, such as striatonigral degeneration, progressive supranuclear palsy, and Shy-Drager's syndrome. Parkinson's disease may even result from the use of certain drugs, including neuroleptic (antipsychotic) drugs, especially haloperidol; antihypertensives, such as reserpine, metyrosine, and methyldopa; antiemetics, such as prochlorperazine and trimethobenzamide hydrochloride; and gastric motility regulators, such as metoclopramide hydrochloride. It also can result from carbon monoxide poisoning.

HEALTH HISTORY FINDINGS

In a health history interview, the client may report or the nurse may detect many of these findings:
• tremors in one arm at rest that improve with purposeful movement
• mild rigidity on one side, interrupted in a cogwheel fashion
• akinesia of the arm
• mild, generalized slowness (bradykinesia)
• postural abnormalities
• use of neuroleptic medications or antiemetics
• difficulty performing fine-motor activities
• altered social activity
• inappropriate skin flushing
• seborrhea
• dysphagia
• constipation
• anorexia
• urinary incontinence
• urinary frequency and urgency
• decreased libido
• impotence
• generalized slowing of movements
• muscle cramps or spasms, especially in the feet
• arm, shoulder, neck, and lower back pain

- instability
- paresthesias, numbness, or coldness
- behavioral changes
- occupational exposure to toxins
- history of lethargic encephalitis, Alzheimer's disease, or Creutzfeldt-Jakob disease
- family history of Parkinson's disease
- history of sleep disturbances
- history of falls
- history of drug abuse

PHYSICAL FINDINGS

In a physical examination, the nurse may detect many of these findings:

Neurologic
- shuffling gait
- festinating gait (retropulsion)
- loss of postural reflexes
- Myerson's sign (positive glabellar reflex)
- palmomental reflex

Integumentary
- eczematous eruptions
- anhidrosis (lack of perspiration)

Cardiovascular
- orthostatic hypotension

Gastrointestinal
- abdominal distention
- excess salivation (sialorrhea)

Musculoskeletal
- loss of arm swing while walking
- micrographia (progressively smaller script when writing)

- difficulty initiating first step
- difficulty getting out of chair
- freezing phenomenon (occasional inability to move)
- lack of facial expression (masklike facies)
- propulsive walking

Psychological
- slow thinking (bradyphrenia)
- depression

Other
- weakness and fatigue
- decreased blinking
- inaudible or mumbled speech
- low, monotonous voice
- gradually accelerated speech
- uncontrolled repetition of syllables

DIAGNOSTIC STUDIES

Diagnostic studies are not helpful in diagnosing or evaluating Parkinson's disease. Diagnosis is made through a detailed history and physical examination.

POTENTIAL COMPLICATIONS
- ineffective airway clearance
- traumatic injury
- infection
- impaired swallowing
- constipation
- immobility
- self-care deficits
- dementia
- impaired speech
- ineffective coping by client and family

Nursing diagnosis: *Ineffective airway clearance related to rigidity of truncal muscles and aspiration pneumonia*

NURSING GOAL: To provide optimal ventilation

Signs and symptoms
- history of frequent upper respiratory infections and choking episodes
- decreased breath sounds
- dyspnea
- tachypnea
- fever
- change in mental status (such as confusion or disorientation)

Interventions

1. Assess the client's respiratory rate and effort, and auscultate his breath sounds.

2. Encourage the client to cough deeply whenever he is sedentary.

Rationales

1. Intercostal muscle rigidity can restrict chest wall expansion.

2. Coughing promotes airway clearance and counteracts hypokinesia and rigid respiratory muscles.

3. Consult a physical therapist for exercises to improve the client's eating and chewing.

3. Teaching the client to improve his digestion of saliva, food, and fluids decreases the risk of aspiration pneumonia.

4. Instruct the client to sleep with his head turned to the side.

4. This position helps prevent aspiration.

OUTCOME CRITERIA
• The client will cough effectively.
• The client will have normal breath sounds and unlabored respirations.

Nursing diagnosis: *Impaired swallowing related to delayed swallowing time and dysphagia*

NURSING GOAL: To promote effective swallowing and management of oral secretions

Signs and symptoms
• slow eating
• drooling
• choking
• red or excoriated skin around mouth
• inadequate secretion clearance
• diminished gag reflex
• weight loss

Interventions

1. Assess the client during meals for chewing and swallowing difficulties.

2. Massage the client's face and neck muscles before meals.

3. Teach the client to manage and minimize saliva by making a conscious effort to swallow regularly, eating sour candy, and keeping his head upright so that saliva will collect in the back of his throat.

4. Serve soft rather than pureed or solid food.

5. Instruct the client to take small bites and to chew thoroughly.

6. Teach the client to consciously move his tongue back and up before swallowing.

7. Avoid conversing with the client while he is eating.

8. Consider consulting a speech therapist.

Rationales

1. Pharyngeal and facial muscle rigidity causes difficulties with chewing and swallowing.

2. Muscles used for swallowing tend to become rigid, making swallowing difficult. Massaging these muscles before meals helps to relax them, thereby facilitating swallowing.

3. Consciously swallowing saliva prevents drooling; a sour taste stimulates swallowing; and a collection of saliva in the back of the throat facilitates automatic swallowing.

4. Soft foods are typically easier to swallow.

5. Small food boluses are easier to swallow than large ones.

6. An awareness of necessary tongue movement facilitates swallowing.

7. Talking during eating can precipitate choking, drooling, or aspiration.

8. Therapy for dysphagia can improve swallowing.

OUTCOME CRITERIA
• The client will maintain an adequate nutritional intake.
• The client will eat without difficulty.

Nursing diagnosis: *Impaired verbal communication, related to problems with pronunciation and enunciation, the inability to move facial muscles, and the inability to write*

NURSING GOALS: To detect communication deficits and to help the client effectively communicate his wants and needs

Signs and symptoms
• slurred speech with omitted word endings
• social withdrawal
• low voice volume
• fading voice
• monotone voice
• rapid speech
• uncontrolled repetition of sounds or words
• poor articulation
• variations in voice quality (such as breathy, tremulous, hoarse, strident, or high-pitched)
• inability to move facial muscles

Interventions

1. Assess the client's speaking ability by engaging him in conversation and his writing ability by asking him to write his name, short phrases, and then sentences.

2. Encourage the client to practice facial muscle exercises, such as making faces in front of a mirror; grimacing, smiling, or frowning; and extending his tongue to touch his chin, nose, and cheeks.

3. Instruct the client to face the listener when speaking, to speak slowly and distinctly, and to speak loudly as if the listener is hard of hearing.

4. Teach the client to pronunciate by taking a breath before starting to speak, to pause every few words or between words, and by forcing his tongue, lips, and jaw to work hard as he speaks.

5. Suggest that the client finish the final consonant of a word before starting the next word.

6. Recommend that the client speak in short, concise phrases or sentences.

7. Encourage the client to take his time when speaking.

8. Recommend that the client who cannot speak loudly use a hand-held, electronic larynx.

9. Suggest that the client with unintelligible speech use gestures and cues, such as pointing to objects or using a communication board.

10. Provide the client who is unable to write with a typewriter.

11. Consider consulting a speech therapist if the client cannot develop a way to communicate.

Rationales

1. Parkinson's disease results in a low, monotonous voice and inaudible or mumbled speech. Handwriting typically grows progressively smaller until it becomes illegible.

2. Such exercises help to improve diminished expressive facial movement, which can lead to a fixed, mask-like stare with reduced blinking.

3. Voice volume may decline to the point of inaudibility, and rigid vocal chords and associated structures cause hypophonia and difficult articulation. These measures should help improve communication.

4. The client with Parkinson's disease has difficulty coordinating the expiration of breath with articulation.

5. Precise word endings help differentiate word meanings.

6. The client will have difficulty making a long, involved sentence understandable.

7. Bradykinesia delays reaction time during speech, and stress and increased effort may slow movement further.

8. This device intensifies sound when speech volume is inadequate.

9. Visual, auditory, and proprioceptive cues facilitate communication.

10. Typing improves fine motor function and allows the client to communicate.

11. A speech therapist can reinforce previous teaching and suggest other ways to facilitate communication.

OUTCOME CRITERION
• The client will speak intelligibly or will develop an alternative method of communication.

Nursing diagnosis: *Potential for injury related to propulsive and retropulsive gaits, rigidity, akinesia, frequent falls, and orthostatic hypotension*

NURSING GOALS: To ensure the client's safety, to prevent traumatic injury, and to help the client to ambulate

Signs and symptoms
• history of frequent falls or loss of balance
• gait disturbance
• loss of arm swing
• loss of postural reflexes
• evidence of recent injuries
• stooped body posture

Interventions

1. Assess the client for orthostatic hypotension.

2. Remind the client to maintain an upright position when ambulating.

3. Teach the client with poor balance to walk and turn cautiously. Instruct him to lift his toes with each step and to touch his heels down first; to walk in a wide arc instead of pivoting to turn; to avoid crossing his legs while turning; to choose a clear path; to avoid crowds; and to stop occasionally to slow his walking speed.

4. Assess the client's environment for safety hazards, such as throw rugs or misplaced furniture, and remove them.

5. Refer the client to a physical therapist for gait training, appropriate exercises, and evaluation for a walker or cane.

Rationales

1. Orthostatic changes commonly occur in the elderly client and increase the risk of falling.

2. The client with Parkinson's disease tends to flex his knees and hips excessively, which pushes the body forward and increases the chance of a fall.

3. The client with parkinsonism typically has trouble initiating walking and controlling involuntary movements. Lifting the toes and touching the heels first helps the client with gait disturbances, including shuffling, taking short steps, and stepping in place without progressing forward. Walking in a wide arc helps improve balancing and turning. Avoiding crossing the legs while walking is especially important for the client whose rigidity prevents him from selectively relaxing or activating muscles for particular movements, as difficulty in uncrossing legs can precipitate a fall. Choosing a clear path and avoiding crowds is advisable for the client who has trouble stopping after taking a backward step. Stopping occasionally while walking is especially important for the client who walks with rapid, small steps.

4. The client with Parkinson's disease may suddenly halt or freeze when confronted with a minor obstacle. Eliminating hazards decreases the client's risk for injury.

5. A physical therapist can help the client learn techniques to overcome akinesia and the loss of postural reflexes.

OUTCOME CRITERIA
• The client will not fall or experience other trauma.
• The client and caregiver will identify and eliminate safety hazards in the client's environment.

Nursing diagnosis: *Impaired physical mobility related to bradykinesia, tremors, and rigidity*

NURSING GOAL: To maintain maximum mobility and independence in self-care

Signs and symptoms
• tremors
• rigidity
• chorea
• decreased postural reflexes

Interventions

1. Assess the client who suffers frequent falls or complains of poor balance for levodopa toxicity. Report significant findings to the physician.

2. Teach the client ways to improve mobility, such as stepping over an imaginary line or rocking from side to side to initiate leg movement.

3. Instruct the client to rise from a sitting position by moving to the edge of the chair, placing his hands on the chair's arm supports, bowing his head slightly and bending his knees, placing his feet flat on the floor 12" to 15" (30.5 to 38 cm) apart, then slowly and rhythmically rocking forward in the chair and rising on the count of three.

4. Provide helpful equipment or devices, such bed pulls, overbed trapezes, and night lights, to ensure safety and ease mobility.

5. Initiate a daily exercise program that includes active range-of-motion exercises, stretching, and massage as soon as the client is positively diagnosed. Schedule the exercise periods to coincide with the peak levels of medications.

6. Refer the client to a physical therapist for individualized exercise and mobility training and for ongoing therapy.

7. Refer the client to an occupational therapist, as needed, for help with dressing, bathing, cooking, and adapting household equipment and furnishings.

8. Refer the client to the American Parkinson's Disease Association for literature on handling activities of daily living (ADLs) and exercises.

Rationales

1. Long-term levodopa treatment can cause marked postural instability (the "on/off" phenomenon). In this phenomenon, sudden akinetic spells interrupt periods of total functional ability and immobilize the client.

2. Rigidity prevents the client from selectively relaxing or activating muscles for a particular movement.

3. Rigidity prevents the client from selectively relaxing or activating muscles, which makes certain activities, such as standing up, more difficult. Rhythmic rocking may facilitate movement.

4. Bed pulls, usually located at the sides or end of the bed, can help the client sit up or turn in bed. Overbed trapezes can help the client change positions in bed. Night lights, placed near the bedroom door, in the hallway leading to the bathroom, and in the bathroom, can help prevent accidental falls and injuries at night.

5. Regular exercise counteracts the effects of the disease and helps the client to maintain function. Scheduling exercise periods during medications' peak levels ensures that the client will be functioning at his optimum level.

6. A physical therapist can help the client with gait training, regaining postural stability, relearning fine motor skills, increasing mobility, and regaining his self-confidence, thereby helping to decrease his risk of falling.

7. An occupational therapist can teach the client and caregiver techniques to compensate for loss of motor function, order adaptive equipment, and train the client and caregiver to use adaptive devices to maximize independence.

8. Written information can reinforce teaching and help the client to adapt to his disease.

OUTCOME CRITERIA
• The client will be free of contractures.
• The client will maintain independence.

Nursing diagnosis: *Altered thought processes related to dementia*

NURSING GOALS: To identify and treat the reversible causes of dementia and to assess the client for possible drug toxicity

Signs and symptoms
• confusion
• paranoia
• depression
• argumentative behavior
• wandering
• altered level of consciousness (such as confusion or forgetfulness)
• altered mood and affect (such as irritability or hostility)
• diminished memory and judgment
• disturbances in sleep-wake cycles
• impaired abstract thinking

Interventions

1. Assess the client for changes in behavior or orientation, such as forgetfulness or hostility.

2. Assess the client for signs and symptoms of depression, and discuss possible interventions with the physician.

3. Review the client's antiparkinsonian medications and discuss possible changes with the physician.

4. Assess the client for adverse reactions to medication, including confusion, tardive dyskinesia, hallucinations, dystonia, and reversed sleep-wake patterns. Report any adverse reactions to the physician, and discuss the possibility of dosage reductions, if necessary.

5. Provide a safe, secure environment.

6. Refer the client to an adult day-care program, if possible.

7. Refer the caregiver to a community support group.

Rationales

1. An assessment will help rule out treatable causes of altered thought processes.

2. Depression can mimic, or coexist with, dementia and may require psychotherapy or antidepressant medication. Successful treatment for depression can markedly improve mental functioning.

3. Many antiparkinsonian medications, such as levodopa, can contribute to mental status changes. Medication readjustments can help improve mental functioning in many cases.

4. Levodopa and anticholinergic toxicity may result with long-term use. Reduced dosages may improve the symptoms; however, the medications may need to be temporarily discontinued.

5. The client with mental status changes may have an altered perception of himself and his environment and requires careful monitoring and a sense of security.

6. A good adult day-care program can monitor the client's mental status and provide activities appropriate for the client's level of functioning. Day care also relieves the caregiver.

7. Coping with the client's mental status changes can be difficult; talking with others in similar situations provides emotional support and a forum for sharing ideas.

OUTCOME CRITERION
• The client will receive a complete assessment for dementia and the causes will be identified and eliminated.

Nursing diagnosis: *Self-care deficit: dressing, bathing, and toileting, related to bradykinesia, rigidity, and tremors*

NURSING GOAL: To foster as much independence in ADLs as possible

Signs and symptoms
• noticeable decline in appearance
• change in usual activities
• inability to bathe or brush teeth
• inability to dress
• inability to perform self-toileting measures
• need for assistive devices

Interventions

1. Assess the client's ability to bathe, eat, and dress.

2. Provide an unhurried, stress-free atmosphere, and allow sufficient time for the client to complete tasks.

3. Enhance the client's bathing capabilities by attaching nonskid strips to the tub or shower floor or using a rubber mat; covering the bathroom floor with a large area rug; using tub seats or shower chairs; installing an inexpensive, flexible shower hose; encouraging the client to use soap on a rope instead of conventional bar soaps; installing grab bars throughout the bathroom; and encouraging the client to use an electric razor to shave.

4. Help the client to dress himself by providing clothing with hook and loop (Velcro) closures instead of buttons, zippers, or ties; a dressing stick or hook for pulling trousers and underclothing over feet and legs; and a reaching stick for grabbing needed clothing articles.

5. Help the client to feed himself by placing guards on plates and by using silverware with thick plastic handles or tubular foam padding.

Rationales

1. The functional abilities of the client with Parkinson's disease often fluctuate. ADLs require repeated movements, which diminish the client's strength with each successive trial.

2. A hurried, tense environment will increase the client's level of dysfunction.

3. Nonskid materials and a large area rug decrease the client's risk of falling or tripping. A shower chair makes bathing easier and safer. Soap on a rope is more convenient for the client to reach. Grab bars provide support and help the client to walk. An electric razor helps prevent cuts caused by tremors.

4. The client with Parkinson's disease often has impaired hand strength and coordination, which makes buttoning or zipping clothing difficult. A dressing or reaching stick allows the client to remain seated while dressing and reduces his risk of falling.

5. Plate guards prevent spills and help the client to manipulate food. The client who suffers from tremors tends to handle thick-handled utensils better than conventional utensils.

OUTCOME CRITERION
• The client will maintain maximal independence in performing ADLs.

Nursing diagnosis: *Ineffective individual and family coping related to the disease*

NURSING GOALS: To maximize the client's control over his life and help the family to cope with the client's deteriorating condition

Signs and symptoms
• fatigue
• depression
• irritability or anger
• social isolation and withdrawal
• anxiety
• fear
• marital or other family problems

Interventions

1. Help the client to establish realistic goals.

2. Encourage the client and caregiver to clarify their expectations of each other.

3. Carefully monitor the client's changes in function, and intervene early to maintain his maximal independence.

4. Respect the client's intelligence by offering intellectually stimulating activities, such as reading or music, depending on the client's interests; speaking to the client as an adult; showing patience; allowing the client to express himself; and reminding the client's family and caregiver of his true intellectual abilities.

5. Each night, discuss the activity plan for the next day with the client.

6. Encourage the client to maintain social contacts and family and occupational responsibilities to counter his tendency toward immobility and apathy.

7. Refer the client and the client's family to a social worker or psychotherapist, as needed.

8. Refer the client and the client's family to appropriate support groups, such as the local chapter of the American Parkinson's Disease Association or local hospitals specializing in Parkinson's disease.

9. Suggest that the client use adult day care, if available and affordable.

Rationales

1. The attainment of realistic goals can enhance the client's self-esteem.

2. Knowing what is expected can decrease frustration.

3. Timely interventions can minimize the disabling aspects of Parkinson's disease.

4. Parkinson's disease rarely affects intellect. Recognizing the client's intelligence enhances self-esteem and instills confidence in the client's ability to maintain control over personal affairs and interests.

5. The discussion should give the client a greater sense of control and decrease his anxiety level, which is typically highest in the evening.

6. These measures will help preserve the client's independence and help him cope with a chronic, progressive, disabling disease.

7. A social worker or psychotherapist can evaluate the client's psychosocial situation and determine his need for further interventions, such as counseling. He can also encourage communication among the client, caregiver, and the client's family.

8. Such groups or organizations can provide the client and family with the latest information on the disease, answer any specific questions, and foster a supportive social environment.

9. An adult day-care program reduces the client's sense of isolation, provides an opportunity for him to participate in worthwhile activity, and decreases his feelings of uselessness. The client typically copes better knowing that others have the same problems; the family typically copes better when it has a break from full-time caregiving.

OUTCOME CRITERION
• The client and the client's family will develop effective coping mechanisms, such as increased socialization, support-group involvement, and the establishment of mutually attainable goals.

NURSING ACTIONS IN VARIOUS SETTINGS

Nursing actions for a client with Parkinson's disease depend on the setting in which care is provided. This section identifies which actions are appropriate in all settings and which pertain to acute care, extended care, or home care situations.

All settings

• Explain the rationale behind the therapy, such as why the client will receive no medications initially. Emphasize that medications treat symptoms but do not cure the disease.
• Encourage the client to exercise during all stages of the disease.
• Help the client and caregiver distinguish between the disease and normal aging.
• Recommend that the client see his physician or nurse at least once every 3 to 6 months, even in the absence of specific complaints.

Acute care

• Act as an advocate for the Parkinson's client receiving treatment for another illness.
• Coordinate the client's activities with his medication schedule, since disease symptoms may worsen shortly before the next dose.
• Coordinate the interventions of all health care providers to avoid overtiring the client.
• Maintain or decrease the client's activity level.
• If levodopa needs to be stopped, prepare the client and the client's family for the severe symptoms that may result.

Extended care

• Teach the nursing staff the principles of caring for a client with Parkinson's disease. Review the most difficult aspects of the disease, such as end-of-dose failure and the on-off phenomenon, which can prevent the client from performing a task he could do hours earlier.
• Maximize the client's level of functioning.
• Encourage the client and nursing staff to use safety precautions.
• Consult physical, occupational, and speech therapists as needed.
• Assess the client's diet, and consult a dietitian to develop meals that avoid excess protein, which can interfere with the client's metabolism of levodopa.
• Keep the physician informed of any changes in the client's symptoms that could signal a need for medication adjustments

Home care

• Explain the effects of Parkinson's disease to the client's family and caregiver. Emphasize that the disease, not the client, caused the client's behavior to change.
• Help the client and caregiver establish a safe environment.

• Teach the client and caregiver which signs and symptoms to report to the physician.
• Teach the client and caregiver about the client's medications, including their purpose, side effects, principles of administration, and signs and symptoms of failure.

SELECTED REFERENCES

Delgado, J.M., and Billo, J.M. "Care of the Patient with Parkinson's Disease: Surgical and Nursing Interventions," *Journal of Neuroscience Nursing* 20(3):142-50, June 1988.

DeLong, M., et al. "Common Disorders of Movement: Tremor and Parkinson's Disease," in Barker, L., et al. *Principles of Ambulatory Medicine.* Baltimore: Williams & Wilkins Co., 1986.

Goetz, C.G., et al. "Update on Parkinson's Disease," *Patient Care* 23(7):124-62, April 15, 1989.

Koller, W.C. "Diagnosis and Treatment of Parkinson's Disease," *Modern Medicine* 57:114-29, May 1989.

Koller, W.C. *Handbook of Parkinson's Disease.* New York: Marcel Dekker, 1987.

Lannon, M.C., et al. "Comprehensive Care of the Patient with Parkinson's Disease," *Journal of Neuroscience Nursing* 18(3):121-31, June 1986.

McDowell, F., and Cedarbaum, J. *Manual for Persons with Parkinson's Disease.* New York: The American Parkinson's Disease Association, 1987.

Norberg, A., and Athlin, E. "The Interaction Between the Parkinsonian Patient and His Caregiver During Feeding: A Theoretical Model," *Journal of Advanced Nursing* 12:545-50, September, 1987.

Topp, B. "Toward a Better Understanding of Parkinson's Disease," *Geriatric Nursing* 8(4):180-82, July/August 1987.

Van Oteghen, S. "An Exercise Program for Those with Parkinson's Disease," *Geriatric Nursing* 8(4):183-84, July/August 1987.

NEUROLOGIC SYSTEM

Delirium

Delirium, an organic brain disorder common among older adults, is characterized by a clouded state of consciousness that impairs the ability to correctly perceive stimuli and to shift or sustain attention. It may accompany almost any physical illness and has a variable rate of onset, depending on the course of the underlying problem. It may manifest periodically during an illness, with the client vacillating between periods of confusion and lucidity; in some cases, it persists for a few days to a week.

Prompt treatment of delirium may restore the client to his previous level of cognitive functioning. However, when left untreated, delirium may permanently impair the client's cognitive ability. Clients at increased risk for delirium include those who are cognitively impaired, suffer from numerous or severe chronic illnesses or stress, or use multiple medications.

ETIOLOGY

Almost any illness can cause delirium in older adults. For example, vascular disease, brain damage or disease, impaired vision or hearing, reduced cerebral blood flow, and impaired glucose metabolism predispose the client to hypoxia and may precipitate delirium. The most common precipitating factor, however, is the use of multiple medications or alcohol, which causes drug-induced delirium from slow or impaired drug metabolism. Neurochemical imbalances, psychosocial stressors, inability to interpret sensory input, and impaired cerebral metabolism may also cause delirium in elderly clients.

HEALTH HISTORY FINDINGS

In a health history interview, the client may report or the nurse may detect many of these findings:
• altered level of consciousness (such as confusion or irritability).
• fluctuating symptoms that worsen at night
• disorientation to place and time
• confabulation
• agitation or stupor
• insomnia
• nightmares
• fecal impaction
• urine retention
• depression
• use of anticholinergic, antispasmodic, mydriatic, antipsychotic, tricyclic antidepressant, psychotropic, sedative, analgesic, or diuretic medications
• use of digitalis
• history of cerebrovascular accident, cerebral damage, or a metabolic or endocrine disorder
• history of cardiovascular disease

• history of cholecystitis, pneumonia, urinary tract infections, or uremia
• recent general anesthesia
• recent burns
• history of poor food and fluid intake
• history of alcohol use
• social isolation
• recent location change
• recent bereavement

PHYSICAL FINDINGS

In a physical examination, the nurse may detect many of these findings:

Neurologic
• asterixis
• coarse tremors

Cardiovascular
• tachycardia
• increased blood pressure

Psychological
• disorientation or confusion
• short-term memory loss
• altered sensory input (such as diminished sight or hearing)
• auditory or visual hallucinations
• paranoia
• apprehension
• irritability
• combativeness

DIAGNOSTIC STUDIES

The following studies may be performed to evaluate the client's health status:
• mental assessment—to diagnose dementing diseases; the preferred tool is the Folstein Mini-Mental State Examination
• complete blood count (CBC) and differential—to identify abnormalities that may cause delirium; an elderly client may have an infection without leukocytosis
• erythrocyte sedimentation rate (ESR)—to identify an infection or tumor; may normally be elevated in elderly clients
• blood urea nitrogen (BUN), creatinine, electrolyte, calcium, phosphate, T_3, and T_4 levels—to determine metabolic disturbances
• serum drug levels—to identify drug toxicity
• electrocardiogram (ECG)—to isolate a possible myocardial infarction
• chest X-ray—to identify infection, emboli, or a neoplasm

• EEG—to differentiate delirium from pseudodelirium and intracranial from systemic diseases
• computed tomography (CT) scan—to identify tumors or hemorrhages

POTENTIAL COMPLICATIONS
• confusion or disorientation
• anxiety or fear
• hallucinations, delusions, or illusions
• incontinence
• falls
• pneumonia

Nursing diagnosis: *Altered thought processes related to confusion, hallucination, medication interaction, or drug toxicity*

NURSING GOALS: To maximize the use of intact cognitive functioning, to improve cognitive function, and to prevent complications

Signs and symptoms
• disorientation
• short-term memory loss
• decreased attention span
• inability to follow directions or perform tasks
• dry mouth
• blurred vision
• stupor
• nausea
• vomiting
• diarrhea or constipation
• neuromuscular instability
• tachycardia

Interventions

1. Assess the client's temperature, pulse rate, respiration rate, and blood pressure every 4 hours while he is delirious.

2. Frequently assess the client's cognitive level using a mini-mental status examination (see *Folstein mini-mental state examination,* page 228).

3. Continually orient the client to the date, time, place, and familiar objects.

4. Assess the client's fluid and electrolyte balance, and monitor it closely when withdrawing medications.

5. Maintain consistency with caregivers.

6. Identify all medications, including over-the-counter drugs, that the client has been taking. Ask the client's family or caregiver to help in compiling the list.

7. Discuss with the physician the possibility of discontinuing all medications.

8. Give the client clear, simple instructions.

Rationales

1. Drug toxicity may alter the client's vital signs; careful monitoring of vital signs helps ensure the client's safety.

2. Frequent assessment of cognitive level is essential because gradually changing levels indicate increasing confusion and delirium.

3. Such reinforcement should help the client to remember information and to decrease or prevent agitation and irritability.

4. Fluid and electrolyte balance affects physical and cognitive function.

5. Familiarity comforts the delirious client and puts fewer demands on his memory.

6. A previously prescribed medication, or an interaction with an over-the-counter drug, may cause delirium.

7. Discontinuing medications helps to isolate toxicity as a cause.

8. The cognitively impaired client sometimes cannot perform complex tasks but can follow simple directions.

9. Provide the client with a nutritious diet, and administer food supplements when necessary.

9. Proper nutrition promotes cognitive function and ensures that the client receives enough food and nourishment while delirious.

10. Evaluate the client's need for sensory aids, such as eyeglasses and hearing aids. Keep the client's room well lit during the day.

10. Sensory deprivation can cause confusion and impaired cognition. The client with twilight confusion may become delirious if isolated in a dark room during the day.

11. Hang written signs in the client's room to identify the date, the location of the room, and specific areas within his visual field, such as the bathroom.

11. Environmental cues decrease the client's need to rely on memory for information that is frequently lost during delirium.

12. Help the client to perform self-care by organizing his clothing, reminding him to use the toilet, helping him to bathe, and assisting him with meal preparations.

12. Promoting activities of daily living allows the client to gain control and a sense of independence over performing self-care and lessens the stressful impact of his delirium.

13. Allow the client to move about the floor or room freely, when appropriate.

13. Increased mobility decreases agitation, provides purposeful activity, and promotes independence.

14. Encourage the client's family to bring familiar objects from home, such as family photographs, and to visit the client regularly.

14. Familiar objects and frequent family visits may help relax the client and increase his orientation and cognitive functioning.

OUTCOME CRITERION
• The client will recover from his delirious state within 1 week, as manifested by orientation to person, time, and place; restful nights without hallucinations or nightmares; and decreased anxiety and agitation.

Nursing diagnosis: *Sensory-perceptual alteration: visual, auditory, and tactile, related to delirium*

NURSING GOAL: To provide sensory stimulation through environmental and verbal cues

Signs and symptoms
• hallucinations
• illusions or delusions
• anxiety or fear
• disorientation
• sleep deprivation

Interventions

1. If the client experiences illusions, delusions, or hallucinations, allow him to express his thoughts, continue talking with him and expressing concern while maintaining eye-to-eye contact, and remain close by until he is calm.

Rationales

1. Comforting a delirious client helps to alleviate his illusions, delusions, or hallucinations. Allowing the client to express himself, making eye-to-eye contact, and remaining nearby convey concern and help to comfort the client.

2. Administer haloperidol, as ordered, to calm the agitated or psychotic client. Discontinue the medication when the client becomes lucid.

2. High-potency neuroleptics, such as haloperidol, effectively calm the client yet have fewer sedative, cardiotoxic, and hypotensive side effects than do low-potency neuroleptics, such as chlorpromazine.

3. Keep a clock or calendar in the client's room; if available, also incorporate the use of a softly playing radio or television.

3. These items provide an appropriate level of sensory stimulation for the delirious client.

FOLSTEIN MINI-MENTAL STATE EXAMINATION

The Folstein Mini-Mental State Examination is the preferred tool for assessing the mental status of an elderly client with suspected cognitive impairment. To perform the examination, the nurse asks the client to follow a series of simple commands that test the client's ability to understand and perform cognitive functions. The nurse awards a designated point value for successful completion of each instruction, then totals the scores to determine the client's mental status. Scores of 26 to 30 indicate that the client is normal; 22 to 25, mildly impaired; and less than 22, significantly impaired.

	Client instructions	Maximum score	Actual score
Orientation	Ask the client to name the year, season, date, day, and month. (Score one point for each correct response.)	5	( )
	Ask the client to name his state, city, street, and house address, and the room in which he is standing. (Score one point for each correct response.)	5	( )
Comprehension	State the name of three objects, pausing 1 second between each name. Then ask the client to repeat all three names. (Score one point for each correct response.) Repeat this exercise until the client can correctly name all three objects (the client will be tested on his ability to recall this information later in the examination).	3	( )
Attention and calculation	Ask the client to count backward by sevens, beginning at 100; have him stop after counting out five numbers. Alternatively, ask the client to spell "World" backward. (Score one point for each correct response.)	5	( )
Recall	Ask the client to restate the name of the three objects previously identified in the examination. (Score one point for each correct response.)	3	( )
Language	Point to a pencil and a watch. Ask the client to identify each object. (Score one point for each correct response.)	2	( )
	Ask the client to repeat "No ifs, ands, or buts." (Score one point for a correct response.)	1	( )
	Ask the client to take a paper in his right hand, then fold the paper in half, then put the paper on the floor. (Score one point for each correct response to this three-part command.)	3	( )
	Ask the client to read and obey the written instruction "Close your eyes." (Score one point for a correct response.)	1	( )
	Ask the client to write a sentence. (Score one point for a correct response.)	1	( )
	Ask the client to copy the following design. (Score one point for a correct response.)	1	( )

Adapted with permission from Folstein, M.F., et al. "Mini-Mental State: A Practical Method for Grading the Cognitive State of Patients for the Clinician," *Journal of Psychiatric Research* 12:196-97, 1975.

4. Keep a night light on in the client's room, and have a familiar person remain with the client at night. Raise the bed side rails, as needed.

4. Agitation and hallucinations may worsen at night because of perceptual distortions. Using a night light and having a familiar person stay with the client can be especially soothing to a delirious client. Keeping the side rails up promotes a feeling of security.

5. Remove extraneous stimuli, such as televisions and radios, from the client's environment, if necessary.

5. Extraneous stimuli may initiate visual, auditory, or tactile hallucinations or may impair the client's ability to receive important stimuli.

6. Use restraints only if the staff cannot calm the client. Use extreme caution when applying restraints.

6. Restraints usually increase the client's agitation.

7. Express concern and caring for the agitated client. Remain close by until the client becomes calm.

7. These measures provide support and help to relieve the client's fears.

OUTCOME CRITERIA
• The client will be oriented to person, place, and time.
• The client will not become agitated and anxious as his delirium improves.

NURSING ACTIONS IN VARIOUS SETTINGS

Nursing actions for a delirious client depend on the setting in which care is provided. This section identifies which actions are appropriate in all settings and which pertain to acute care, extended care, or home care situations.

All settings
• Inform the client and the client's family or caregiver that the delirium is transient and temporary. Teach the client's family and caregiver ways to improve the client's cognitive functioning.
• Teach the caregiver and nursing staff the prodromal symptoms of delirium, such as insomnia, nightmares, fleeting hallucinations, and anxiety.
• Teach the night staff to observe for early warning signs, since delirium commonly occurs at night.
• Identify clients at high risk for delirium, such as those who are extremely old, have impaired vision and hearing, and receive multiple medications (especially several different anticholinergic agents).

Acute care
• Assess the client for orientation to person, place, and time and for his ability to concentrate.
• Recognize the phenomenon of intensive care unit (ICU) psychosis, which commonly occurs in elderly hospitalized clients.
• Discuss the signs and symptoms of delirium with clients in or recently returned from the ICU, because such clients may equate delirium with psychosis.
• Initiate a psychiatric consultation to further evaluate delirium.
• Assess the client who recently underwent surgery for a fractured femoral neck for signs of delirium, which commonly occurs after this procedure.

Extended care
• If the client becomes acutely delirious, contact the physician or transfer the client to a hospital for diagnosis of an underlying cause.
• Evaluate the client's cognitive level daily.
• Keep the client away from others who are agitated.

Home care
• If the client's delirium worsens, contact the physician or transfer the client to the hospital for an evaluation of an underlying cause.

SELECTED REFERENCES

Campbell, E.B., et al. "After the Fall—Confusion," *American Journal of Nursing* 86(2):151-54, February 1986.

Carnevali, D.L., and Patrick, M. *Nursing Management for the Elderly.* Philadelphia: J.B. Lippincott Co., 1986.

Easton, C., and MacKenzie, F. "Sensory-Perceptual Alterations: Delirium in the Intensive Care Unit," *Heart & Lung* 17(3):229-34, March 1988.

Folstein, M.F., et al. "Mini-Mental State: A Practical Method for Grading the Cognitive State of Patients for the Clinician," *Journal for Psychiatric Research* 12:189-98, 1975.

Gomez, G.E., and Gomez, E.A. "Delirium," *Geriatric Nursing* 8(6):330-32, November/December 1987.

Gomez, G.E., and Gomez, E.A. "Dementia? or Delirium?" *Geriatric Nursing* 10(3):141-43, May/June 1989.

Lipowski, Z.J. "Delirium in the Elderly Patient," *New England Journal of Medicine* 320(9):578-81, March 2, 1989.

Sullivan, N., and Fogel, B.S. "Could This Be Delirium?" *American Journal of Nursing* 86(12):1359-63, December 1986.

NEUROLOGIC SYSTEM

Sensory Deprivation

Sensory deprivation refers to the loss of, or decreased or denied stimulation to, any of the five senses. Such deprivation, which is common among older adults, can compound other health problems, threatening the client's well-being. Those with sensory deficits typically require more time to process information and have a diminished capacity to process simultaneous, complex stimuli. In many cases, such deficits result in sensory overload, confusion, difficulty concentrating, or environmental withdrawal.

Most adults begin to experience loss of vision at about age 40. Presbyopia, the loss of vision resulting from advancing age, is most apparent when an older adult has difficulty reading small print. Many older adults have visual deficits that lead to peripheral vision impairment, far-sightedness, and an intolerance for light and glare. The ability to perceive blues, greens, and violets diminishes with age, but elderly clients retain the ability to visualize orange, yellow, and red.

An estimated 8.5 million Americans, including 30% of those over age 65, suffer some degree of hearing loss, making hearing loss the most common chronic health problem. Hearing loss may be conductive or sensorineural in origin. Conductive hearing losses typically affect those who have difficulty transmitting sound through the external or middle ear, such as from otosclerosis. Sensorineural hearing losses, which involve inner-ear impairment, typically affect those with damage to cranial nerve VIII, such as from medication use, Ménière's disease, tertiary syphilis, hypothyroidism, or Paget's disease. Many elderly clients suffer both types of hearing loss. Presbycusis, the inability to hear high-pitched sounds, also occurs with aging.

The sense of smell typically diminishes with age, most adults completely losing their capacity to smell by age 80. The sharpest decline in the ability to smell usually occurs during middle age in both sexes; however, women tend to retain their sense of smell longer than men.

Hypogeusia, the complete loss of taste or the inability to taste certain flavors, is a common age-related condition. In many cases, older adults lose their ability to distinguish sweet and salty tastes sooner than their ability to distinguish sour and bitter tastes.

The loss of tactile sensitivity commonly diminishes with age, the degree of loss depending on the individual. Such loss, which typically begins with diminished sensation on the nonhairy body surfaces, such as the palms and soles, affects the client's ability to localize and react to stimuli. Difficulty in localizing stimuli is best exemplified in the client's inability to differentiate coins, fasten buttons, or grasp small objects. Elderly clients also have a diminished sense of vibration, which is most apparent in the legs and feet.

ETIOLOGY

Sensory deprivation in the elderly client can result from numerous causes, depending on the sense affected. For example, visual deficits can result from certain physiologic changes to the pupils and iris that occur with aging. Also, the lens, cornea, and vitreous humor become less permeable to light with age, impairing night vision and the ability to adjust from lightness to darkness. Certain diseases and disorders can also lead to visual deficits in older adults. For example, transient ischemic attacks can produce transient blindness. Cerebrovascular accident, diabetes, or primary ophthalmic problems can result in diplopia. Glaucoma, macular degeneration, and vitamin A and D deficiencies can also cause visual deficits.

The amount of time required to process sound increases with age. Consonants are particularly difficult to distinguish because they are typically of a short duration and high frequency, which makes them harder to hear. Rapid speech or background noise can also interfere with an elderly client's ability to hear. Acoustical nerve trauma, ototoxic medications, infections, and malignant tumors also can cause hearing loss in the older adult.

Hearing deficits in older adults can also begin during middle age from degenerative changes in the ear, resulting in progressive atrophy of the sensory brain cells and related supporting cells. Later, the neurons of the vestibulocochlear nerve and the higher auditory pathways atrophy, which causes a sensorineural hearing loss.

The leading cause of the loss of the sense of smell is accidental injury. About 1 in 16 clients with head trauma permanently loses the ability to smell. Influenza, brain tumors, allergies, smoking, environmental factors, and aging contribute to the problem.

Because the sense of taste is closely tied to the sense of smell, the loss of the sense of smell typically interferes with the ability to taste. As a person ages, the total number of taste buds decline and the taste buds themselves deteriorate, which decreases taste sensitivity. Smoking, vitamin D deficiency, decreased saliva production, dentures, and certain medications also dull the sense of taste.

Loss of tactile sensitivity may result from neuropathy, disease, injury, or circulatory insufficiency.

HEALTH HISTORY FINDINGS

In a health history interview, the client may report or the nurse may detect many of these findings:

Vision
- decreased tolerance of glare
- night blindness
- vision difficulties, such as the inability to read small print or to identify objects or people
- diplopia
- eye pain and fatigue
- headaches
- history of diabetes, glaucoma, hypertension, cerebrovascular accident, transient ischemic attacks, or cataracts
- history of head trauma, frequent falls, or car accidents

Hearing
- unusual voice quality or loud speech
- diminished ability to hear high-pitched voices
- exaggerated sensitivity to loud sounds
- difficulty understanding speech, especially with increased background sounds
- epistaxis
- tinnitus
- ear drainage and cerumen accumulation
- depression or paranoia
- dizziness
- history of tertiary syphilis, hypothyroidism, Ménière's disease, or Paget's disease
- history of frequent ear or upper respiratory tract infections
- previous ear surgery
- history of head trauma
- use of aspirin or other ototoxic drugs
- history of occupational exposure to loud noises

Smell
- anorexia
- history of chronic sinusitis, brain tumor, or rhinorrhea
- history of head trauma or allergies
- history of tobacco use

Taste
- history of preference for sweets or high-carbohydrate foods
- anorexia
- rhinorrhea
- dry mouth
- poor-fitting dentures
- history of food allergies
- use of multiple drugs or anticholinergic medications
- decreased appetite
- lactose intolerance
- use of smoking or chewing tobacco

Touch
- leg ulcers or skin tears
- tingling or numbness in the arms and legs
- history of diabetes, Ménière's disease, Alzheimer's disease, or gastrointestinal disease
- history of peripheral vascular disease, cardiac disease, osteoarthritis, or rheumatoid arthritis
- history of head trauma or frequent burns

PHYSICAL FINDINGS
In a physical examiniation, the nurse may detect many of these findings:

Vision
- decreased function of cranial nerves II, IV, V, and VI
- macular degeneration
- homonymous hemianopia
- intraocular implants
- tearing, crustation, irritation, or redness of outer eye
- increased intraocular pressure
- lens opacity

Hearing
- Positive Rinne and Weber test for perceptive or conductive hearing loss
- redness, swelling, drainage, lesions, or scales on the outer ear
- cerumen accumulation and discharge in the inner ear
- tenderness of the external and inner ear
- nose discharge
- nasal polyps

Smell
- diminished ability to identify such odors as alcohol and lemon
- malnourished appearance

Taste
- mouth tears and ulcerations
- mouth burns or bruising
- weight loss
- hair loss
- missing teeth
- stomatitis
- diminished swallow and gag reflexes
- thrush
- ulcerations on the tongue and soft palate
- inability to discern sweet and sour tastes

Touch
- decreased position sense
- abnormal stereognosis
- diminished tactile stimulation
- decreased facial sensation
- increased pain tolerance
- hypothermia

DIAGNOSTIC STUDIES
The following studies may be performed to evaluate the client's health status:
- Snellen eye examination—to evaluate visual impairment
- comprehensive audiology examination—to identify hearing imparment; screening techniques include a self-estimate of hearing loss by the client, pure tone audiometry, speech perception tests, and pure-tone air (Weber) and bone conduction (Rinne tuning fork) tests

• scratch and sniff test—to identify smelling impairment; scents tested include vinegar, coffee, and perfume; smelling-impaired client can typically identify only one scent
• taste tests—to identify sweet, bitter, sour, and salty taste deficits; client sips a mixture of sucrose, quinine, hydrochloric acid, or sodium chloride and water
• computed tomography (CT) scan—to rule out secondary causes for changes in sensation, such as a brain tumor

POTENTIAL COMPLICATIONS
Vision
• presbyopia
• night blindness
• glaucoma
• macular degeneration
• retinitis pigmentosa

• conjunctivitis
• cataracts

Hearing
• sensory deprivation
• impaired communication

Smell
• inability to detect toxins or environmental hazards

Taste
• malnutrition
• dehydration

Touch
• sensory overload
• skin trauma

Nursing diagnosis: *Sensory-perceptual alteration: visual, related to impaired vision, presbyopia, recruitment, or night blindness*

NURSING GOALS: To restore visual function with an optimal level of independence and to help the client adapt environmentally to compensate for normal age-related vision changes

Signs and symptoms
• inability to read small print
• trauma
• poor communication skills
• frequent falls
• refusal to drive at night

Interventions

1. Assess the client's degree of visual deficit by having him read a newspaper using only one eye. Allow him to wear corrective lenses during testing.

2. Assess the client's need for glasses or contact lenses.

3. Wash the client's eyeglasses with soap and water, and dry them thoroughly with a nonlint-gathering fabric.

4. Advise the client to make use of nonoptical devices, such as a reading stand, colored acetate filter sheets or other contrast enhancers, higher-watt light bulbs, telephone dialing attachments with enlarged numbers, and large-print books.

5. Adapt the client's environment to accommodate his vision loss. For example, arrange his personal effects in a specific manner, and never alter their placement; arrange his food in a clockwise pattern on his plate, and inform him of the location of the food.

6. Provide the client with prescribed magnification devices, such as a telescope, magnifier, or projection device.

Rationales

1. Such assessment should help the nurse to determine the adequacy of the client's vision in relation to his daily living needs.

2. Eyeglasses and contact lenses can dramatically improve visual acuity, particularly in aphakic clients.

3. Dirty glasses hinder clear vision.

4. Nonoptical devices can help the visually impaired client to see more clearly.

5. Adapting the client's environment allows for mobility while preventing injury. Arranging his personal effects helps to ensure that the client knows the exact location of objects. Placing food in a designated pattern on the client's plate facilitates independent eating.

6. Low-vision optical devices help the client to see better by magnifying a portion of an object.

7. Encourage the client to walk with another person to maintain mobility. Instruct him to place his hand on the guide's upper arm when walking and to walk beside but slightly behind the guide when walking down halls or stairs.

7. This technique helps the visually impaired client negotiate his environment while avoiding injury.

8. Ensure that the client's environment is well lighted. Provide additional lighting for detailed work and a night light in the client's bathroom and bedroom. Avoid fluorescent lighting.

8. Concentrated light illuminates small objects; a night light prevents injury by helping the client locate switches at night. Fluorescent lighting produces glare and should therefore be avoided.

9. Teach the client to reduce glare by wearing sunglasses, a visor, or a wide-brimmed hat or by using an umbrella.

9. The elderly client is sensitive to glare, which can impair vision and cause discomfort.

10. Use stimulating colors, such as burgundy, red, yellow, and orange in the client's environment; avoid poorly visualized colors, such as blue, green, and violet.

10. The elderly client may find bright colors stimulating to the senses and dark colors difficult to differentiate.

11. Refer the client to a support group or an agency that serves elderly clients.

11. Support groups and agencies provide information on various medical, surgical, optical, and rehabilitative treatments that can prevent vision loss or aid functional independence.

OUTCOME CRITERIA
- The client will function safely within his environment.
- The client will function within his environment through the use of optical devices.

Nursing diagnosis: *Impaired verbal communication, related to hearing loss*

NURSING GOALS: To maintain the client's hearing acuity, to screen for and remove impacted cerumen, and to adapt the client's environment to facilitate communication

Signs and symptoms
- poor communication skills
- inappropriate behavior
- increased accumulation of cerumen
- poor attention span
- agitation
- withdrawal
- confusion

Interventions

1. Test the client's hearing using a voice test, ticking watch, Rinne tuning fork test, or Weber test.

2. Use an otoscope to inspect the client's ear for cerumen buildup and to observe the condition of the tympanic membrane. If impacted cerumen is noted, use a peroxide-containing agent and a lubricant to prevent dryness. Use carbamide peroxide (Debrox) to remove wax pulp, and irrigate the client's ear with an ear syringe or water pick set on a low pulsation. Avoid using cotton-tipped applicators in the client's ears.

Rationales

1. These tests estimate the client's hearing acuity.

2. Impacted cerumen is the most common cause of hearing loss in the elderly client. It contains a large amount of keratin, which cannot be removed easily with ordinary irrigations. Medications, such as Debrox, emulsify and disperse accumulated cerumen. Cotton-tipped applicatiors can push cerumen further into the ear canal, causing further impaction, and should therefore be avoided.

3. Help the client communicate by sitting directly across from him at eye level; avoiding speaking directly in the client's ear; keeping your lips within the client's view; providing appropriate lighting; speaking in a well-modulated, normal tone; asking the client whether he can hear while you are speaking; using appropriate gestures or pointing; giving simple, one-step commands; avoiding exaggerated lip movements; ensuring the client's hearing aid is in place and operational; and explaining any environmental noises the client can hear.

3. All of these measures help to improve the client's ability to comprehend and communicate.

4. Avoid using an intercom to communicate with the client.

4. Background sound from an intercom device diminishes the client's ability to hear.

5. Instruct the client with a hearing aid to remove the device weekly for cleaning. Also instruct him to clean his ears when not using the device. Teach the client how to maintain the device and to troubleshoot any problems (see *Troubleshooting hearing aids*, pages 238 and 239).

5. A hearing aid acts as a foreign substance in the client's ear and promotes cerumen production. Weekly cleaning of the hearing aid and the client's ears is recommended.

6. Evaluate the client for possible use of a hand-held assistive hearing device.

6. Such adaptive equipment may be appropriate for the hearing-impaired client in an extended-care setting.

7. Reduce any glare in the client's environment.

7. Glare decreases visualization and interferes with lip reading.

8. Seat the client at a small four-person square table to eat.

8. A small square table promotes hearing, whereas a round or oblong tables decreases hearing capacity.

OUTCOME CRITERION
• The client will communicate effectively with others.

Nursing diagnosis: *Potential for injury related to loss of sense of smell*

NURSING GOAL: To prevent injury

Signs and symptoms
• inability to recognize gas leaks, smoke, or spoiled food
• inattention to bathing
• strong body odor

Interventions

1. Assess the client's sense of smell by having him identify the aromas of alcohol and coffee.

Rationales

1. These two substances emit strong odors, and a client with an adequate sense of smell should be able to identify them.

2. Monitor the client's nutritional status, and weigh him weekly.

2. Typically, a client with anosmia (loss of the sense of smell) also suffers hypogeusia (loss of the sense of taste) and may lose interest in eating.

3. Encourage communal dining.

3. A social environment may enhance the client's interest in eating.

4. Advise the client's family or caregiver to check the client's refrigerator for spoiled food.

4. A client with anosmia may be unable to detect spoiled food. The problem may be compounded if the client has poor vision.

5. Teach the client specific strategies to prevent gas leaks, such as installing spring safety caps for gas jets and avoiding air currents that could extinguish the flame on a gas stove.

6. Install smoke detectors with loud buzzers or flashing lights in the client's home.

7. If the client has a pet, monitor his environment for droppings.

5. The elderly client with a reduced sense of smell is at increased risk for asphyxia from gas leaks.

6. The client may be unable to smell faint traces of smoke.

7. The client may be unable to detect the pet's droppings, which could pose a health hazard.

OUTCOME CRITERION
• The client will be free from injury.

Nursing diagnosis: *Altered nutrition: less than body requirements, related to diminished sense of taste*

NURSING GOAL: To identify and correct malnutrition and nutritional deficiencies

Signs and symptoms
• weight loss
• anorexia
• skin breakdown

Interventions

1. Assess the client's sense of taste by having him identify the tastes of salt and sugar.

2. Provide frequent meticulous mouth care, including brushing the client's mouth and tongue and cleaning his dentures.

3. Use a soft-bristled or sponge toothbrush to clean the client's mouth.

4. If the client's mouth is coated with debris, such as food particles, have the client rinse his mouth with papaya juice.

5. Encourage the client to get out of bed for meals whenever possible.

6. Encourage the client to eat in a communal setting whenever possible.

7. Allow the client to smell cooking odors, such as by preparing toast in dining room.

8. Remove all negative stimuli, such as the radio and television, and all distracting odors, such as cleaning chemicals or soiled sheets, during meals.

9. Encourage the client to drink four to ten 8-oz glasses (1,000 to 2,500 ml) of fluid a day, if not contraindicated.

10. Serve visually appealing foods.

Rationales

1. Because routine assessments often fail to test for taste sensation, the nurse should remember to test the client's ability to distinguish salty and sugary tastes, typically the elderly client's only remaining taste senses.

2. Keeping the client's mouth clean enhances taste and helps prevent anorexia.

3. Such devices prevent tissue damage in the client's mouth.

4. Papaya juice contains a natural enzyme that removes debris and, when swallowed, acts as a natural digestive aid.

5. Exercise and activity enhance digestion and stimulate the appetite.

6. Socialization may enhance the appetite.

7. The sense of smell enhances the sense of taste and promotes appetite.

8. Obnoxious stimuli and odors will depress the client's appetite.

9. Adequate hydration keeps the client's mouth moist, which enhances his sense of taste.

10. Pleasantly arranged foods enhance the appetite.

11. Serve finger foods instead of pureed foods.

11. Pureed foods have no texture and little appeal.

12. Serve the client with dysphagia and impaired mobility first, and pick up his tray last.

12. This allows the client more time to eat.

13. Provide adaptive eating utensils when indicated, such as when the client has arthritis in his hands.

13. These utensils enhance dexterity and prevent pain.

14. Encourage the client to feed himself; explain to the client's family the reasons for doing so.

14. Encouraging the client to feed himself provides stimulation, allows the client to maintain some control over his environment, and promotes self-esteem.

15. Ensure an adequate supply of zinc by including green vegetables in the client's diet.

15. Zinc enhances the acuity of taste.

16. Serve the client his meals only when he is hungry.

16. This allows the client to maintain a sense of control over his needs.

17. Encourage the client's family to bring some of the client's favorite foods from home, provided they fit into the overall diet plan.

17. Food from home may stimulate the client's appetite.

18. Provide a diet high in fiber. Explain to the client the importance of a high-fiber diet, and reassure him that the initial side effects, such as bloating, will fade within 2 weeks.

18. A diet high in fiber prevents constipation, which may depress the client's appetite.

19. Supplement the client's diet with a multiple vitamin when prescribed.

19. Multiple vitamins help prevent vitamin deficiencies.

20. Encourage the client to save meal menus to use as a reference after discharge.

20. Hospital menus are a teaching aid for home menu planning, especially for those who must adhere to a therapeutic diet.

OUTCOME CRITERIA
• The client will maintain optimal weight.
• The client will continue to enjoy food.

Nursing diagnosis: *Sensory-perceptual alteration: kinesthetic and tactile, related to diminished sense of touch*

NURSING GOAL: To prevent skin injury

Signs and symptoms
• sensory overload
• frequent burns
• skin breakdown
• pressure sores
• withdrawal
• agitation
• confusion

Interventions

1. Assess the client's tactile sense by lightly touching his arms, legs, and forehead with a cotton ball and a safety pin.

2. Carefully assess the client for pain, especially cardiac pain or pain from a hip fracture or fall.

Rationales

1. These tests help the nurse to determine whether the client has diminished tactile sensitivity.

2. The client may be unable to feel the intense pain that usually signals a severe injury or ischemia.

3. Take necessary measures, such as turning the client or giving back rubs, to prevent pressure sores. If needed, use a special preventive mattress, such as a convoluted foam mattress, to reduce unrelieved pressure when all other measures to manage pressure sores fail.

3. Clients with kinesthetic deprivation are at highest risk for pressure sores while immobilized.

4. Set the controls on the client's tub or shower so that the water temperature is no higher than 120° F (49° C). If using a bath thermometer, make sure the bath water does not exceed 115° F (46° C).

4. The client's decreased ability to sense pain could precipitate a thermal burn.

OUTCOME CRITERION
• The client will remain free from skin injuries.

NURSING ACTIONS IN VARIOUS SETTINGS
Nursing actions for a client with sensory deprivation depend on the setting in which care is provided. This section identifies which actions are appropriate in all settings and which pertain to acute care, extended care, or home care situations.

All settings
Vision
• Instruct the client and the client's family to make necessary environmental changes to prevent injuries.
• Provide the client and the client's family with information about appropriate support groups and associations.
• Encourage all clients over age 65 to have a medical eye examination, including a refraction test, at least every 2 years and more frequently if the client has a history of diabetes or eye problems.

Hearing
• Teach the client and the client's family techniques to enhance hearing and communication.
• Encourage the client to recieve regular audiologic examinations.
• Teach the client and the client's family how to use and care for a hearing aid.

Smell
• Encourage the client to bathe regularly, and instruct the caregiver to promote bathing.

Taste
• Explain to the client's caregiver the importance of presenting appetizing foods, enhancing the client's sense of smell, and serving foods with various textures.

Touch
• Teach the client and the client's family to prevent injury by implementing appropriate safety precautions.

Acute care
Vision
• Provide a safe, clutter-free environment.
• Arrange objects in the client's environment consistently, and inform him of the arrangement.
• Keep a night light on in the client's bedroom and bathroom.
• Keep visual aids available and within the client's reach.

Hearing
• Reduce background sounds, and identify environmental noises for the client.
• Encourage the client to use his hearing aid and to maintain its proper functioning.
• Ensure that the client has heard all instructions, especially those relating to informed consent.
• Avoid rapid I.V. administration of ototoxic medications, such as furosemide (Lasix).

Smell
• Identify odors for the client.
• Provide food that is visually appealing to compensate for the client's loss of the sense of smell.

Taste
• Provide foods with various textures that are visually appealing.

Touch
• Monitor subtle changes in behavior, such as confusion, that may indicate a serious illness.
• Reduce the dosage of pain medication, but do not avoid giving the confused client analgesics as needed.

Extended Care
Vision
• Adapt the elderly client's environment so that it is visually stimulating.
• Provide talking books or reading material with large print.

(Text continues on page 240.)

TROUBLESHOOTING HEARING AIDS

Below is a listing of some of the most common problems encountered by clients with hearing aids, along with practical information on probable causes and easily implemented interventions.

Problem	Probable cause	Intervention
Whistling or howling noise	• Excessively high volume	• Reduce the volume when wearing the hearing aid, and keep the device in the "Off" position when removed from the ear (this is especially important if the client has a pet living in the house, as high-pitched whistling attracts animals).
	• Cerumen	• Use an otoscope to examine the client's ear for cerumen buildup. Use carbamide peroxide (Debrox), as needed, to clean the ear.
	• Water or moisture in ear mold or tubing	• Dry out the ear mold or tubing by flushing with air from an empty syringe. Instruct the client to avoid exposing the device to water or perspiration.
	• Improper ear mold positioning	• Readjust the ear mold so that it fits properly under the ear helix. Contact the manufacturer or a hearing aid suply company as necessary.
	• Cracked tubing	• Replace the plastic tubing. Keep a replacement kit with extra parts (wires, plastic tubing, batteries) in the client's home or on the unit.
	• Bad connection between ear mold and amplifier	• Replace the wire.
	• Improperly selected hearing aid	• Help the client to select the proper hearing aid from the four available types: behind-the-ear aid (standard model), in-the-ear aid (typically reserved for mild hearing loss), body aid (typically reserved for significant hearing loss), or eyeglass aid (least popular).
Absence of whistling noise during functional checks (checks are performed by holding the hearing mold outside of the ear before insertion; whistling indicates normal functioning)	• Hearing aid switched to "Off" position	• Turn the switch to the "On" position.
	• Dead battery	• Shut off the hearing aid and replace the battery. Remind the client to change the batteries frequently (weekly when used 10 to 12 hours/day) and to use only batteries recommended by the audiologist. Advice him to store the batteries in a cool, dark place when not in use to extend their wear.
	• Loose wires	• Tighten all wires.
Redness, irritation, pain, or inflammation in ear canal	• Allergic reaction to soft material in ear mold	• Instruct the client to stop using the hearing aid immediately and to seek medical attention. Typically, allergic reactions (redness and irritation) occur shortly after the start of wearing a hearing aid; a harder ear mold material may be needed.
	• Cracked or rough edges on the hearing aid	• Replace worn or damaged parts.
	• Perspiration from hot weather	• Avoid exposing the hearing aid to hot weather.
Inadequate amplification	• Hearing aid turned to "Off" position or volume set too low	• Readjust the volume so that a normal speaking voice can be heard about 3' to 4' (0.9 to 1.2 m) away.
	• Weak or dead battery	• Replace the battery.
	• Cerumen or other material in ear mold	• Check the ear mold daily for cracked or rough edges that can accumulate cerumen or other debris. Instruct the client to clean the ear mold (except an in-the-ear model) weekly.
	• Cerumen in ear canal	• Remove cerumen with Debrox, as necessary.
	• Improperly fitting ear mold	• Assess the client for changes in skin resiliency, tissue structure, and muscle tonicity; refer him to an audiologist as necessary.
	• Disconnected tubing or wire	• Replace the wire or tubing.

TROUBLESHOOTING HEARING AIDS (continued)

Problem	Probable cause	Intervention
Intermittent sound loss	• Dirt lodged in the switch	• Clean the switch using a dry cotton-tipped applicator to remove dirt or debris. Instruct the client to avoid using agents that may clog the microphone, such as hair spray.
	• Loose connection between the amplifier and tubing	• Replace the wires.
	• Poor battery contact	• Rub the connection points of the battery and amplifier with cotton-tipped applicator, pencil eraser, or fine-grade sandpaper to remove dirt, corrosion, or debris.

• Educate the nursing staff about how to properly maintain and clean eyeglasses, contact lenses, and eye prophylaxes.
• Keep extra magnification devices available for the client's use.

Hearing
• Provide an environment that facilitates hearing.
• Maintain the client's hearing aid and encourage him to use it.
• Teach the nursing staff how to clean a hearing aid.
• Schedule all clients for annual audiology examinations.
• Closely monitor the client for ototoxicity to medications.
• Employ someone adept at sign language to communicate with the client.

Smell
• Closely monitor the client's nutritional status.
• Promote communal dining.
• Provide visually appealing food.
• Minimize obnoxious odors in the client's environment.

Taste
• Closely monitor the client's nutritional status.
• Promote communal dining.
• Provide visually appealing food.

Touch
• Monitor the client for subtle changes in behavior, such as confusion, that may indicate a serious illness.
• Reduce dosages of pain medication, but administer analgesics, as necessary.
• Provide diversional activities.
• Create a homelike environment by placing familiar objects in the client's room, such as pictures or a favorite chair.
• Provide pet therapy.
• Promote outside community activities.
• Provide activities that promote sensory stimulation but not pain, such as swimming.

Home care
Vision
• Help the client and the client's family to identify potential safety hazards.
• Help the client and the client's family to obtain adaptive aids.
• Encourage the client to participate in community programs that screen for glaucoma and check visual acuity.

Hearing
• Teach the client and the client's family about adaptive aids, such as a telephone attachment that flashes when the phone rings.
• Provide the client and the client's family with information about appropriate hearing support groups and associations.
• Suggest the use of a person adept at sign language for a companion.

Smell
• Help the client's family to check the home for safety hazards, especially faulty appliances, electric outlets, and plumbing.
• If the client lives alone, ask the fire department or local government to install smoke detectors; ask the gas company to periodically inspect for leaks.
• Help the client learn to prevent foods from spoiling by dating products that spoil quickly and checking the dates periodically.

Taste
• Monitor the client's nutritional status.
• Help the client to obtain the resources necessary to purchase, prepare, and store food (such as through charitable organizations or food stamp programs) or contact Meals On Wheels.

Touch
• Teach the client and the client's family to assess the home for safety hazards.
• Teach the client, especially the diabetic client, to check the insides of his shoes for protruding objects or

rough material before putting them on, because the soles of the foot may have diminished sensation.
• Teach the client and the client's family about hypothermia; emphasize that it can occur in a relatively comfortable environment.

SELECTED REFERENCES

Dornhard, L., ed. *Manual of Clinical Problems in Adult Ambulatory Care.* Boston: Little, Brown & Co., 1985.

Heckheimer, E.F. *Health Promotion of the Elderly in the Community.* Philadelphia: W.B. Saunders Co., 1989.

Mahoney, D.F. "One Simple Solution to Hearing Impairment," *Geriatric Nursing* 8(5):242-45, September/October 1987.

Mendelsohn, S., et al. "Assessment Protocols for Acute Medical Conditions," *Journal of Gerontological Nursing* 12(7):17, July 1986.

Monamaney, T. "Are We Lead by the Nose?" *Discover* 48-56, September 1987.

Smith, A.J., and Aston, S.J. "The Use of Activity in Rehabilitation of Elders with Vision Impairments," *Topics in Geriatric Rehabilitation* 4(4):45-52, July 1989.

NEUROLOGIC SYSTEM

Aphasia

Aphasia, the impaired or lost ability to comprehend or communicate through language because of a brain injury, is a common disorder among older adults. Aphasia typically affects one of four language areas—verbal expression, written expression, auditory comprehension, or reading comprehension—and, in many cases, causes some degrees of deficit in all four areas. These deficits may range from extremely subtle changes to dramatic impairments, depending on the degree and location of brain damage.

Aphasia is usually classified as one of two types—nonfluent or fluent—depending on the client's fluency of verbal expression. In nonfluent aphasia, the client's speech is totally lost or limited to only the use of single words (commonly nouns or verbs) or short phrases. In fluent aphasia, the client's speech is a compilation of words strung together, conveying little or no meaning; in many cases, the words are nonsense or jargon. In both types of aphasia, the client's writing skills tend to parallel his verbal skills and his auditory and reading comprehension may be impaired.

Frequently, those with aphasia have other concomitant conditions that can affect treatment. For example, dysarthria, the inability to move or control the muscles used to speak, can make articulation difficult. Apraxia, the inability to plan and sequence voluntary muscle movement, may affect the muscles involved in speech (verbal apraxia), further impairing the ability to speak, or the muscles of the arms and legs (limb apraxia), impairing the ability to gesture.

ETIOLOGY

Most clients with aphasia have suffered some damage to the major speech centers in the dominant (left) hemisphere of the brain. The most common cause of aphasia in elderly clients is a cerebrovascular accident involving the left hemisphere. In about 25% of all left-handed clients, however, the major speech centers are housed in the nondominant (right) hemisphere; in these instances, aphasia results from damage to the right hemisphere. Aphasia may also result from damage to the subcortical areas of the brain, such as the thalamus, caudate, putamen, and internal capsule.

Other conditions that can cause aphasia include tumors, head injuries, brain abscesses, encephalitis, exposure to toxins, electrolyte imbalance, and anoxia. Clients with early or advanced dementia may have a type of aphasia called anomia.

HEALTH HISTORY FINDINGS

In a health history interview, the client may report or the nurse may detect many of these findings:
• weakness or paralysis
• diminished or absent sense of touch, sight, or hearing
• blurred vision, diplopia, or loss of visual field
• depression
• dementia
• use of antidepressant, hypnotic, sedative, or analgesic medications

PHYSICAL FINDINGS

In a physical examination, the nurse may detect many of these findings:

Neurologic
• dysarthria or verbal apraxia
• diminished sensation on one side of body

Psychological
• decreased alertness and shortened attention span
• confusion

Other
• decreased auditory acuity
• poorly-fitting dentures
• edentia

DIAGNOSTIC STUDIES

The following studies may be performed to evaluate the client's health history status:
• language function screening—to detect fluent or nonfluent aphasia; performed at the client's bedside
• Boston Aphasia Evaluation (BAE), Western Aphasia Battery (WAB), and Porch Index of Communication Ability (PICA)—to determine the client's strengths and weaknesses in specific language areas
• psychological evaluation—to detect depression or dementia, if suspected
• computed tomography (CT) scan, magnetic resonance imaging (MRI) scan, positron emission tomography (PET) scan, or cerebral blood flow studies—to localize the causative lesion and form a prognosis

POTENTIAL COMPLICATIONS
• impaired verbal and written communication
• decreased comprehension
• ineffective coping
• disturbed self-esteem and body image

Nursing diagnosis: *Impaired verbal communication, related to aphasia*

NURSING GOALS: To establish a means of functional communication and to encourage verbalization when possible

Signs and symptoms
• sparse or slurred speech
• anomia or word-selection problems
• unusual speech rhythm
• frequent gesturing
• excessive meaningless speech
• use of nonsense words or jargon
• inappropriate grammar or verb tenses

Interventions

1. Use a calm, positive approach with the client.

2. Pay close attention to the client's attempts to speak.

3. Allow extra time for the client to speak.

4. Encourage the client to speak by not interrupting or prematurely supplying the correct word.

5. Cue the client by providing the initial sound or phoneme of the word or by providing the context.

6. Do not demand perfection or continually correct the client.

7. Ensure your understanding by reflecting the client's message and requesting confirmation.

8. Do not pretend to understand the client when you cannot. Explain that you are having difficulty understanding, and institute other communication strategies.

9. Provide time to practice oral and written exercises as recommended by the speech pathologist, such as saying the alphabet, naming items in a category, or copying letters, words, or phrases.

10. Enhance the client's articulation by encouraging him to wear dentures, if applicable. Advise him to use an adhesive, or to see a dentist to ensure a proper fit.

11. Instruct the client to speak slowly and to pronounce each sound of each word.

12. Encourage the client to practice mouth and tongue exercises as recommended by the speech pathologist, such as frowning, smiling, protruding the tongue and moving it from side to side, and making sounds, such as "la,la,la" or "k,k,k."

Rationales

1. Communication improves when the client is relaxed and perceives empathy and confidence in the listener.

2. The client's body language or inflection may contain clues about what he is trying to say.

3. The client may need time to formulate responses or to retrieve elusive words.

4. If the client anticipates help, he may no longer attempt word retrieval.

5. This technique may facilitate immediate or future word retrieval.

6. The client may feel as though he has failed and stop attempting to speak. The client should begin to monitor his own speech as he improves.

7. This prevents misinterpretation of the client's message.

8. This prevents ignoring a potentially important message.

9. Practice will enhance future performance. The nurse should be careful, however, to challenge the client without consistently frustrating him. If a speech pathologist is unavailable, the nurse should begin with simple exercises and gradually introduce more difficult ones.

10. Edentia or poorly fitting dentures may mimic or contribute to dysarthria.

11. This encourages the client to monitor his speech for clarity.

12. These exercises strengthen and increase the coordination of the muscles of the lips, palate, and tongue.

13. Discourage the staff and the client's family from having the client write messages.

13. This technique usually is limited to the client with dysarthria. It is rarely useful for aphasia; in fact, the client with true aphasia commonly loses the ability to write.

14. Ask "Yes" and "No" questions, beginning with a general category and gradually become more specific.

14. "Yes" and "No" questions allow the client to give simple responses. Even if the client gives inconsistent "Yes" and "No" responses, he may indicate a correct response through body language.

15. Instruct the client to spell messages by pointing to letters on a communication board. Say the letters with the client as he points.

15. A communication board is useful if the client can recognize letters. Saying the letters with the client reinforces speech and may enhance the nurse's understanding.

16. Instruct the client to point to pictures on a communication board or booklet. Make sure the pictures are simple black-and-white line drawings that depict common needs; ensure that the related word is printed below the picture.

16. This method provides stimulation through more than one means, such as through hand signals and pointing and may be effective even in the client with severe aphasia.

17. Encourage gesturing, pantomime, or pointing.

17. Unless the client has severe limb apraxia, gesturing is useful.

18. Document effective gestures and techniques in the client's care plan.

18. Documentation enhances future communication and ensures consistency with new caregivers.

OUTCOME CRITERIA
• The client will communicate effectively using techniques developed in the nursing care plan.
• The client will be able to communicate with the nursing staff and his family.

Nursing diagnosis: *Sensory-perceptual alteration: visual and auditory, related to decreased language comprehension*

NURSING GOALS: To promote independent function through compensatory techniques and to increase language comprehension

Signs and symptoms
• inability to follow oral or written instructions
• inappropriate responses to questions
• inconsistent "Yes" or "No" responses
• inability to recognize pictures, letters, or words

Interventions

1. Provide the client with a quiet environment.

2. To capture the client's attention, stand within the client's visual field and call his name.

3. Allow only one person to speak to the client at a time.

4. Allow extra time for the client to respond.

5. Repeat instructions once, if necessary.

Rationales

1. Minimizing distractions will enhance the client's understanding.

2. This method helps gain the client's attention.

3. Multiple messages make comprehension more difficult.

4. The client may need additional time to process information.

5. Repeating instructions helps to ensure that the client has heard correctly; repeating them only once prevents excessive repetition that can annoy the client.

6. If the client appears not to have understood a question, consider rephrasing the question. For example, if the client fails to respond to "Are you thirsty?", rephrase the question as "Is your mouth dry?"

6. Frequently, a change in wording can provide additional clues to enhance the client's comprehension.

7. Discuss only one subject at a time, and always inform the client when you change the subject.

7. The aphasic client frequently has difficulty processing more than one idea or distinguishing a change in the focus of conversation.

8. Provide visual cues, such as pictures, pantomime, or pointing.

8. Visual cues provide additional information and increase the likelihood that the client will understand.

9. Show the client what you want by demonstrations or by physically taking the client through the motions while providing a simple explanation.

9. Demonstrations provide auditory, visual, and tactile stimulation, which help to increase the client's comprehension.

10. When providing care, be sure to follow an established routine that is familiar to the client.

10. Providing a consistent pattern (time structuring), enables the client to predict at what time each day an event will occur. In time, the client should learn to anticipate the task and may perform the activity automatically.

11. Simplify the client's activities by giving one-step commands.

11. Simplifying activities improves the client's understanding and enhances his performance.

OUTCOME CRITERION
• The client will understand the form of communication developed by the nurses.

Nursing diagnosis: *Ineffective individual coping, related to the inability to communicate needs*

NURSING GOAL: To meet the client's immediate needs while provoking minimal frustration

Signs and symptoms
• sighing
• cursing
• angry outbursts
• crying

Interventions

1. Anticipate the client's emotional outbursts; express understanding, and avoid chastising him.

2. Attempt to consistently assign the same caregivers to the client.

3. When planning the client's activities, try to intersperse challenging or new tasks with familiar tasks the client has already mastered.

4. Consider temporarily changing a subject if the client is having difficulty comprehending. Request the client's permission before changing the subject.

Rationales

1. The client who has suffered brain injury may have difficulty controlling emotions. Nurses should learn to anticipate outbursts and should try to be supportive.

2. Consistency may minimize both the client's and the staff's frustration by allowing the caregiver to learn to anticipate some of the client's needs.

3. The client will tolerate failures better if they are tempered by successes.

4. This may decrease the client's frustration and allow the caregiver time to plan a new approach.

OUTCOME CRITERION
• The client will develop effective coping mechanisms for handling his communication impairment.

Nursing diagnosis: *Self-esteem disturbance related to depression and the inability to speak clearly*

NURSING GOALS: To provide support and to promote the client's willingness to attempt speech

Signs and symptoms
• decreased initiation of speech
• apathy
• decreased interest in personal appearance
• social withdrawal

Interventions

1. Assess the client's strengths, and encourage him to incorporate them in conversation.

2. Set short-term goals and praise the client for his progress.

3. Inform the client that progress is possible, but that it may be a gradual process.

4. Praise the client's desirable behaviors.

5. Keep the complexity of the conversation geared toward the client's comprehension level.

6. Avoid speaking loudly unless the client has a hearing deficit.

7. Do not force the client to speak against his will.

8. Avoid talking about the client when he is within earshot.

9. Schedule pleasurable activities at regular intervals.

Rationales

1. Success and positive feedback increase self-esteem and performance.

2. This provides positive feedback and evidence of the client's progress.

3. This allows the client to have a realistic but positive attitude.

4. Rewards of acceptance, support, and encouragement permit the client to accept his disability and to concentrate on his remaining abilities.

5. Although an aphasic client is not necessarily less intelligent, he may require some simplification to understand.

6. Speaking loudly will not increase the client's understanding and may only frustrate him.

7. Speech requires the client's cooperation; not forcing the client to speak shows respect for his feelings.

8. Talking about the client when he is within earshot conveys a lack of respect.

9. This provides the client with something positive to anticipate.

OUTCOME CRITERION
• The client will develop self-esteem through an improved ability to communicate.

Nursing diagnosis: *Impaired social interaction related to communication impairment*

NURSING GOALS: To encourage participation in group conversations and to stimulate communication

Signs and symptoms
• reluctance to participate in conversation
• avoidance of social events
• withdrawal from family or friends

Interventions

1. Engage the client in conversation whenever possible, and encourage the client's family and friends to do the same.

2. Choose topics of conversation that are familiar or relevant to the client.

3. Provide stimulation through the controlled use of radio, television, tapes, and records.

Rationales

1. Even if the client can only say "Yes" and "No" or gesture, he can participate in appropriately structured conversations.

2. The client may be more willing to participate if the topic has personal significance.

3. The client should benefit from hearing conversational speech; however, he should be protected from sensory overload.

OUTCOME CRITERION
• The client will begin interacting socially with other clients or groups.

NURSING ACTIONS IN VARIOUS SETTINGS
Nursing actions for a client with aphasia depend on the setting in which care is provided. This section identifies which actions are appropriate in all settings and which pertain to acute care, extended care, or home care situations.

All settings
• Evaluate the client at the bedside for aphasia.
• Explain that aphasia is a communication problem that may involve speaking, writing, reading, and understanding speech.
• Explain the relationship between aphasia and the client's underlying condition.
• Teach the client's family effective communication techniques.
• Encourage family participation in speech therapy sessions.
• Inform the family what to expect in terms of recovery.
• Provide the client and the client's family with written materials concerning aphasia.

Acute care
• Establish appropriate communication methods as advised by the speech pathologist.
• Reinforce skills the client learns in speech therapy.
• When planning the client's discharge, consider his need for continued speech therapy, periodic reevaluation, and intensive family instruction.

Extended care
• Establish a method of functional communication.
• Perform speech exercises with the client.
• Periodically reevaluate the client's progress and strengths.
• Involve the family in the client's treatment whenever possible.

Home care
• Perform the same interventions listed for extended care.
• Provide ongoing support and direction to ensure family involvement.
• Suggest an attendant, respite care, or a medical alert system to ensure the client's safety when the family is unavailable.

SELECTED REFERENCES
Albert, M.L., and Helm-Estabrooks, N. "Diagnosis and Treatment of Aphasia: Part 1," *Journal of the American Medical Association* 259(7):1043-47, February 19, 1988.
Albert, M.L., and Helm-Estabrooks, N. "Diagnosis and Treatment of Aphasia: Part 2," *Journal of the American Medical Association* 259(8):1205-10, February 26, 1988.
Flicker, C., et al. "Implications of Memory and Language Dysfunction in the Naming Deficit of Senile Dementia," *Brain & Language* 31(2):187-200, 1987.
MacKay, S., et al. "Methods to Assess Aphasic Stroke Patients," *Geriatric Nursing* 9(3):177-179, May/June 1988.
Pimental, P.A. "Alterations in Communication: Biopsychosocial Aspects of Aphasia, Dysarthria, and Right Hemispheric Syndromes in the Stroke Patient," *Nursing Clinics of North America* 21(2):321-37, February 1986.
Tanner, D.C., et al. "Guidelines for Treatment of Chronic Depression in the Aphasic Patient," *Rehabilitation Nursing* 14(2): 77-80, March/April 1989.

ENDOCRINE SYSTEM
Diabetes Mellitus

Diabetes mellitus, a metabolic disorder caused by insulin deficiency or the ineffective use of insulin and characterized by hyperglycemia and glycosuria, affects nearly 20% of those over age 65. Almost 30% of all older adults have impaired glucose tolerance, a condition characterized by plasma glucose levels that are higher than normal but too low to fit the diagnostic criteria for diabetes, and are sometimes labeled "borderline diabetic." The incidence of both diabetes mellitus and impaired glucose tolerance increases with age.

Most elderly diabetic clients are classified as having Type II noninsulin-dependent diabetes (formerly called adult-onset diabetes), which constitutes about 80% of all the diagnosed cases of diabetes mellitus in the United States. In this type, which typically presents in obese clients over age 40 who have relatively few of the classic symptoms (thirst, weight loss and polyuria), onset is gradual; the client may have a significant carbohydrate intolerance that remains undetected for years. When positively diagnosed, this type of diabetes is usually controlled through dietary adjustments, exercise, and the administration of oral hypoglycemic agents; in some cases, however, insulin may be necessary.

Diseases and conditions associated with diabetes mellitus and impaired glucose tolerance that may affect the elderly client include chronic pancreatitis, pheochromocytoma, and Cushing's disease.

ETIOLOGY
Although glucose tolerance deteriorates with age, the exact reason for this is unknown. Researchers, however, have been able to identify some of the causes of impaired glucose tolerance and thus diabetes mellitus in the elderly client, the most significant of which include altered insulin action at the receptor, postreceptor, or intracellular level; and reduced synthesis or secretion of insulin by the pancreas. Contributing factors include decreased muscle mass and increased fat deposits, poor nutrition, genetic tendancy toward obesity, reduced physical activity, acute illness, and medication use.

HEALTH HISTORY FINDINGS
In a health history interview, the client may report or the nurse may detect many of these findings:
• extreme fatigue
• depressive psychosis
• polydipsia
• polyphagia
• diarrhea or constipation
• nausea and vomiting
• polyuria
• numbness and tingling in extremities
• impotence

• calf pain with exercise
• syncope
• headache
• drowsiness
• use of diuretics, antihypertensives, corticosteroids, phenytoin, estrogen, beta blockers, or antianxiety agents
• recurrent skin, intertriginous, or urinary tract infections
• history of renal disease, hyperthyroidism, carcinoma, or pernicious anemia
• history of peripheral vascular disease, coronary artery disease, or congestive heart failure
• history of frequent infections, accidents, or burns
• family history of diabetes

PHYSICAL FINDINGS
In a physical examination, the nurse may detect many of these findings:

Integumentary
• lesions on the soles of the feet and between the toes
• ischemic ulcers
• cool extremities

Gastrointestinal
• ill-fitting dentures
• loose, brittle, or missing teeth
• periodontal disease
• palpable and percussable bladder
• fecal impaction

Neurologic
• absent knee and ankle reflexes
• sensory loss
• decreased peripheral pulses

Other
• obesity
• blurred vision
• senile cataracts
• macular degeneration and edema
• opacification of the lens or cornea
• proliferative or hemorrhagic retinopathy

DIAGNOSTIC STUDIES
The following studies may be performed to evaluate the client's health status:
• random blood glucose screening—to detect abnormal levels indicating hyperglycemia; a level of 200 mg/dl or greater is considered positive
• fasting plasma glucose test—to detect abnormal levels indicating hyperglycemia; a level of 140 mg/dl on at least two separate occasions is considered positive

• 2-hour oral glucose tolerance test (HbgA₁C)—to diagnose impaired glucose tolerance; a level between 140 and 200 mg/dl is considered positive; however, the test is expensive and unreliable
• glycosylated hemoglobin test (HgA₁C)—to reveal the average percentage of total hemoglobin linked to glucose over the previous 4 to 10 weeks; performed every 2 to 3 months to reveal the degree of glycemic control over time

POTENTIAL COMPLICATIONS
• depression
• hypoglycemia
• diabetic ketoacidosis

• hyperglycemia or hyperosmolar nonketotic syndrome (HNKS)
• cardiovascular disease or myocardial infarction
• cerebrovascular accident
• retinopathy
• senile cataracts
• neurogenic bladder
• impotence
• pain
• constipation or diarrhea
• foot lesions

Nursing diagnosis: *Potential for injury related to hypoglycemia secondary to oral hypoglycemic agents or insulin therapy*

NURSING GOAL: To prevent injury by identifying and preventing low blood glucose levels

Signs and symptoms
• shakiness
• sweating
• palpitations
• blurred vision
• tachycardia
• confusion
• loss of consciousness

Interventions

1. Assess the client for the symptoms of hypoglycemia, including fatigue, weakness, headache, sweating, shakiness, palpitations, or slurred speech.

2. If the client becomes hypoglycemic, take the following measures:
• Provide a safe environment, encourage the client to rest, institute seizure precautions, and notify the physician.

• Give the conscious client 10 to 15 g of a fast-acting carbohydrate (such as 6 oz of orange juice, five or six pieces of hard candy, or four sugar cubes); wait 15 minutes, then repeat if necessary. Follow up with a meal.

• Give the unconscious client 1 mg of glucagon S.C. or an I.V. bolus of dextrose 50%.

3. Monitor the client's normal eating habits. Identify whether financial constraints, ill-fitting dentures, tooth loss, medication side effects, or cognitive disorders are contributing to the client's hypoglycemia.

4. Monitor the client's alcohol consumption.

5. Review the client's physical activity and suggest changes as necessary.

Rationales

1. Early detection of hypoglycemia can prevent a mild reaction from becoming severe.

2. Immediate action is necessary to prevent the client from going into hypoglycemic shock.
• Safety measures are important, as severe hypoglycemia can cause the client to lose consciousness and have a seizure.

• Rapidly absorbed carbohydrates elevate the blood glucose and reverse hypoglycemic symptoms.

• Glucagon stimulates the liver to release glycogen, thus raising the blood glucose level.

3. These problems may cause the client to miss, skip, delay, or cut back on meals, causing his blood sugar level to drop.

4. Alcohol causes the liver to release glucose and can result in hypoglycemia overnight.

5. Exercise causes the muscles to take up glucose and reduces the blood glucose level.

6. Consider whether the client's use of oral hypoglycemic agents is a possible cause of hypoglycemia, and consult the physician about necessary dosage adjustments.

6. Oral hypoglycemic agents, such as chlorpropamide, have long-acting metabolites and can cause severe hypoglycemia in clients with renal or hepatic disease.

7. Determine whether the client has any visual, cognitive, or physical impairments that are interfering with his ability to accurately draw up insulin doses.

7. Errors in dosage can cause hypoglycemia.

8. Encourage the client with poor vision to use a glucose meter instead of reading glucose test strips.

8. Glucose meters provide more accurate results than those obtained by comparing test strips to a color chart. The client may misread the color chart, take too much insulin, and develop hypoglycemia.

9. Review the client's medication regimen for possible causes of hypoglycemia.

9. Highly protein-bound medications, such as warfarin sodium, sulfonamides, or nonsteroidal anti-inflammatory agents, compete with protein-binding sites. This causes an increase in circulating sulfonylurea, which results in hypoglycemia. Such drugs as beta blockers, aspirin, or alcohol may mask or induce hypoglycemia by blocking the production of glucose by the liver or displacing sulfonylurea.

10. Consider contacting the client's family, a neighbor, a nutritional service, Meals On Wheels, homemaker services, or an adult day-care center to ensure that the client receives properly balanced meals.

10. Community resources can help the client to obtain adequate nutrition while maintaining independence.

11. Teach the client at high risk for hypoglycemia to monitor his blood glucose level. The client with unstable diabetes who receives multiple daily insulin injections, has a tendency to develop severe ketosis or hypoglycemia, and who typically experiences hypoglycemic episodes without the usual warning symptoms (such as anxiety, trembling, and hunger) is at high risk.

11. Self-monitoring blood glucose tests help the client to control his blood glucose level, which may help reduce the risk of acute and chronic complications.

OUTCOME CRITERION
• The client will maintain normal blood glucose levels by following a proper diet and by monitoring for signs and symptoms of hypoglycemia.

Nursing diagnosis: *Fluid volume deficit related to abnormal fluid loss associated with HNKS*

NURSING GOALS: To restore normal plasma volume, to reduce the client's blood glucose level, and to maintain fluid and electrolyte balance

Signs and symptoms
• elevated blood glucose level
• serum osmolality greater than 350 mOsm/kg
• decreased blood pressure
• increased pulse rate
• elevated serum creatinine level
• hyponatremia
• acute confusion, delirium, stupor, or coma
• profound dehydration

Interventions

1. Assess the client for signs and symptoms of hyperglycemia, including frequent urination, headache, drowsiness, stomach pain, rapid breathing, fruity breath smell, and nausea and vomiting.

2. Obtain specimens for laboratory studies (such as blood glucose, serum osmolality, electrolyte, blood urea nitrogen, creatinine, hematocrit, and hemoglobin levels and urine specific gravity and arterial blood gas studies), as ordered.

3. Test the client's urine for ketones.

4. Institute fluid replacement therapy, as ordered. Administer 4 liters or more of I.V. fluids over 12 to 24 hours, beginning with normal saline solution, then switching to a dextrose solution as the client's blood glucose level stabalizes.

5. Assess the client for signs and symptoms of congestive heart failure (such as orthopnea, dyspnea, anxiety, neck vein distention, and S_3 gallop heart sounds) during fluid replacement. Notify the physician if such symptoms are noted.

6. Administer regular insulin intravenously, titrated according to blood glucose levels and other laboratory data, or as ordered.

7. Observe the client for complications of hyperglycemia and ketoacidosis, including hypokalemia, cardiac irregularities, hypotension, renal insufficiency, and thrombotic events (such as myocardial infarction, cerebrovascular accident, or transient ischemic attack).

8. Identify factors that may have precipitated severe hyperglycemia and HNKS, such as administration of a new medication (specifically a diuretic or beta blocker), an acute illness, a documented increase in glucose or ketone levels, or an infection.

Rationales

1. Severe hyperglycemia in an elderly client with insulin-dependent diabetes can lead to the breakdown of body fat for energy when insufficient insulin is available to convert blood glucose into energy.

2. These laboratory values reflect the client's state of hydration and tissue and renal perfusion.

3. During episodes of severe hyperglycemia, acetone, one of the ketone substances, is excreted in urine.

4. Polyuria leads to intracellular dehydration and to HNKS. Sufficient I.V. fluids increase intravascular fluid volume; the specific fluid ordered usually depends on the degree of hypotension and the client's electrolyte values.

5. The elderly client may develop congestive heart failure with rapid fluid replacement because of reduced cardiac reserves.

6. Insulin forces glucose into the cells and liver, thereby decreasing the degree of hyperglycemia. Because the severely dehydrated client with poor peripheral circulation absorbs S.C. or I.M. insulin poorly, insulin is administered I.V.

7. Hyperglycemia and ketoacidosis can cause dehydration and salt depletion. Serum potassium levels can plummet when insulin therapy causes the cells to take up glucose. This can be lethal in the client who has underlying cardiac disease. The client who takes nonpotassium-sparing diuretics is especially at risk. Cardiac irregularities may result from potassium abnormalities and rapid rehydration. Severe dehydration causes hypotension and decreased renal blood flow, which can result in renal failure in the elderly client. Exacerbation of hyperglycemia may lead to a greater fluid loss, a thrombotic event, and postural hypotension.

8. Timely identification of the causative factor may prevent recurrent severe hyperglycemia and HNKS. The client receiving diuretics or beta blockers may not be receiving adequate fluids; an acute illness can cause glucose, and possibly ketone, levels to rise; a documented increase in glucose or ketones may signal an unrecognized illness. Infection is the chief cause of hyperglycemia in the elderly client.

OUTCOME CRITERIA
• The client will not develop HNKS.
• The client's blood glucose level will return to normal after institution of appropriate interventions.

Nursing diagnosis: *Sensory-perceptual alteration: visual, related to diabetic retinopathy and cataracts*

NURSING GOALS: To delay or prevent visual impairment, when possible, and to help the client adapt to his visual impairment

Signs and symptoms
- microaneurysm
- blurred vision, "floaters," or "cobwebs" in the client's visual field
- sudden and painless loss of vision
- reduced visual acuity
- inability to perform insulin self-injection, foot care, or glucose self-monitoring
- glare intolerance
- corneal opacity

Interventions

1. Examine each of the client's eyes, noting the pupil's size and reaction to light and any opacity of the crystalline lens.

2. Assess the client's visual acuity by checking his ability to read newspaper print or a Snellen eye chart.

3. Teach the client about the importance of obtaining an annual visual examination, including pupil dilatation and an ophthalmoscopic examination.

4. Assess to what degree the client's vision loss affects his ability to function; determine whether visual aids, such as magnifiers or large print materials, would be helpful.

5. Instruct the client to follow his physician's recommendations to control hypertension.

6. Maintain tight control of the client's blood glucose levels by having the client monitor his own values.

7. Determine whether the client can differentiate between the green and brown tones used in urine glucose monitoring.

8. Teach the client and caregiver about the various treatments for diabetic retinopathy, such as photocoagulation (laser treatment) and vitrectomy.

9. As cataracts progress, refer the client to an ophthalmologist for evaluation.

Rationales

1. The diabetic client is at high risk for developing senile cataracts, a condition found in over 40% of all elderly clients. As cataracts mature, the pupil undergoes mydriasis and exhibits a diminished reaction to light. The red reflex typically disappears.

2. An assessment will quantify the degree of visual loss.

3. Early detection and treatment of eye changes can prevent proliferative retinopathy and blindness. Diabetic retinopathy commonly occurs without symptoms, necessitating a retinal examination through dilated pupils.

4. An assessment should identify the need for support services. Visual aids will help the client maintain independence.

5. Hypertension may accelerate diabetic retinopathy and retinal hemorrhages.

6. Normalization of blood glucose levels may reduce or delay retinal changes.

7. Such monitoring is useless if the client cannot discern green and brown tones. He may need to monitor his blood glucose using another testing method, such as an electronic blood glucose monitor.

8. Teaching reduces anxiety, enhances knowledge, prepares the client for potential side effects, and promotes an optimal outcome. Laser treatments prevent the progression of retinopathy to a proliferative stage and may delay or prevent hemorrhage and blindness; however, vision typically does not improve and may worsen slightly. Vitrectromy, which is performed when the client has had a retinal hemorrhage and loses his vision, removes hemorrhagic tissue from the vitreous; it may restore vision and prevent retinal detachment.

9. Cataract surgery on the elderly diabetic client is controversial because surgical trauma may accelerate retinopathy. Alternative therapies, such as the use of aldosereductase to reduce the amount of sugar alcohol in the lens, may be suggested.

10. Promote maximum independence by teaching the client self-care skills to compensate for his visual impairment, such as using a magnifier for syringe calibrations or using monitoring and injection devices designed for visually impaired or blind clients.

10. Clients with visual impairment or motor neuropathy need assistance to prepare and administer insulin.

11. Refer to the client to appropriate vocational rehabilitation programs and other support services, such as the American Diabetes Association.

11. Various formal community and national organizations can provide supportive services to the elderly diabetic client.

OUTCOME CRITERION
• The client will demonstrate an ability to perform self-care measures that require visual acuity, such as administering insulin and performing blood glucose self-monitoring.

Nursing diagnosis: *Potential for injury related to autonomic and peripheral neuropathies*

NURSING GOALS: To prevent falls and disability and to decrease pain

Signs and symptoms
• observable trauma
• decreased sense of touch, pain, and temperature sensation
• decreased vibration in legs and hands
• pale, cold extremities with scant hair
• decreased mobility
• impaired performance of activities of daily living
• pain or burning in legs
• diminished or absent deep tendon reflexes
• diminished or absent pedal, popliteal, and femoral pulses

Interventions

1. Assess the client's extremities for diminished peripheral pulses and ulcers.

2. Assess the client for postural hypotension.

3. Assess the client for nighttime pain; advise the client take a mild analgesic, such as acetaminophen, or to go for a walk.

4. Perform a neurologic examination, testing for postural control (such as a righting reflex, proprioception, orthostatic hypotension, and swaying), balance tests (such as the Romberg test; guard the client during this manuever), and sensation (such as touch, pain, temperature, and vibration).

Rationales

1. The basement membranes of smaller blood vessels throughout the body gradually thicken in the diabetic client, causing the lumens of the veins to narrow, reducing their ability to carry blood. Decreased circulation to the peripheral vessels can lead to ulcerations and skin breakdown.

2. Autonomic neuropathies affect the vagal and sympathetic nerves, causing postural hypotension that can precipitate falls.

3. Pain results when blood supply and stimulation of the blood vessels decreases. Analgesics relieve pain, and walking increases the movement of blood through the vessels.

4. High glucose levels over months or years can damage nerves and cause numbness, tingling, burning, or pain in the lower legs and feet. The diabetic client should be tested for postural control, as an alteration (such as that in orthostatic hypotension) can precipitate falls. The diabetic client also has reduced reflex activity and should be tested for balance. Vibratory sense decreases by as much as 50% in the elderly client, primarily because of an increased threshold for vibration. In the diabetic client, the loss of the sense of vibration begins in the legs and progresses upward.

5. Ask the client if he has suffered any recent falls. Observe him for unusual behavior, such as a reluctance to undress during the examination.

5. The elderly client frequently does not report injuries suffered from falls because he fears hospitalization or institutionalization. Also, because the elderly client commonly has diminished sensation, pain may not be apparent; therefore, the nurse must ask the client about recent falls and observe him for unusual behavior.

6. Observe the client's ability to ambulate and whether the client uses an assistive device.

6. The client who clings to furniture as he ambulates may have an unsteady gait. Also, the use of an assistive device indicates that the client has difficulty walking.

7. Observe the client's ability to climb and descend stairs.

7. Because of autonomic dysfunction, the diabetic client has difficulty judging the height of stairs. Also, the elderly client has a tendency to not lift his legs high enough when climbing stairs.

8. Advise the client wear elastic stockings, if not contraindicated.

8. Elastic stockings increase venous return and decrease the effects of neuropathies.

9. Instruct the client to wear low-heeled, well-fitting shoes that offer good support.

9. Improper shoe fit can result in accidental falls.

10. Caution the client against wearing tight garments, such as girdles, and sitting with crossed legs.

10. Tight clothing and crossed legs constrict already compromised blood vessels.

11. Teach the client to check the temperature of his bath water with his elbow before bathing and to use potholders when cooking.

11. Peripheral neuropathy reduces the client's temperature sensitivity, placing him at risk for burns.

OUTCOME CRITERIA
• The client will identify the symptoms of peripheral neuropathies and describe appropriate measures to prevent resultant trauma.
• The client will be free from neuropathic pain.

Nursing diagnosis: *Potential for impaired skin integrity related to diminished sensitivity*

NURSING GOAL: To enhance the client's knowledge of specific foot-care measures

Signs and symptoms
• foot drop or Charcot's joint
• hyperesthesia
• foot blanching upon elevation and ruboring when dependent
• dryness and fissuring on the heels and interdigital spaces
• atrophic skin changes on legs
• leg ulcers or gangrene
• cold feet, intermittent claudication, or nocturnal cramps
• calluses, corns, or ingrown nails
• absent or diminished hair growth
• slow or nonhealing leg or foot wounds

Interventions

1. Check the client's feet, including between the toes, for soft-tissue injuries, dryness, cracked skin, color or temperature changes, or corns and calluses.

Rationales

1. Neuropathies can cause changes in the skin and soft tissues of the feet.

2. Assess the client's feet for a hammertoe deformity.

2. A hammertoe deformity results from toe muscle weakness and tendon shortening because of neuropathies. This deformity increases the client's risk for skin breakdown.

3. Teach the client to inspect his feet daily for ingrown, sharp, or jagged nails, reactive hyperemia (a Stage 1 pressure sore), signs of foot trauma, and calluses, corns, or bunions.

3. A proper foot examination can identify injuries that may otherwise go undetected.

4. Teach the client and caregiver proper diabetic foot care.

4. Early detection and intervention can reduce the risk of serious foot complications.

5. Teach the client to avoid soaking feet regularly unless prescribed by a physician or podiatrist.

5. Regular, routine soaking can dry the skin excessively and cause cracks that act as portals of entry for bacteria.

6. Instruct the client in proper foot care. Advise him to avoid walking barefoot, even when indoors; to routinely care for toe nails through self-care or by visiting a podiatrist; to avoid using over-the-counter medications or chemical agents to treat corns, calluses, or warts; to wear only thick-soled, wide-toed shoes made of soft leather; to break in new shoes gradually; and to routinely inspect the insides of shoes for sharp objects, rough areas, and thick seams.

6. Foot neuropathy reduces the client's sensitivity to injury. Wearing shoes protects the feet from injury. Proper, routine foot care prevents breaks in the skin, the possibility of infection, and serious complications that can lead to gangrene and possible amputation. Avoiding over-the-counter foot medications prevents injury from harsh chemicals that can burn the epidermis. Wearing thick-soled, wide-toed shoes redistributes pressure points; soft leather promotes shoe flexibility and allows the foot to breath. Gradually breaking in new shoes prevents blister formation. Routine shoe inspection can prevent injuries, as the client with neuropathy commonly has impaired sensitivity and may be unable to feel sharp or rough objects.

7. Advise the client to stop smoking, if applicable.

7. Smoking causes vasoconstriction, and the diabetic client already has a compromised vascular system.

OUTCOME CRITERION
• The client will describe and demonstrate appropriate skin and foot care and will have no evidence of skin breakdown.

Nursing diagnosis: *Altered nutrition: more than body requirements related to uncontrolled hyperglycemia or glucose intolerance*

NURSING GOAL: To help the client control or modify his diet to facilitate weight loss

Signs and symptoms
• body weight 20% greater than ideal weight
• high-fat diet
• uncontrolled hyperglycemia

Interventions

1. Place the client on a weight loss program, if necessary. Weigh him weekly, and record the results.

2. Advise the client to keep a food diary that details moods and events immediately preceding meals and snacks.

Rationales

1. Weight loss increases the number of insulin receptors, thereby reducing insulin resistance and improving blood glucose control.

2. Behavior modification helps remold eating habits. A food diary can help the client identify and control the causes of eating binges.

3. Teach the client to restrict dietary fat to no more than 30% or 35% of his total calorie intake and to use only polyunsaturated fat. Also caution him to limit his sodium intake.

3. Researchers have identified a strong correlation between diabetes and cardiovascular disease. Hyperlipidemia can exacerbate the macrovascular complications of diabetes.

4. Recommend that the client participate in a regular exercise program, such as walking, golfing, gardening, or swimming.

4. Exercise improves glucose tolerance, decreases insulin resistance, and increases the number of insulin receptors. Exercise also helps the client to reduce weight and lower lipid levels, which reduces the cardiac risk factors.

5. Advise the client to eat a diet that includes 40 mg of fiber per day. Inform him that common sources of fiber include bran cereals, vegetables, fruits, and whole grain breads.

5. Fiber delays carbohydrate absorption, which reduces the speed at which glucose enters the bloodstream. Fiber also improves the efficiency of endogenous insulin, promotes weight loss, and reduces the client's need for insulin or oral hypoglycemic medications.

6. Advise the client to space his meals about 5 hours apart.

6. Approximately 5 hours are needed for blood glucose levels to return to a baseline level after a meal. Additional food intake during that interval abnormally elevates glucose levels.

7. Refer the client to a dietician for teaching about exchange lists, calorie counting, and diet plans.

7. Proper diet is the cornerstone of diabetes management. Individualized teaching can provide support, encouragement, and simplified instructions.

8. Teach the client that he can tolerate a large amount of carbohydrates only if he controls calorie intake. Explain that carbohydrates must come from complex carbohydrates, such as rice, corn, or potatoes, and not from simple sugars.

8. Because the body digests complex carbohydrates slower than simple sugars, these carbohydrates cause less of a rise in blood glucose levels.

9. Advise the client to avoid alcohol completely or to drink only small amounts of alcohol with meals.

9. Heavy drinking can precipitate painful diabetic neuropathy and hyperglycemia. If the client drinks alcoholic beverages without eating or drinking nonalcoholic beverages, the alcohol can cause hypoglycemia by decreasing blood glucose, diminishing the action of insulin, and interfering with the body's ability to produce glucose in response to falling blood glucose levels.

OUTCOME CRITERIA
- The client will adhere to a therapeutic, diabetic diet.
- The client will maintain his weight, or lose weight, according to established goals.

Nursing diagnosis: *Potential for infection related to vaginal candidiasis*

NURSING GOAL: To prevent vaginal infections

Signs and symptoms
- intense vulval or vaginal itching
- dysuria or incontinence
- dyspareunia
- erythematous or edematous external genitalia
- thick, white, curdy vaginal discharge

Interventions

1. Assess the perineum of the client at high risk for vaginal infections daily during bathing. The client who is obese, has poor hygiene, are under stress, or is immunosuppressed is at greatest risk.

2. Inspect the client's external genitalia, noting erythema, edema, or lesions.

3. Assess the client and the client's sexual partner for symptoms of infection, and note the onset and duration of the symptoms as well as aggravating or alleviating factors.

4. Obtain blood glucose levels as necessary; provide immediate treatment to correct hyperglycemic episodes.

5. Insert a moistened saline swab into the client's vagina, and culture any drainage. Roll the swab onto a clean glass slide for bacteriologic studies, as ordered.

6. Recommend the use of boric acid douches (2 tablespoons of boric acid crystals in 1 pint of warm water), as needed.

7. Teach the client correct perineal hygiene. Advise the client to avoid perineal sprays and powders, to always wipe from the front to back after voiding or defecating, and to avoid nylon garments and tight clothing.

8. Instruct the client to relieve irritating symptoms until a diagnosis is confirmed by applying a water-soluble lubricant or cool compresses to the vaginal orifice daily.

9. Instruct the client in the proper use of vaginal antibiotic creams or suppositories, if prescribed. Advise the client to use the medication for 3 to 7 nights, to instill the medication while recumbent, and to avoid coitus until therapy is complete.

Rationales

1. Vision loss may prevent the client from observing leukorrhea, and she may attribute dyspareunia to atrophic changes of the vagina. Also, the vaginal pH becomes alkaline with age, placing the elderly female client at high risk for infection.

2. Infection may cause intense vulval inflammation and bleeding. Satellite lesions may also occur.

3. The elderly female client is particularly prone to candidal vulvovaginitis because of postmenopausal changes in the vagina.

4. Uncontrolled diabetes prevents the control or cure of vaginitis.

5. Vaginal culturing is necessary to confirm a fungal infection.

6. The diabetic female is at high risk for candidal infections. Boric acid douches are an economical prophylactic.

7. These measures help prevent infection.

8. Cool compresses and lubricants help soothe irritated mucosa.

9. Proper use of vaginal medication will ensure direct treatment to the infected area.

OUTCOME CRITERIA
- The client will have controlled blood glucose levels.
- The client will institute appropriate measures to treat vaginal infections.

Nursing diagnosis: *Knowledge deficit related to the disorder, glucose monitoring, and usual treatments*

NURSING GOALS: To teach the client and caregiver about diabetes, including its treatment and complications, and to instruct the client and caregiver in the various methods of glucose monitoring

Signs and symptoms
- newly diagnosed diabetes mellitus
- expressed lack of knowledge about diabetes or glucose monitoring

Interventions

1. Identify any barriers to learning, such as visual, hearing, or cognitive impairments or low literacy.

2. Limit teaching sessions to 10 minutes each.

3. Ask the client to demonstrate or repeat instructions for diet, exercise, and medications.

4. Promote a positive attitude and encourage the active participation of the client and the client's family in setting goals.

5. Teach the client and caregiver about the benefits of and the steps for blood glucose self-monitoring. Instruct the client to prick the sides of his finger pads with a needle, using a different finger each time; apply a drop of blood to a chemically treated strip; and insert the prepared strip into a glucose meter.

6. Teach the client who is unable or unwilling to perform blood glucose self-monitoring to test his urine using tablets or a dipstick. Instruct him to obtain one specimen 30 to 60 minutes before bedtime and another specimen within 30 minutes before eating a meal.

7. Teach the client and caregiver about the use of oral hypoglycemic agents.

8. Explain to the client and the client's family the importance of avoiding stress.

9. Instruct the client taking insulin to rotate injection sites between the upper arms, abdomen, and thighs. Instruct the obese client to use a long 18G needle, pinch the skin, then insert the needle at a 90-degree angle. Instruct the thin client to use a small needle, pinch the skin, then inject the needle at a 45-degree angle.

10. Assess the client's need for home follow-up.

11. Use available resources, such as dietitians, nurse specialists, and audiovisual and printed educational aids, when teaching the client.

12. Teach the client and the client's family about hypoglycemia, including its causes, symptoms, treatment, and prevention. Emphasize the importance of wearing a diabetes identification bracelet or necklace and carrying a fast-acting carbohydrate (such as orange juice, hard candy, or sugar cubes) at all times.

Rationales

1. Identifying such barriers helps the nurse to develop effective teaching strategies. Effective strategies might include having a family member or neighbor sit in on teaching sessions, using written instructions with large print, or providing magnification devices.

2. This will prevent information overload.

3. This will ensure that the client understands the instructions.

4. Participation and mutual goal setting increases understanding of, and adherence to, instructions.

5. Blood glucose self-monitoring allows the client to see firsthand how his blood glucose level is responding to treatment; it also provides an immediate incentive for adhering to his diet and exercise programs.

6. Although this type of testing provides limited information, urine glucose testing can be performed fairly easily and can be useful. Since the elderly client has a high renal threshold for glucose, he may be hyperglycemic before glucose appears in the urine.

7. Oral hypoglycemic agents stimulate the beta cells of the pancreas to produce insulin and increase the receptivity to insulin by the cells.

8. Stressful situations cause storage sites to release glucose, which elevates blood glucose levels.

9. Because the elderly client typically has a lesser amount of fatty tissue, rotating sites prevents tissue trauma. Pinching the skin separates the subcutaneous tissue from the underlying muscle and allows the injection to occur in the subcutaneous tissue. Using a long needle and a 90-degree angle ensures that the medication will reach the subcutaneous area; a short needle and a 45-degree angle, that the needle does not extend below subcutaneous fatty tissue into the muscle.

10. An assessment will determine the client's ability to adequately care for himself.

11. These resources enhance learning.

12. Instruction reduces the incidence of hypoglycemia.

OUTCOME CRITERIA
• The client and the client's family will verbalize an understanding of the disorder, prescribed regimen, and complications.
• The client will effectively demonstrate diabetes-related tasks.

Nursing diagnosis: *Noncompliance related to the inability to administer insulin and to maintain a proper diet*

NURSING GOALS: To evaluate the client's ability to inject insulin and to determine the reason for noncompliance with the diet

Signs and symptoms
• failure to return for follow-up
• exacerbations of diabetes symptoms
• inability to perform proper skin care, exercise, select appropriate foods, or administer medication
• increased blood glucose level
• increased HgA$_1$C level
• weight gain

Interventions

1. Determine whether that client is unable to understand the directions or is afraid, anxious, or depressed about his situation.

2. Evaluate the client's urine and blood glucose readings. Isolate particularly high or low readings, and correlate the readings with the client's activities at that time.

3. Ask the client receiving insulin to demonstrate his self-administration technique.

4. Advise the client with visual problems to arrange for a family member, neighbor, or visiting nurse to prefill syringes with insulin for later use.

5. Advise the client who uses two different types of insulin to use a premixed solution containing 70% NPH insulin and 30% regular insulin instead.

6. Explain to the client the rationale for adhering to a diabetic regimen.

Rationales

1. Any of these problems can impair the client's ability to learn and to comply with therapy.

2. This should help identify any activities contributing to the client's hypoglycemia or hyperglycemia, such as undereating or overeating, improper food selection, or inactivity.

3. This will enable the nurse to assess the client's ability to administer insulin. Assessment may reveal that the client's noncompliance is caused by impaired vision or dexterity, which can hinder his ability to properly administer medications.

4. The client may not be complying with the treatment regimen because he cannot see clearly enough to fill the syringe.

5. The client's noncompliance may be related to his inability to mix solutions.

6. The client needs to understand how compliance improves health and reduces the incidence of acute and chronic complications.

OUTCOME CRITERION
• The client will comply with treatment as evidenced by having controlled blood and urine glucose levels and an absence of profound hypoglycemic or hyperglycemic episodes.

NURSING ACTIONS IN VARIOUS SETTINGS

Nursing actions for a client with diabetes mellitus depend on the setting in which care is provided. This section identifies which actions are appropriate in all settings and which pertain to acute care, extended care, or home care situations.

All settings

• Educate the client and caregiver about the causes, symptoms, treatment, and prevention of hypoglycemia and hyperglycemia.

• Teach the caregiver to assist the client, as needed, with meal preparation and daily foot care and with scheduling preventive eye, podiatric, and dental evaluations.

• Teach the client and caregiver the skills necessary to perform blood and urine glucose monitoring and how to interpret and respond to the results.

• Teach the client actions to take during an acute illness, such as monitoring of blood glucose levels more frequently and contacting the physician to learn insulin requirements.

Acute care

• Determine risk factors that place the client at high risk for hyperglycemia, such as recent surgery, total parenteral nutrition, peritoneal dialysis, medication use, and infection. Intervene as appropriate.

• Begin discharge planning with the client or caregiver.

• Assess all elderly clients for nosocomial infection; implement preventive measures, such as performing mouth care on clients receiving enteral feedings.

Extended care

• Observe the client for signs of hypoglycemia, hyperglycemia, or infection, including any changes in mental status, activity level, appetite, fluid consumption, or urine output.

• Avoid inserting indwelling urinary catheters or applying external urinary drainage devices whenever possible; use bladder retraining instead.

• Protect the client's skin and legs from injury and infection. Avoid overusing incontinence pads, which contribute to skin maceration and infection. Assign one staff member to inspect the client's feet and skin daily.

• Consult the dietitian and use exercise groups, medications, and meal plans to help control the client's diabetes. Assess the client's response through urine and blood glucose monitoring or routine HgA$_1$C levels.

Home care

• Protect the client's skin and legs from injury and infection by implementing home safety measures.

• Encourage the client to be as independent as possible with his diabetes-related tasks, such as monitoring urine and blood glucose levels, preparing meals, taking medication, inspecting his feet, and performing proper skin care.

• Educate the client's family or friends to assist the client, or to help him access community resources, nutrition centers, or transportation services.

• Emphasize the importance of wearing a diabetes identification bracelet or necklace, carrying fast-acting carbohydrates, informing the physician of hypoglycemic or hyperglycemic episodes, and establishing a means of accessing the emergency medical care.

• Promote early detection and treatment of diabetes complications by encouraging the client to visit the ophthalmologist every 6 to 12 months and to obtain regular dental and podiatric evaluations.

SELECTED REFERENCES

Bartholomew, G., et al. "Oral Candidiasis in Patients with Diabetes: A Thorough Analysis," *Diabetes Care* 10(5):607-11, September/October 1987.

Dillon, R. "Management of Soft-Tissue Infections in Elderly Persons with Diabetes," *Geriatric Medicine Today* 6(10):21-35, October 1987.

Hendricks, J., and Hendricks, C. *Aging in Mass Society: Myths and Realities.* Boston: Little, Brown & Co., 1986.

Hollander, P. "Diabetes, An Overview," *Caring* 7(11): 4-9, November 1988.

Huzar, J.G., and Cerrato, P.L. "The Role of Diet and Drugs," *RN* 52(4):46-50, April 1989.

Lima, J.S. "Lessening the Risk: Preventive Diabetes Foot Care," *Caring* 7(11):42-45, November 1988.

Rosenthal, M., et al. "UCLA Geriatric Grand Rounds: Diabetes in the Elderly," *American Geriatric Society* 35(5):435-45, May 1987.

Tomky, D. "A Three-Pronged Approach to Monitoring," *RN* 52(3):23-30, March 1989.

ENDOCRINE SYSTEM

Hypothyroidism and Hyperthyroidism

Hypothyroidism, which results from failure of the thyroid gland to secrete a sufficient amount of thyroid hormone, is characterized by generalized fatigue, sensitivity to cold, forgetfulness, unexplained weight gain, and constipation. Primarily affecting women between ages 50 and 70, this disorder can progress to life-threatening myxedema coma if neglected or undiagnosed. About 50% of all cases of myxedema coma occur in hospitalized clients who are treated with hypnotics; however, sedatives, cold weather, stress, and acute illness can also trigger the coma.

Hyperthyroidism, which results from excessive thyroid hormone secretion, is characterized by thyroid gland enlargement (goiter), nervousness, heat intolerance, unexplained weight loss, sweating, diarrhea, tremor, and palpitations. It occurs in about 10% to 30% of all elderly clients, 75% of whom exhibit classic signs and symptoms.

Thyroid storm (thyroid crisis), a life-threatening manifestation of hyperthyroidism, typically results from increased hypermetabolism, increased hyperactivity of the thyroid gland, or abrupt withdrawal from antithyroid agents. Although thyroid storm occurs in only a small percentage of clients with hyperthyroidism, it accounts for many of the deaths associated with the disorder and, for this reason, is considered a medical and nursing emergency.

Although all elderly clients are at increased risk for hypothyroidism because of age-related antithyroid antibody production, an estimated 40% remain undiagnosed. Researchers think this is because hypothyroidism can mimic other diseases, physicians sometimes confuse clinical manifestations of the disorder with the aging process, and thyroid tests can be difficult to interpret. Hyperthyroidism may also remain undiagnosed because many elderly clients present with atypical symptoms. The disorder is easier to detect in a hospital setting, where abnormal thyroid functioning can be observed.

ETIOLOGY
Hypothyroidism is caused by inadequate thyroid hormone production resulting from dysfunction of the thyroid gland, possibly from autoimmune thyroiditis (a condition in which the body develops an immunologic reaction to the thyroid) or from medical or surgical treatment for hyperthyroidism. Hyperthyroidism commonly results from toxic multinodular goiter, autonomous nodules, and Graves' disease; in some cases, it results from exposure to iodine.

HEALTH HISTORY FINDINGS
In a health history interview, the client may report or the nurse may detect many of these findings:

Hypothyroidism
• lethargy
• fatigue
• dry, flaky skin
• hair loss
• edema of the face, hands, arms, and legs
• cold intolerance
• constipation
• seizures
• syncope
• slow mentation with memory loss

Hyperthyroidism
• recent angina
• palpitations or tachycardia
• apathy
• hypertension
• severe weight loss
• heat intolerance
• anorexia
• depression
• history of congestive heart failure
• history of diabetes

PHYSICAL FINDINGS
In a physical examination, the nurse may detect may of these *hypothyroidism* findings:

Integumentary
• edema of the face, hands, arms, or legs

Respiratory
• wheezing
• dry cough
• dyspnea or shortness of breath

Cardiovascular
• diastolic hypertension
• tachycardia

Gastrointestinal
• ascites
• fecal impaction

Neurologic
• gait disturbances

Other
• raspy voice
• hearing loss

In a physical examination, the nurse may detect many of these *hyperthyroidism* findings:

Cardiovascular
• atrial fibrillation
• tachydysrhythmia

Respiratory
• shortness of breath

Gastrointestinal
• abdominal pain or tenderness

Musculoskeletal
• generalized muscle wasting

Neurologic
• tremors or nervousness

Other
• placid, staring face
• infraorbital edema

DIAGNOSTIC STUDIES
The following studies may be performed to evaluate the client's health status:

Hypothyroidism
• creatinine phosphokinase study—to determine abnormalities; levels may be elevated

• complete blood count (CBC)—to reveal macrocytic anemia, which responds to thyroid hormone replacement, or pernicious anemia
• serum thyroid-stimulating hormone studies—to help confirm diagnosis; will be elevated
• serum thyroid (T_4) concentration and free thyroxine index—to determine abnormalities; levels will be low
• electrolyte studies—to indicate hyponatremia and hyperuricemia
• chest X-ray—to identify cardiomegaly

Hyperthyroidism
• serum alkaline phosphatase—to determine abnormalities; may be elevated
• thyroid studies—to help confirm diagnosis; results include elevated serum T_4 concentration, resin T_3 uptake, serum free T_4, and thyroidal radioactive iodide uptake
• thyrotropin-releasing hormone stimulation test—to determine abnormalities; performed if T_4 and T_3 are only slightly elevated
• electrocardiogram (ECG)—may reveal atrial fibrillation

POTENTIAL COMPLICATIONS
• myxedema coma
• Graves' disease
• thyroid cancer

Nursing diagnosis: *Knowledge deficit related to the thyroid dysfunction and treatment*

NURSING GOALS: To help the client avoid the adverse effects of hypothyroidism and to identify and appropriately care for the client with myxedema coma

Signs and symptoms
Hypothyroidism
• easy fatigability
• change in mental status (such as confusion)
• increasing lethargy
• diminished hearing
• constipation and abdominal distention
Myxedema coma
• neck scar
• hypothermia
• delayed relaxation of tendon reflexes
• respiratory failure and apnea

Interventions

1. Before beginning thyroid replacement therapy, determine whether the client has had a thyroidectomy.

Rationales

1. This will help the nurse assess the client's need for continual thyroid replacement. About 17% of clients who undergo thyroidectomy develop hypothyroidism within 2 years.

2. Teach the client about thyroid replacement therapy, explaining his need for such medications as sodium L-thyroxine (T_4) or liothyronine sodium (T_3). Emphasize that therapy begins slowly and that the dosage will be increase at 1- to 3-week intervals.

3. Advise the client to maintain a warm, comfortable environment, and suggest that he dress warmly when outdoors.

4. Teach the client with neurologic abnormalities and his caregiver appropriate safety measures, such as keeping the bed side rails elevated, keeping a tongue blade available at the bedside, and keeping a call bell or other alarm system within the client's reach.

5. Instruct the client and his caregiver to monitor bowel activity patterns and to institute a bowel regimen if constipation occurs (see "Constipation and Fecal Incontinence," pages 97 to 104).

6. Recommend that the client avoid using sedatives, hypnotics, and analgesics.

7. Teach the client and caregiver about myxedema coma. Emphasize that the client would require hospitalization in intensive care with possible intubation and mechanical ventilation.

2. Thyroid hormone preparations elevate serum thyroid levels to reverse hypothyroidism. Gradual increases are necessary, however, because rapid correction of hypothyroidism can cause adverse cardiac effects.

3. A client with hypothyroidism typically has an intolerance to cold because of his decreased metabolic rate and inability to perspire.

4. Syncope, seizures, and dementia may occur in the client who has severe, undetected hypothyroidism and may continue to occur even after treatment is started, until serum thyroid levels rise. Therefore, safety precautions are necessary.

5. Constipation commonly occurs in the client with hypothyroidism, usually resulting from reduced intestinal motility.

6. The client with hypothyroidism metabolizes these drugs slowly, which may result in respiratory complications or myxedema coma.

7. Myxedema coma is a medical emergency with a high mortality rate. Death, when it occurs, commonly results from hypercapnia and respiratory failure.

OUTCOME CRITERIA
- The client will understand the treatment for and complications associated with hypothyroidism.
- The client and caregiver will understand the severity of myxedema coma.

Nursing diagnosis: *Altered cardiopulmonary tissue perfusion related to hyperthyroidism and thyroid storm*

NURSING GOALS: To recognize hyperthyroidism, to institute appropriate treatment, and to prevent adverse effects

Signs and symptoms
- unexplained weight loss, anorexia, or constipation despite increased appetite
- unexplained heart failure
- chest pain and palpitations
- muscle wasting and weakness
- lethargy

Interventions

1. Assess the client for cardiovascular manifestations of hyperthyroidism by weighing the client daily, monitoring fluid intake and output, checking for peripheral edema, noting complaints of chest pain, and monitoring for increased pulse rate and blood pressure.

2. Assess the client during treatment for a slowly rising temperature, marked apathy, tachycardia, prominent muscle weakness, and coma.

Rationales

1. Hyperthyroidism commonly causes angina and congestive heart failure.

2. These signs and symptoms signal apathetic thyroid storm, a form of hyperthyroidism that may affect the elderly client. Severe stress, illness, injury, or abrupt withdrawal of iodine therapy can precipitate the condition.

3. If the client becomes febrile, apply warm blankets and administer sponge baths and acetaminophen.

3. These measures will help decrease the client's temperature. Avoid using aspirin as it can raise thyroxine levels.

4. Institute the prescribed treatment for hyperthyroidism, as ordered. Short-term treatment may include the use of propranolol, inorganic iodide, propylthiouracil, methimazole, or glucocorticoids. Long-term treatment usually involves the administration of radioactive iodide.

4. Proper treatment will prevent complications of thyrotoxicosis.

5. Monitor the client's serum liver function tests, and assess the client for signs and symptoms of jaundice while he is receiving treatment.

5. Drugs used to treat hyperthyroidism may cause liver damage and jaundice.

6. Explain to the client and the client's family that treatment consists of medications and radiation and that surgery is usually not an option.

6. Thyroidectomy is used only in the client who has a malignancy or an obstruction in the neck.

7. Consult a dietitian, if necessary, about supplemental feedings for the client who has experienced significant weight loss.

7. Hyperthyroidism causes weight loss in over 70% of all clients. The weight loss may be severe, especially if the client is already anorectic.

OUTCOME CRITERIA
- The client will be free from cardiac complications related to hyperthyroidism.
- The client will receive prompt treatment for hyperthyroidism.

NURSING ACTIONS IN VARIOUS SETTINGS

Nursing actions for a client with a thyroid disorder depend on the setting in which care is provided. This section identifies which actions are appropriate in all settings and which pertain to acute care, extended care, or home care situations.

All settings
- Educate the client and the client's family about possible drug interactions, including prescribed and over-the-counter medications.
- Stress to the client and caregiver the need for frequent follow-up.
- Review all previous teaching with the client and caregiver to keep the client's knowledge current and accurate.

Acute care
- Monitor the client's thyroid function studies to determine effectiveness of treatment and to prevent a medication overdose.
- Be aware of conditions that may accompany hypothyroidism, such as cirrhosis, severe hepatitis, renal failure, cancer, and diabetic acidosis.

Extended care
- Monitor the client's medication use.
- Ask the physician about what follow-up care the client needs.
- Assess the client for signs and symptoms of thyroid dysfunction, such as increasing depression or confusion.

Home care
- Evaluate the effectiveness of treatment.
- Determine whether the client and the client's family understand the need for continued treatment.
- Periodically obtain laboratory studies to monitor the effectiveness of treatment and to prevent adverse effects.
- Give the client and caregiver written information concerning the signs and symptoms of hypothyroidism and hyperthyroidism.

SELECTED REFERENCES

Felicetta, J.V. "Thyroid Changes with Aging: Significance and Management," *Geriatrics* 42(1):88, 90-91, January 1987.

Mattewson, M.K. "Thyroid Disorder," *Critical Care Nurse* 7(1):74-78, January 1987.

Patel, P.H., and Thomas, E. "Gastrointestinal Dysfunction in the Elderly Patient with Thyroid Disease," *Geriatric Medicine Today* 6(7):88-89, 93, 95-96, July 1987.

Rossman, I. *Clinical Geriatrics.* Philadelphia: J.B. Lippincott Co., 1986.

Schroffner, W.G. "The Aging Thyroid in Health and Disease," *Geriatrics* 42(8):41-52, August 1987.

Depression

Depression, a state of lowered self-esteem accompanied by feelings of hopelessness and helplessness, is a common disorder among older adults. About 20% of all clients over age 65 have clinically significant depression, while an estimated 40% have a milder form of the disorder. Acute depression, which occurs suddenly after a crisis, is most common among those aged 55 to 70.

Three types of depression—endogenous, reactive, and secondary—are most common among elderly clients. In the endogenous type, the client is typically depressed because of some internal biochemical process, not because of a metabolic disease or drug reaction. In the reactive type, the client's depression evolves from a precipitating event or major loss. In the secondary type, the client's depression stems from trauma or illness. Depression may also occur as a medication side effect or a symptom of certain diseases, such as hypothyroidism.

Many nurses presume that depression is a natural reaction to a client's disease or diagnosis. Although this may be true on a short-term basis, prolonged depression is never a normal response to chronic illness or pain. Nurses should keep in mind that those who suffer depression, especially elderly white men, are at high risk for suicide and that older adults commit 25% of all suicides.

ETIOLOGY
Endogenous depression commonly results from a biochemical change in brain metabolism, specifically a decrease in the secretion of the neurotransmitters serotonin and dopamine. This decrease results in slowed responses and thought processes, the classic symptoms of depression in elderly clients. Because of these symptoms, endogenous depression is commonly known as pseudodementia and is usually treated with tricyclic antidepressants.

Reactive depression occurs in response to a stressful situation or major loss. Clients can easily identify the onset of the depression, and the precipitating event usually is obvious. Those with this type of depression are still able to care for themselves and usually respond to psychotherapy. Such depression typically improves within 3 months of the precipitating event. If no improvement is noted at the end of this period, or if no particular event or situation is found to have triggered the depression, the client may be developing a major depression that requires professional intervention and treatment, such as psychotherapy, electroconvulsive therapy, or drug therapy.

Secondary depression may follow a trauma or an illness, such as a head injury, Parkinson's disease, cerebrovascular accident, thyroid dysfunction, a neoplasm, or alcoholism. If the depression is triggered by a loss of function, such as urinary incontinence, vegetative symptoms and somatic complaints may result.

HEALTH HISTORY FINDINGS
In a health history interview, the client may report or the nurse may detect many of these findings:
• dysphoric mood
• hypochondriasis
• loss of energy
• social withdrawal
• sleep disturbances
• anorexia or weight gain
• sinus pain and congestion
• palpitations or chest pain
• abdominal pain or constipation
• decreased libido
• headaches
• mood change and inability to concentrate
• inappropriate feelings of guilt
• suicidal ideation
• use of nonsteroidal anti-inflammatory, cardiac, antiparkinsonian, antihistamine, anticonvulsant, analgesic, antihypertensive, or antimicrobial medications
• use of cytoxic agents, hormones, or immunosuppresive agents
• history of rheumatoid arthritis, gout, or lupus
• history of Alzheimer's disease, multiple sclerosis, diabetes, or Parkinson's disease
• history of hypothyroidism or hyperthyroidism, Addison's disease, Cushing's disease, cancer, pneumonia, or anemia
• history of depression or psychiatric problems
• recent use of a new medication
• history of alcohol use
• family history of suicide or psychiatric illness
• recent family upheaval
• recent change in body image
• recent change in health status

PHYSICAL FINDINGS
In a physical examination, the nurse may detect many of these findings:

Psychological
• agitation
• withdrawal
• dull affect

Integumentary
• rashes or increased psoriasis

Respiratory
- wheezing
- crackles
- decreased bibasilar breath sounds

Cardiovascular
- increased blood pressure
- rapid or irregular heartbeat

Gastrointestinal
- hyperactive or hypoactive bowel sounds
- abdominal pain or tenderness
- fecal impaction

Musculoskeletal
- decreased flexibility and joint mobility
- increased pain with movement

Neurologic
- slowed reflexes
- decreased attention span

DIAGNOSTIC STUDIES
The following studies may be performed to evaluate the client's health status:
- serum blood urea nitrogen (BUN), glucose, potassium, calcium, and magnesium studies—to determine the metabolic cause; levels may be abnormal
- liver function studies—to determine the metabolic cause; levels may be abnormal
- dexamethasone suppression test (DST)—to support the diagnosis of depression; a positive result occurs if a client does not have a suppresed morning cortisol level after receiving an 11:00 p.m. dose of dexamethasone; has a 50% specificity rate
- computed tomography (CT) scan—to rule out reversible causes of dementia
- drug levels—to rule out drug toxicity as a cause of depression
- thyroid levels—to rule out thyroid disease as a cause of depression

POTENTIAL COMPLICATIONS
- immobility
- institutionalization
- social isolation
- suicide

Nursing diagnosis: *Potential for self-directed violence related to the inability to cope with chronic illness*

NURSING GOALS: To help the client identify effective coping measures for depression and to prevent him from attempting suicide

Signs and symptoms
- suicidal ideation
- thoughts of escape
- detailed plan for suicide
- sudden increase in energy after severe depression
- giving away personal objects
- feelings of hopelessness and helplessness

Interventions

1. Ask the client the following questions to assess his suicide potential: "Do you think of suicide?" "Have you ever, recently or in the past, thought of ending your life?" "Do you have a method or plan for suicide?" and "What prevents you from committing suicide?"

2. Establish a contract with the client that states he will not commit suicide without first notifying his therapist or a suicide hot line.

Rationales

1. Every depressed client should be assessed for his suicide potential. Suicide risk increases in proportion to the specificity of the plan. The elderly male client commonly chooses a more violent method of suicide, such as drug overdose, hanging, jumping off high places, or using firearms and explosives. The female client might choose drawn-out destructive behavior, such as refusing food or medications, drinking excessively, or refusing treatment.

2. This allows the client an opportunity to change his mind, if he so desires.

3. Refer the client to a psychotherapist or geropsychotherapist.

3. A therapist can help the client to identify and use appropriate defense mechanisms, understand his depression, and recognize the changes that result from treatment.

4. Teach the client's family to recognize subtle suicide cues, such as the client's suddenly paying all bills or talking about getting his affairs in order.

4. The elderly client may give little warning before carrying out suicide plans.

5. Take all suicide threats seriously.

5. The elderly client is more likely to succeed at suicide than a younger client. Nurses need to recognize more subtle but equally destructive behaviors, such as medication misuse, starvation, ignoring dietary restrictions, or refusing therapy.

6. Institute safety precautions, such as closely observing the client and removing objects that could be used as suicidal implements, such as guns, razors, or medications.

6. These measures help ensure the client's safety.

7. Encourage the client to express feelings of anger, guilt, and frustration.

7. Expression of feelings may help prevent suicide.

8. Carefully monitor the client whose depression seems to have lifted.

8. A sudden change may indicate that the client has gathered enough energy to carry out the suicide.

9. Help the client to identify and evaluate the events and feelings surrounding the suicidal ideation.

9. This crisis-intervention model helps the client work on acute problems and helps him to identify the causes of his suicidal ideation.

10. Encourage reminiscence therapy by exposing the client to familiar scents, foods, music, and pictures.

10. Reminiscence therapy encourages the client to review his life experiences, to draw on assets that he may have overlooked, and to come to terms with unresolved issues.

11. Identify the client's significant other, and enlist that person's support if possible.

11. A significant other can help the depressed client socialize and carry out activities of daily living and can also assist during illnesses and crises.

12. If suicide appears imminent, discuss with the physician the possibility of hospitalizing the client on a 72-hour, involuntary basis (where legal).

12. Hospitalization may be the treatment of choice for the client at risk of harming himself.

OUTCOME CRITERIA
• The client will identify support mechanisms.
• The client will receive emergency life-saving measures, if necessary.

Nursing diagnosis: *Dysfunctional grieving related to recent family loss or life-style change*

NURSING GOALS: To help the client cope with severe reactive depression and to assist him through the grieving process

Signs and symptoms
• somatic complaints
• grief lasting more than 6 months
• dysfunctional life-style
• weight and sleep loss

Interventions

1. Assess the client for a recent life loss, such as the loss of a spouse, retirement, the loss of health, or a recent cerebrovascular accident.

2. Assess the client's ability to cope with everyday tasks, such as paying bills, shopping, and banking. Suggest the services of a home health aide, if necessary.

3. Instruct the client on the usual progression of the grieving process. Explain that mild to moderate depression and normal grieving are usually self-limiting and treatable.

4. Treat the client's somatic complaints conservatively by avoiding the use of medications.

5. Refer the client for behavioral therapy.

6. Encourage the client to attend social activities.

7. Refer the client to appropriate support groups.

Rationales

1. These events frequently precipitate stress and depression.

2. The client suffering from depression may not complete these tasks.

3. Such instruction can help relieve the client's fears about lack of control and the problems associated with depression.

4. Reactive depression is usually unresponsive to medications.

5. Behavioral therapy teaches the client to identify problems and to develop a reasonable plan for solving them. It aims to increase the number of positive experiences in the client's daily life.

6. Depressed elderly clients need to interact with others to distract them from self-absorbing thoughts.

7. Support groups provide counseling. Interactions with these groups provide socialization opportunities, furnish role models, help with coping, and facilitate the grieving process.

OUTCOME CRITERIA
- The client will identify appropriate methods of handling his dysfunctional grieving.
- The client will cope effectively with feelings of loss.

Nursing diagnosis: *Altered health maintenance related to depressive state*

NURSING GOALS: To help the client assume responsibility for self-care and activities of daily living and to teach the client and caregiver about various treatments for depression

Signs and symptoms
- extremely slow movements
- inability to follow a daily routine or to complete personal hygiene
- anorexia and weight loss

Interventions

1. Ask the following questions to assess the client's nutritional status: "What have you eaten in the past 24 hours?" "Who regularly fixes your food?" "Who shops for your food?"

2. Assess the client for secondary physical problems, such as malnutrition, poor hygiene, constipation, and fatigue.

3. Establish a daily routine for the client to follow.

Rationales

1. An assessment enables the nurse to identify areas in which the client needs assistance.

2. Such assessment identifies the physiologic effects of the client's depression and allows for treatment.

3. A structured plan allows the client to focus on things other than his depression. Completing the tasks outlined on the plan can help to enhance the client's self-esteem.

4. Refer the client for counseling, or implement a cognitive group therapy program.

4. Psychotherapy can help the elderly client identify interpersonal assets and coping skills for adapting to different situations in later life. Cognitive group therapy can prevent depression, withdrawal, and isolation. Empathetic, genuine, warm, and consistently accepting forms of psychotherapy produce the best results.

5. Discuss with the client the possible use of individual, group, or family therapy.

5. Therapy focuses on the client's strengths to maximize his functional ability.

6. Refer the client to appropriate support services, such as home health aides.

6. Home health aides can assist the client with activities of daily living until the client can resume these activities on his own.

7. Determine whether the client feels isolated or unsafe in his home. Identify his safety and security needs; instruct him in ways to meet those needs, such as through a mental health professional, a telephone help line, or a visitor.

7. Helping the client identify where to obtain help strengthens the client's support system.

8. Administer tricyclic antidepressant medications (such as amitriptyline, imipramine, doxepin, nortriptyline, desipramine, protriptyline, trazodone, or maprotiline), as ordered.

8. Tricyclic antidepressant medications, which appear to selectively block presynaptic reuptake of serotonin and norepinephrine, are used to treat depressions unresponsive to environmental manipulation or psychotherapy.

9. Inform the client and caregiver that antidepressant medication may require 4 to 6 weeks to take effect.

9. Although individual symptoms, such as sleep disturbances, may respond rapidly to medication, a maximal therapeutic effect may require several weeks of therapy.

10. Assess client for medication side effects, such as drowsiness, tachycardia, blurred vision, dry mouth, or urine retention. Discuss with the physician the possibility of altering the dosage schedule to alleviate these effects.

10. Medications require careful adjustment to maximize effectiveness and minimize side effects. Many side effects decrease after a few days' use; however, some clients may require a reduced dosage, a compound substitution, or a change in administration.

11. Assess the client for neurovegetative symptoms, such as sleep and appetite disturbances or psychosomatic changes. If any are noted, discuss with the physician the possibility of electroconvulsive therapy. Also consider electroconvulsive therapy for clients with life-threatening symptoms, such as refusal to eat or marked suicidal ideation.

11. Electroconvulsive therapy is the treatment of choice for the severely depressed client or the client who cannot take, or is unresponsive to, tricyclic antidepressants. Although the reason for its effectiveness is unknown, it may be effective because brain activity is stimulated. Nurses should know that unipolar electroconvulsive therapy may cause temporary memory loss.

OUTCOME CRITERIA
- The client will enlist the aid of others to meet his physical needs until treatment for depression is effective.
- The client will understand the rationale for the therapies instituted.

NURSING ACTIONS IN VARIOUS SETTINGS

Nursing actions for a client with depression depend on the setting in which care is provided. This section identifies which actions are appropriate in all settings and which pertain to acute care, extended care, or home care situations.

All settings
- Encourage the proper diagnosis and treatment of depression in elderly clients by suggesting evaluation, when appropriate.

- Teach the client and the client's family the signs and symptoms of depression and the course of the disease.
- Teach the client about the medications prescribed for depression.

Acute care
- Prepare the client and the client's family for scheduled tests and evaluations.
- Evaluate the client for suicidal ideation, and institute safety precautions or transfer the client to a psychiatric unit.

• Prepare the client for discharge by helping him to set up appropriate community support services.

Extended care
• Evaluate the client's response to drug therapy, and consult the physican about the use of alternative drugs if the client shows no response.
• Weigh the client weekly.
• Assess the newly admitted or newly disabled client for reactive depression.
• Assess the client who has frequent somatic complaints for depression.

Home care
• Suggest that the client participate in social activities, such as senior citizen clubs or support groups.
• Provide for home services, such as Meals On Wheels, a homemaker, or a home health aide service, during the client's severe vegetative states.
• Assess the client's suicide potential and the feasibility of his plan.

SELECTED REFERENCES
American Psychiatric Association Task Force. "The Dexamethasone Suppression Test: An Overview of Patient's Current Status in Psychiatry," *American Journal of Psychiatry* 144(10):1253-61, October 1987.
Ben-Arie, O., et al. "Depression in the Elderly Living in the Community," *British Journal of Psychiatry* 150:169-74, 1987.
Boxwell, A.O. "Geriatric Suicide: The Preventable Death," *Nurse Practitioner* 13(6):10-11,15,18-19, June 1988.
Copeland, J., et al. "Range of Mental Illness Among the Elderly in the Community," *British Journal of Psychiatry* 150:815-23, 1987.
Dryfus, J. "The Prevalence of Depression in Women in an Ambulatory Care Setting," *Nurse Practitioner* 12(4):34-50, April 1987.
Parsons, C. "Group Reminiscence Therapy and Levels of Depression in the Elderly," *Nurse Practitioner* 11(3):68-76, March 1986.
Ronsman, K. "Therapy for Depression," *Journal of Gerontological Nursing* 13(12):18-25, December 1987.
Todd, B. "Depression and Antidepressants," *Geriatric Nursing* 8(4):203-04, July/August, 1987.
Zorumski, C.F., et al. "Electroconvulsive Therapy for the Elderly: A Review," *Hospital and Community Psychiatry* 39(6):643-47, June 1988.

Disruptive Behavior

Disruptive behavior constitutes any behavior that disrupts or upsets others in a living or working environment. In many cases, the behavior occurs in the form of agitation, aggression, violence, or physical or verbal abuse. Although disruptive behavior is possible in any setting, it most frequently occurs in extended care facilities and commonly involves exchanges between clients and nurses.

Agitation involves the use of inappropriate words or actions not explained by the client's apparent needs or confusion. This type of behavior can lead to aggression and violence in which the client becomes dangerous to himself and others. Agitation commonly occurs in elderly clients with organic brain changes.

Aggression typically occurs when the client feels that he has lost control or that his rights have been violated. This type of behavior is most common among males and frequently serves as an outlet for feelings of powerlessness and frustration.

Violence may occur when a client expresses aggressive behavior toward himself or others. Dementia, confusion, disorientation, drug toxicity, or acute illness places the client at high risk for developing this type of behavior.

Physical or verbal abuse of caregivers, chiefly nurses, by residents in extended care facilities is a prevalent problem that has not been thoroughly studied or documented. Common behaviors include hitting, pinching, biting, and shoving as well as the use of obscenities and racial slurs.

ETIOLOGY

Agitation may occur in elderly clients because of physiologic or psychological reasons, including drug intoxication, drug withdrawal, organic brain syndrome, and functional disorders. Agitation may also result from sensory impairment, physical discomfort, communication problems, environmental isolation, and overstimulation.

A loss of environmental control, limited social support, and certain personality characteristics place clients at risk for exhibiting disruptive behaviors. The most frequent causes of aggression include sensory loss, limited mobility, frustration over lost control, feelings of invasion of personal space, others' behavior, confusion, loneliness, and depression.

Clients who are dependent upon others for their activities of daily living are most inclined to be abusive or violent. Violent episodes most often occur when clients are restrained or placed in seclusion or when they are fed or toileted in a nonprivate setting.

HEALTH HISTORY FINDINGS

In a health history interview, the client may report or the nurse may detect many of these findings:
• pruritus
• multi-infarct dementia
• aphasia
• emotional difficulties
• poor coping patterns
• history of brain disease, epilepsy, Alzheimer's disease, or Parkinson's disease
• history of psychosis or a suicide attempt
• history of a head injury or a burn
• history of alcohol or drug abuse
• history of exposure to environmental pollutants
• history of multiple losses, such as family members or money

PHYSICAL FINDINGS

In a physical examination, the nurse may detect many of these findings:

Psychological
• flat, inappropriate, or labile affect

Integumentary
• multiple bruises, lacerations, or burns
• dry, flaky skin

Neurologic
• pacing, agitation, or wandering
• changes in posture or facial expression

DIAGNOSTIC STUDIES

The following studies may be performed to evaluate the client's health status:
• serum electrolyte levels—to determine imbalances that may cause behavior changes; blood glucose levels are particularly important in diabetic clients
• electrocardiogram (ECG)—to identify cardiac dysrhythmias as a cause of disruptive behavior
• computed tomography (CT) scan—to determine reversible causes of agitation, such as hydrocephalus or tumors

POTENTIAL COMPLICATIONS
• violence
• wandering
• sleep-pattern disturbances
• self-care deficit
• malnutrition
• depression
• falls
• skin lacerations or infection

Nursing diagnosis: *Potential for impaired skin integrity related to pruritus and scratching secondary to self-inflicted aggressive behavior*

NURSING GOAL: To promote skin integrity by preventing dryness and itching

Signs and symptoms
• poor nutritional status
• dehydration
• infection
• allergies
• infestation
• bruises or scratches

Interventions

1. Assess the client's skin daily, and observe for lacerations, bruises, or burns.

2. Assess how frequently the client needs to bathe.

3. Use tepid, not hot, water, ensuring that the temperature does not exceed 110° F (43.3° C).

4. Add baby oil or mineral oil to the client's bath water, and help the client get into and out of the tub.

5. Add about 1 cup of oatmeal to the client's bath water, and encourage the client to soak for 20 to 30 minutes.

6. Instruct the client to use mild soaps, such as Dove, or soaps with lanolin. Discourage the use of deodorant soaps.

7. Gently pat, do not rub, the client's skin when drying him after the bath.

8. After drying the client's skin, apply cornstarch to skin folds, being careful not to cake the cornstarch.

9. Discourage the client from scratching.

10. Administer antihistamines, as ordered.

11. Trim the client's nails.

12. Avoid applying perfumes and scented lotions to the client's skin.

13. Instruct the client to avoid excessively warm or cool temperatures and dry air.

14. Attach a bed cradle to the client's bed.

Rationales

1. An assessment will determine the cause of itching and scratching. Tissue trauma may indicate overt, self-injurious behavior.

2. Frequent bathing removes natural oils and dries the skin. The elderly client may need a complete bath only once weekly.

3. Hot water dries the skin and can lead to itching and eventual breakdown.

4. Oils lubricate the skin but make the tub slippery.

5. Oatmeal baths sooth and decrease itching.

6. Soaps with lanolin moisturize the skin.

7. Rubbing damages the skin.

8. Cornstarch is inexpensive, soothing, and absorbs moisture.

9. Scratching and increased itching becomes a cycle and may be a sign of self-directed violence.

10. Antihistamines help control itching but should not be used in the client with respiratory problems.

11. Trimming the client's nails reduces the risk of injury to the skin.

12. These products contain alcohol, which increases pruritus.

13. Temperature extremes irritate the skin; low humidity dries the skin.

14. Bed cradles provide warmth while preventing sheets and blankets from applying direct pressure to the client's skin.

15. Put gloves on the confused or psychotic client who is unable to control scratching.

15. Gloves prevent damage to the skin from scratching.

16. Provide the client with diversional activities.

16. Diversional activities distract the client from scratching.

OUTCOME CRITERIA
• The client will be free from continually itchy skin.
• The client will not scratch obsessively.

Nursing diagnosis: *Potential for violence: self-directed or directed at others, related to the inability to control behavior*

NURSING GOALS: To help the client control his behavior and to help him identity constructive ways to express his feelings

Signs and symptoms
• withdrawal
• demanding of attention
• refusal to go places
• complaining
• treating others as inferior
• committing overtly aggressive acts
• refusing help from others
• accusing others falsely
• crying
• expressing a death wish

Interventions

1. Listen actively to the client; remain honest, calm, clear, and concise during interactions. Be sure to sit near the client, maintain appropriate eye contact, and respond with appropriate facial expressions.

2. Maintain a stable physical environment by decreasing sensory overload and retaining the same room assignment whenever possible.

3. Maintain a safe environment by removing all potentially harmful items from the client's reach.

4. Do not rush the client or overly structure his environment.

5. Share meals with the client whenever possible.

6. Use behavior modification techniques, when appropriate, to reinforce nonviolent behavior.

7. Orient the client to his environment, when necessary.

8. Establish set times to interact with the client, such as 15 minutes every hour. Explain all plans and the purpose behind the plans during this time.

Rationales

1. This method establishes a sense of trust, conveys attention and concern, and facilitates communication.

2. Sensory stimuli can increase agitation and confusion.

3. The client may be unable to control his behavior and may use objects within his environment to injure himself or others.

4. Tension commonly results from feelings of being forced or pushed to act a certain way.

5. Familiar social interaction can improve rapport.

6. These techniques work by rewarding the client for positive behaviors and discouraging negative outbursts.

7. Unfamiliar sights and sounds may result in misconceptions, fear, and agitation.

8. Aggressiveness occurs when the client feels threatened because of an inability to control his environment, and these actions foster trust and rapport.

9. Establish familiar, secure routines; encourage the client to do as much for himself as possible.

9. Invading the client's personal space may cause physical aggression.

10. Simplify decisions the client must make or tasks the client must complete; assist him, as necessary. Avoid asking the client why he did a certain thing.

10. Simplification helps the client maintain self-esteem. "Why" questions tend to threaten clients.

11. Assess the client's response to touch; employ therapeutic touch, such as dance therapy, when appropriate.

11. Touch can help bond the client and nurse; however, a client who does not like being touched may find this behavior threatening.

12. Avoid arguing or trying to reason with a client who is exhibiting violent or aggressive behavior.

12. The client cannot appreciate another point of view at such a time.

13. Employ pet therapy if the client likes animals.

13. Pets can provide companionship and enhance self-esteem.

14. Assess whether the client responds better to individual or group activities, and provide appropriate diversional activities.

14. Activities can help to maintain self-esteem and a positive self-image.

15. Promote regular exercise, such as walking.

15. Regular exercise helps control wandering and channels the client's energies.

16. Ensure that caregivers do not use aggression or make threats when dealing with the client.

16. Caregivers need to understand the client's inability to control his behavior and the importance of a calm approach.

17. Establish short-term goals, such as having the client limit yelling to certain places or times during the day.

17. Realistic short-term goals enhance self-esteem.

OUTCOME CRITERIA
- The client will begin to control his behavior with the assistance of others.
- The client will have fewer violent responses.

NURSING ACTIONS IN VARIOUS SETTINGS
Nursing actions for a client with disruptive behavior depend on the setting in which care is provided. This section identifies which actions are appropriate in all settings and which pertain to acute care, extended care, or home care situations.

All settings
- Involve the client in developing a plan of care.
- Help the client and the client's family to recognize and cope with problem behaviors, and help them to understand the underlying causes.
- Help caregivers to access appropriate support groups.

Acute care
- Avoid restraining the agitated client whenever possible.
- Avoid overmedicating the client.
- Provide a safe, nonchaotic environment.

Extended care
- Provide a comfortable, homelike environment.
- Restrain the client only when the possibility of harm is imminent. Reevaluate the need for restraints daily, and discontinue their use as soon as possible.
- Educate and support caregivers, especially nursing assistants.
- Monitor the client closely for signs of abuse from caregivers.
- Help the client's family to recognize the difference between willful and uncontrollable problem behaviors.

Home care
- Help the client's family provide a safe, comfortable environment.
- Monitor the client closely for signs of potential abuse from exhausted or frustrated caregivers.
- Provide information about adult day care, and encourage the client's family to participate.

SELECTED REFERENCES

Bernell, S.L., and Small, N.R. "Disruptive Behaviors," *Journal of Gerontological Nursing* 14(2):8-13, February 1988.

Burgio, L.D., et al. "Behavior Problems in an Urban Nursing Home," *Journal of Gerontological Nursing* 14(1):32-34, January 1988.

McHutchion, E., and Morese, J.M. "Releasing Restraints: A Nursing Dilemma," *Journal of Gerontological Nursing* 15(2):16-21, February 1989.

Mendelsohn, S., et al. "Assessment Protocols for Acute Medical Conditions," *Journal of Gerontological Nursing* 12:17, July 1986.

Mentes, J.C., and Ferrario, J. "Calming Aggressive Reactions: A Preventive Program," *Journal of Gerontological Nursing* 15(2):22-27, February 1989.

Struble, L.M., and Sivertsen, L. "Agitation Behaviors in Confused Elderly Patients," *Journal of Gerontological Nursing* 13(11):40-44, November 1987.

Thomas, D.R. "Assessment and Management of Agitation in the Elderly," *Geriatrics* 43(6):45-50, June 1988.

SECTION III

GENERAL CARE PLANS

Chronic Pain

Chronic pain, a common problem among older adults, typically results from various acute and chronic illnesses that accompany aging. Although pain is subjective and difficult to define, researchers have been able to classify pain according to its various sources: Somatic pain results from nociceptor stimulation in the skin and subcutaneous tissues or in deep somatic tissue, such as the blood vessels, connective tissue, and muscle. Visceral, or organ-type, pain results from the stretching, inflammation, or ischemia of an organ that commonly occurs with cancer. Referred pain, which can accompany visceral pain, occurs in a site distal to the original source or cause. Afferentation pain results from injury to the peripheral or central nervous system and sometimes from cancer.

Chronic pain may begin as acute pain that exacerbates and does not lessen or resolve; it may be debilitating to the client and, in many cases, becomes an important part of the client's life, necessitating long-term adaptation. Such pain can be limiting (occurring because of a disorder or condition and expected to resolve), intermittent (recurring sporadically over a long period), persistent (continuing without interruption), or intractable (occurring uncontrollably, without the hope of relief or a cure).

ETIOLOGY
Sensory receptors (nociceptors), which are found throughout the skin, muscle, connective tissue, organs, and the lining of the thoracic and abdominal cavities, transmit painful stimuli from mechanical, thermal, or chemical stimulation through myelinated and unmyelinated afferent sensory fibers to the dorsal horn of the spinal cord. From there, pain impulses travel up the neospinothalamic and paleospinothalamic tracts. The neospinothalamic tract discriminates between sensations; the paleospinothalamic tract handles the affective components of pain and may also cause motor responses to pain. The cortex may control pain perception, although its exact role is unclear.

Chronic pain syndrome can result from degenerative conditions, such as osteoarthritis or osteoporosis, or from vascular conditions, such as peripheral vascular disease. Pain resulting from vascular conditions is caused by insufficient oxygenation to, and edema of, peripheral tissues. Clients with diabetic neuropathies may have chronic pain because of damaged nerve fibers.

Cancer causes chronic pain from various physiologic factors, including pressure on body structures or on nerve endings or trunks; infiltration of cancer into bones, nerves, blood vessels, or connective tissue; altered circulation; tissue damage; and obstructed or swollen organs. Chronic pain may also develop from trauma or from unknown causes (idiopathic pain).

HEALTH HISTORY FINDINGS
In a health history interview, the client may report or the nurse may detect many of these findings:
• dull, deep, and aching pain
• poorly localized or diffuse pain that changes over time
• continuous or intermittent pain
• muscle spasms
• depression
• use of pain-relieving medications
• special diet to control pain
• recent precipitating loss or stressful event
• altered interpersonal relationships
• inability to perform activities of daily living
• use of adaptive equipment
• use of hot or cold compresses

PHYSICAL FINDINGS
In a physical examination, the nurse may detect many of these findings:

Integumentary
• skin breakdown
• vascular insufficiency and neuropathy in arms and legs

Musculoskeletal
• decreased mobility
• contractures
• muscle spasms

Neurologic
• decreased sensitivity to pain, touch, and temperature

DIAGNOSTIC STUDIES
The following studies may be performed to evaluate the client's health status:
• computed tomography (CT) scan or spinal X-ray—to identify nerve compression
• drug level studies—to monitor the therapeutic blood range for antidepressant medications
• Doppler ultrasonography—to assess peripheral blood flow
• serum glucose levels—to monitor control of blood glucose levels

POTENTIAL COMPLICATIONS
• constipation
• skin breakdown
• depression
• malnutrition
• immobility

Nursing diagnosis: *Chronic pain related to arthritis, peripheral vascular disease, neuropathies, or terminal cancer*

NURSING GOALS: To decrease pain to a tolerable level and to promote the client's and the family's participation in care

Signs and symptoms
• complaints of pain
• complaints of stabbing, aching, or throbbing sensations
• facial grimacing or crying
• anorexia
• inability to perform activities of daily living
• guarding movements
• decreased social interaction
• altered sleep patterns
• altered mood or behavior
• anxiety

Interventions

1. Determine the client's willingness and ability to participate in developing his plan of care.

2. Allow the client to vent anger, denial, sadness, and concerns about living with chronic pain.

3. Evaluate the client's verbal and nonverbal cues to assess the degree and severity of his pain.

4. Assess the client's ability to concentrate by observing him while he listens to music, watches television, engages in conversation, or reads.

5. Encourage the client to use diversional activities, such as watching television, reading, visiting friends, or relaxing through guided imagery or biofeedback.

6. Provide the client with opportunities for rest and sleep. Suggest a sedative, if necessary.

7. Determine the client's need for assistive devices, such as a corset or brace for low-back pain. Use assistive devices when appropriate.

8. Refer the client to a physical therapist.

Rationales

1. Client participation in the decision-making process fosters a sense of control, decreases feelings of helplessness, and increases participation in treatment.

2. This enables the nurse to provide empathy and understanding, which decrease the client's sense of helplessness and helps him tolerate the pain. The elderly client may deny the chronicity of his pain.

3. Pain is subjective, and certain behavioral and psychological expressions, such as facial grimacing, hostility, and withdrawal, verify its presence.

4. The client who is able to concentrate may benefit from diversional activities or relaxation therapy.

5. Distracting activities overload the nerves and, therefore, diminish the pain impulses traveling to the brain. Such activities also stimulate descending inhibitory pathways, thereby reducing the client's perception of pain.

6. Adequate rest can help the client to better tolerate pain and provides him with the energy needed for other activities.

7. Assistive devices improve the client's mobility while conserving his energy. Walkers and canes reduce the pressure on weight-bearing joints and the vertebral column; braces or binders support or splint painful or unstable body parts.

8. Physical therapy can help the client to adapt to his altered life-style, improve his exercise tolerance, and prevent deformities and complications associated with immobility.

9. Use a transcutaneous electrical nerve stimulation (TENS) unit with medication therapy or other interventions for the client with localized pain.

9. A TENS unit delivers a slight electrical current through electrodes placed near the painful area. The current stimulates certain nerve fibers to inhibit the transmission of the pain impulse. The unit rarely produces a dramatic effect on its own, and the relief usually lasts only as long as the area is stimulated. The degree of pain relief varies among individuals.

10. Use noninvasive techniques, such as back rubs or massage, to relieve pain whenever possible.

10. Noninvasive cutaneous stimulation may stimulate endorphin production. It may also bolster the client's confidence in the nurse's ability to relieve discomfort.

11. Discuss with the physician the need for nonnarcotic pain-relieving medications.

11. Acetaminophen, aspirin, and nonsteroidal anti-inflammatory medications inhibit prostaglandin synthesis to decrease inflammation. Although acetaminophen has less of an anti-inflammatory effect than does aspirin, its analgesic properties are comparable. Aspirin has an anticoagulant effect, so it should be avoided in the client who has a low platelet count, is taking an anticoagulant, or who has a bleeding problem. Also, the nurse should be aware that 1,000 mg of acetaminophen every 4 hours can cause liver toxicity.

12. Administer nonsteroidal anti-inflammatory medications, either alone or in combination with other analgesics, to the client with primary or metastatic bone cancer.

12. As cancer invades the dense portions of bones, prostaglandins are released, causing the nerve receptors to sense more pain. Nonsteroidal anti-inflammatory medications inhibit prostaglandin synthesis.

13. Discuss with the physician the client's need for antidepressant medications.

13. Antidepressant drugs enhance analgesia by promoting sleep, reducing anxiety, and alleviating depression. These drugs may also enhance the activity of endogenous opiates, endorphins, and enkephalins.

14. Administer narcotic analgesics (such as codeine, hydromorphone, levorphanol, meperidine, methadone, or oxycodone) as ordered.

14. Analgesics stimulate certain opiate receptors in the brain, spinal cord, and periphery to inhibit the transmission of pain. Narcotic analgesics help to control severe pain.

15. Administer narcotic analgesics around the clock according to their analgesic duration.

15. Dosing on a regular schedule, rather than on an as-needed basis, provides optimal pain control by preventing pain and decreasing the client's anxiety.

16. Administer medications orally, rather than by injection or I.V. bolus, whenever possible.

16. Oral narcotics are easier to administer and help to sustain effective blood drug levels. Intermittent I.M. or I.V. push drugs may cause erratic changes in blood levels.

17. Use equianalgesic equivalents as a guide to determine the comparative analgesic potencies among drugs. Make modifications, as necessary, based on the client's response to the drug.

17. Equianalgesic equivalents are different drugs that produce the same degree of analgesia. When switching the type of narcotic or the route of administration, it is important to maintain an equianalgesic effect.

18. Instruct the client's caregivers to administer pain medication in the early stages of discomfort.

18. Unrelieved discomfort causes anxiety and muscle tension, which may lead to frank pain.

19. Monitor the client for potential side effects of analgesics. If side effects persist, consider an alternative narcotic.

19. Common side effects of narcotic analgesics include nausea, vomiting, constipation, and respiratory or central nervous system depression. The client who develops side effects to one opioid may not develop side effects to another.

20. Consult the physician about the possibility of switching the client to a long-acting opioid.

20. Long-acting opioids, which have an analgesic effect for 4 to 6 hours, are more convenient to administer and prevent the continued cycling of pain. The nurse should always use caution when administering long-acting opioids, since the elderly client has delayed renal clearance of narcotics.

21. Review the possibility of referring the client with intractable chronic pain to a pain clinic.

21. Pain clinics specialize in pain reduction modalities and may be the client's most effective means of coping with intractable pain.

22. Assess whether the client has become physically dependent on pain relievers. Do not confuse physical dependence with addiction.

22. Physical dependence occurs when the body tissues biologically adapt to a narcotic so that the body will react if it is withdrawn abruptly. Addiction describes certain social behaviors indicative of drug abuse, such obtaining drugs from nonmedical sources or using them for psychological regression. Less than 1% of clients receiving medicinal narcotics for pain become addicted.

OUTCOME CRITERIA
• The client will be more comfortable using nonpharmaceutical methods of pain control.
• The client will experience pain relief through the proper administration of analgesics.

Nursing diagnosis: *Potential for impaired skin integrity related to the use of supportive or adaptive devices or immobility*

NURSING GOAL: To prevent skin breakdown

Signs and symptoms
• use of a brace or binder
• reddened areas over pressure points
• immobility
• poor nutritional status

Interventions

1. Assess the client's skin over bony prominences.

2. Assess the client's skin when removing adaptive devices, looking for redness, warmth, breakdown, and dryness.

3. Assess the fit of braces and abdominal binders immediately after application, then again in 15 minutes.

4. Inspect all adaptive devices before using them.

5. Massage generous amounts of body lotion into the client's skin underneath braces or over pressure points.

Rationales

1. Skin integrity over bony prominences may be impaired, especially if the client is edematous, immobilized, or malnourished.

2. Devices worn for prolonged periods can cause insidious skin irritation.

3. The client may have great difficulty applying devices when he is in pain or has decreased mobility. Skin breakdown can occur within a short period if devices are applied incorrectly.

4. Devices with sharp edges or creased linings can damage skin.

5. This helps prevent skin breakdown from the prolonged pressure or rubbing caused by devices.

OUTCOME CRITERION
• The client will use adaptive or assistive devices without developing skin breakdown.

Nursing diagnosis: *Ineffective individual coping related to painful episodes*

NURSING GOALS: To help the client to identify effective coping strategies and to promote a positive attitude

Signs and symptoms
• feeling of hopelessness
• suicidal ideation or death wish
• withdrawal
• lack of motivation
• noncompliance
• crying

Interventions

1. Allow the client to vent anger, sadness, and concerns about living with chronic pain.

2. Work with the client and the client's family to establish realistic goals and expectations.

3. Offer appropriate counseling to help the client and family cope with the problems and needs associated with chronic pain.

Rationales

1. Verbalization allows the nurse to provide empathy and understanding, which helps diminish the client's sense of hopelessness and helps him to better tolerate pain.

2. Achieving realistic goals promotes a sense of accomplishment; conversely, an inability to achieve goals promotes the sense of hopelessness.

3. The elderly client may have preexisting problems or difficulty coping with aging; chronic pain may exaggerate them. Counseling may help to find solutions to the problems or better ways of coping.

OUTCOME CRITERION
• The client will develop effective coping strategies to help him adapt to pain.

NURSING ACTIONS IN VARIOUS SETTINGS
Nursing actions for a client with chronic pain depend on the setting in which care is provided. This section identifies which actions are appropriate in all settings and which pertain to acute care, extended care, or home care situations.

All settings
• Inform the client and the client's family of the need for reassessment by the physician or nurse if pain increases.
• Teach the client and the client's family how to apply and use necessary adaptive devices, such as braces, reachers, walkers, or wheelchairs.
• Develop an individualized medication plan that includes the preferred drug, possible side effects, and indications for administration.
• Inform the client and the client's family that pain tolerance increases when coexisting symptoms (such as

nausea, constipation, insomnia, depression, and restlessness) are eliminated.

Acute care
• Assess the client for signs and symptoms of chronic pain.
• Alert the physician to the client's need for a pain management program.
• Continually evaluate the effectiveness of interventions.
• Consult occupational and physical therapists for necessary adaptive equipment.
• Monitor and treat coexisting symptoms.

Extended care
• Continually assess the effectiveness of pain management.
• Involve occupational and physical therapists in developing adaptive devices.
• Treat coexisting symptoms, such as constipation, nausea, insomnia, restlessness, and depression.

• Suggest that the client's family provide noninvasive interventions, such as supportive listening, distraction, touching, and promoting comfort through hygiene and other personal care measures.

Home care
• Teach the client and the client's family about the need to readjust pain medications as the client's disease or terminal illness progresses.
• Inform the client and client's family of the need to report any increase in pain so that the physician can prescribe stronger medications.
• Review the difference between physical dependency and addiction with clients taking narcotic analgesics.
• Review with the client the importance of noninvasive interventions to decrease pain, such as adequate sleep, supportive listening, and distraction.
• Inform the client and the client's family of the need to alleviate coexisting symptoms, such as constipation, nausea, depression, and restlessness.

SELECTED REFERENCES
Eland, J.M. "Pain Management and Comfort," *Journal of Gerontological Nursing* 14(4):10-15, April 1988.

Gandy, S., and Payne, R. "Back Pain in the Elderly: Updated Diagnosis and Management," *Geriatrics* 41(12):59-72, December 1986.

McGuire, D.B., and Yarbro, C.H., eds. *Cancer Pain Management.* New York: Grune & Stratton, 1987.

Portenoy, R.K., and Farkash, A. "Practical Management of Non-Malignant Pain in the Elderly," *Geriatrics* 43(5):29-47, May 1988.

Sternbach, R. *Pain A Psychophysiological Analysis.* New York: Academic Press, 1986.

Strandness, E.D. "Vascular Diseases of the Extremities," in *Harrison's Principles of Internal Medicine,* 11th ed. Edited by Braunwald, E., et al. New York: McGraw-Hill Book Co., 1987.

Thomas, P.K., and Scadding, J.W. "Treatment of Pain in Diabetic Neuropathy," in *Diabetic Neuropathy.* Edited by Dyck, P.J., et al. Philadelphia: W.B. Saunders Co., 1987.

GENERAL CARE PLAN
Cancer

A leading cause of death among older adults, cancer is a malignant tumor whose natural course is normally fatal. About 50% of all cancers occur after age 65, primarily involving the colon, rectum, breast, lung, and prostate. The incidence increases with age, typically doubling between ages 60 and 80.

Cancers are classified according to their point of cellular origin. Carcinomas, which arise from epithelial tissue, are most common in adults, whereas sarcomas, which arise from mesodermal tissue, are more predominant in children. Squamous cell carcinomas arise from superficial epithelium, or squamous cells; adenocarcinomas arise from glandular tissue. Other cancers, such as leukemias, lymphomas, and neural tissue tumors are classified separately because of their low incidence and origin.

This care plan discusses breast, lung, bladder, uterine, colon, and rectal cancers (for discussions of skin and prostate cancers, see "Skin Cancer," pages 32 to 34, and "Benign Prostatic Hypertrophy and Prostate Cancer," pages 138 to 146).

ETIOLOGY
Aging is the greatest risk factor for developing cancer, possibly because of the prolonged period between the initial exposure to carcinogens and development of disease or because of the decreased efficiency of the immune system to deter the proliferation of errant cells. Also, certain age-related physiologic changes may promote tumor growth.

Cancer arises when normal cells lose their ability to differentiate or mature. The process of carcinogenesis is complex and usually begins with a single change, or multiple changes, in the normal architecture of cellular deoxyribonucleic acid (DNA). Stages of tumor genesis help to explain the multifaceted process of malignant cell transformation.

The first stage of tumor growth (initiation) occurs when the genetic composition of cellular DNA irreversibly alters. The second stage (promotion) occurs when the malignant cell begins to proliferate; this can only occur after the cell has undergone initiation. Eventually, after initiation and promotion, malignant cell transformation progresses and produces an uncontrollable group of cells that can invade normal tissue and cause death. Examples of initiators include carcinogens, such as chemicals, radiation, and viruses; examples of promoters include diet and hormones. Cigarette smoking may be both an initiator and a promotor.

Each type of cancer varies as to its cause and course. Breast cancer may result from a genetic predisposition, an impaired immunologic response, a virus, or estrogen use. Uterine cancer, which typically metastasizes late (commonly to the cervix, fallopian tubes, and other peritoneal structures), may be caused by excess body weight and increased circulating levels of estrogen.

Lung cancers are classified into one of four categories: adenocarcinoma, epidermoid carcinoma, small-cell (oat-cell) carcinoma, and large-cell (anaplastic) carcinoma. Adenocarcinoma, which commonly affects women and sometimes nonsmokers, metastasizes widely, frequently invading the contralateral lung, liver, bones, kidneys, or central nervous system (CNS). Epidermal carcinoma of the lung, which typically occurs in those who smoke, constitute 30% of all bronchogenic tumors; they grow slowly and are usually less invasive than the other tumor types. Small-cell carcinoma is typically aggressive, rapidly growing in clients who smoke; it commonly metastasizes to the contralateral lung, lymph nodes, liver, bones, bone marrow, and CNS. Large-cell carcinoma is the rarest type of bronchogenic cancer.

Bladder cancer may be noninvasive, as in bladder-wall tumors, or invasive, as in bladder-muscle tumors. Tumors seldom invade the surrounding pelvic organs or metastasize systemically. Transitional cell carcinomas constitute about 90% of primary bladder tumors and commonly affect elderly clients. Cigarette smoking and industrial carcinogens may contribute to the development of bladder cancer. Whether artificial sweeteners, such as saccharin and cyclamates, contribute to the development of bladder cancer, is a controversial topic.

Colorectal cancers most likely develop in a multistage process. Many researchers believe that colorectal cancers originate from a benign, edematous polyp that undergoes malignant transformation over a 5- to 10-year period. Other causes include a diet low in fiber and high in fat and concurrent premalignant diseases, such as ulcerative colitis.

HEALTH HISTORY FINDINGS
In a health history interview, the client may report or the nurse may detect may of these findings:

Breast cancer
- history of fibrocystic breast disease
- history of nulliparity or first birth after age 30
- history of menarche before age 12
- history of menopause after age 50
- history of a high-fat diet
- family history of breast cancer
- high socioeconomic status

Uterine cancer
- history of low parity or nulliparity
- history of menopause after age 52
- history of anovulation
- abnormal uterine bleeding

- history of irregular menstrual periods
- history of hypertension or diabetes mellitus
- endometrial adenomatous tumor
- use of estrogen therapy

Lung cancer
- weight loss
- fatigue
- chest pain
- anorexia
- streaky hemoptysis
- dyspnea
- history of persistent upper respiratory infections, tuberculosis, chronic bronchitis, pleural disease, or pulmonary emboli
- family history of lung cancer
- history of heavy or passive cigarette smoking
- history of exposure to asbestos or environmental or occupational pollutants

Bladder cancer
- dysuria
- painless hematuria
- urinary frequency and urgency
- history of cigarette smoking
- history of occupational exposure to carcinogens

Colorectal cancers
- change in frequency, consistency, and color of stools
- blood in stools or rectal bleeding
- constipation
- incomplete bowel evacuation with urgency
- altered bowel habits
- history of inflammatory bowel disease or iron deficiency anemia
- history of female genital, breast, or bladder cancer
- history of a low-fiber, high-fat diet
- family history of colorectal cancer
- familial polyposis syndrome
- history of exposure to occupational carcinogens

PHYSICAL FINDINGS
In a physical examination for *breast cancer*, the nurse may detect many of these findings:

Genitourinary
- recently developed breast asymmetry
- painless mass, lump, or thickening in breast
- redness of skin over breast lump
- change in the contour of the breast or nipple
- crusting or retraction of the nipple
- dimpling ("orange peel" skin)
- breast swelling
- nipple discharge

Other
- obesity

In a physical examination for *uterine cancer*, the nurse may detect many of these findings:

Genitourinary
- pelvic pain
- irritative voiding symptoms (frequency and urgency)
- gross or microscopic hematuria

Other
- overweight by more than 30%

In a physical examination for *lung cancer*, the nurse may detect many of these findings:

Integumentary
- palpable lymph nodes in the neck or axilla

Respiratory
- wheezing or stridor
- cough
- shortness of breath

Cardiovascular
- chest pain

In a physical examination for *bladder cancer*, the nurse may detect many of these findings:

Genitourinary
- bladder pain
- hematuria

Cardiovascular
- lower extremity edema

Gastrointestinal
- lower abdominal pain

In a physical examination for *colorectal cancer*, the nurse may detect many of these findings:

Gastrointestinal
- tenesmus or abdominal pain
- fecal impaction

DIAGNOSTIC STUDIES
The following studies may be performed to evaluate the client's health status:

Breast cancer
- breast examination—to detect breast changes, lumps, or asymmetry; performed monthly by the client and yearly by the physician
- mammography—to detect lesions too small to be detected by palpation; recommended to be performed annually in female clients over age 50

• biopsy—to determine a definitive diagnosis; performed on suspicious lesions or lumps, even if mammogram is normal

Uterine cancer
• endometrial biopsy—to obtain an accurate diagnosis; accurate about 75% of the time; should be performed on women at high risk for developing endometrial cancer at menopause
• Papanicolaou (Pap) smear—to detect abnormal cells; only effective 50% of the time in detecting endometrial cancer; should be performed on women who have never had a Pap smear or who have had dysplasia

Lung cancer
• sputum cytological examination—to recover and identify tumor cells
• chest X-ray—to detect a mass; recommended yearly for clients at risk
• lung biopsy—to identify tumor cells if sputum does not contain pulmonary cells; obtained through bronchoscopy, mediastinoscopy, or thoracentesis or by a lymph node or open-lung biopsy

Bladder cancer
• urinalysis—to detect bacteria and microscopic hematuria or to rule out other sources of inflammation
• cytological studies of urine or bladder wall—to detect cancerous cells
• cystourethroscopy—to obtain a biopsy of bladder mucosa lesions

• intravenous pyelography—to identify a renal mass, stones, urethral obstruction, or lesions in the collecting system or ureters

Colorectal cancers
• stool guaiac test—to detect blood in the stool; a negative result does not rule out cancer; should be performed annually
• digital rectal examination and proctosigmoidoscopy—to diagnose all rectal cancers; elderly clients should have 2 tests a year apart, and then, if negative, every 3 to 5 years
• barium enema with air contrast—to detect growths overlooked by other procedures; detects tumors in the upper colon but cannot easily detect those in the rectum

POTENTIAL COMPLICATIONS
• multiorgan malfunction
• bleeding
• infection
• weight loss
• malnutrition
• cachexia
• fatigue
• nausea
• anorexia
• immobility
• diarrhea
• pain

Nursing diagnosis: *Impaired oral tissue integrity related to the cytotoxic effects of cancer therapy*

NURSING GOALS: To keep the oral mucous membranes free from ulceration and infection and to institute preventive oral measures

Signs and symptoms
• thick, swollen, erythematous oral mucosa
• sensitivity to hot and cold foods
• slight burning sensation in mouth
• ulcerations
• dry mouth (xerostomia)
• oral candidiasis

Interventions

1. Inspect the client's oral mucous membranes daily for ulcerations or lesions, color changes, swelling, or candidiasis.

Rationales

1. Some chemotherapeutic agents, as well as radiation therapy to the head and neck, damage the cells of the oral mucosa and may cause inflammation and ulceration.

2. Teach the client preventive measures, such as brushing his teeth in the morning and at night with a soft brush or oral swabs, using a mild, nonabrasive toothpaste; rinsing his mouth with normal saline solution after meals and at bedtime and avoiding commercial mouthwashes; and removing ill-fitting dentures between meals.

2. Prophylactic oral care helps keep oral mucous membranes and teeth clean, thereby preventing further damage. Commercial mouthwashes contain alcohol and phenol which may also damage oral tissue. Ill-fitting dentures can trap food particles, causing further damage to the oral mucosa.

3. Refer the client to a dentist for devices, such as fluoride trays, or other measures before radiation therapy.

3. Dentists can help protect the client's teeth and oral mucosa from the effects of radiation.

4. Teach the client who suffers dry mouth from chemotherapy to drink fluids frequently, to suck on ice chips, and to apply gravies and sauces to foods.

4. These measures help keep oral tissues moist.

5. Teach the client the early signs and symptoms of stomatitis, including swollen or thick mucous membranes, erythematous or pale membranes, increased sensitivity to hot and cold foods, oral discomfort, and a burning sensation in the mouth.

5. When detected early, treatment can help prevent further oral problems.

6. Institute the following measures to manage stomatitis: discuss with the physician the appropriate solution for oral irrigations or rinses, such as ¼ to ½ strength hydrogen peroxide, ¼ strength modified Dakin's solution, sodium bicarbonate solution, or warm saline rinses or lavage; have the client keep his mucous membranes clean and moist by rinsing frequently or using an artificial saliva solution; and teach the client to avoid alcoholic beverages and smoking.

6. Oral mucous membranes, tongue, and teeth must be kept clean when stomatitis is evident. Oral irrigants remove debris and damaged cells, and some solutions, such as hydrogen peroxide, have an antibacterial effect. One-fourth strength Dakin's solution debrides the oral membranes, while sodium bicarbonate removes the thick mucin that collects in the mouth because of reduced salivation and decreased food intake. Frequent rinsing with an artificial saliva solution can help moisten the oral membranes of the client with decreased saliva flow. Alcoholic beverages and smoking irritate the oral tissues and should therefore be avoided.

7. Administer mycostatic mouth rinses or lozenges, as ordered, to prevent or treat oral candidiasis.

7. Oral candidiasis commonly occurs when chemotherapy, antibiotics, malnutrition, or myelosuppression disrupts the normal flora of the mouth.

8. Administer local anesthetics, milk of magnesia or kaolin mouth rinses, and systemic pain medications, as prescribed.

8. Topical anesthetics and systemic pain medications relieve pain, promote compliance with the regimen, and help maintain adequate nutrition. Milk of magnesia or kaolin mouth rinses coat and protect oral membranes.

OUTCOME CRITERIA
• The client will maintain good oral hygiene practices.
• The client will have minimal or no change to his oral membranes from cancer therapy.
• The client will identify the signs and symptoms of stomatitis, and will report their presence immediately to the physician should they occur.

Nursing diagnosis: *Potential for injury related to bleeding episodes*

NURSING GOALS: To identify clients at risk for bleeding and to monitor blood clotting factors

Signs and symptoms
• active bleeding
• purpura and ecchymosis
• petechiae on skin and mucous membranes
• tarry stools

Interventions

1. Assess the client's oral mucosa and dependent parts daily for petechiae, ecchymosis, purpura, or other signs of bleeding.

2. Check the client's platelet count daily. If the count is abnormal, consult the physician on the need for platelet transfusions.

3. Assess the client with a platelet count of less than 20,000 μl for neurologic changes, such as headaches and blurred vision.

4. Avoid invasive procedures, such as I.M. injections, rectal temperatures, or urinary catheters, if the client's platelet count drops below 75,000 μl.

5. Teach the client with a platelet count of less than 100,000 μl to use an electric razor and a soft toothbrush and to report any bruising or bleeding from the rectum, vagina, gums, or nose.

6. Test the client's urine, stool, emesis, and sputum for blood. Instruct the client to avoid using vitamin C before obtaining a guaiac stool specimen.

Rationales

1. Petechiae, ecchymosis, and purpura signal severe thrombocytopenia.

2. Some chemotherapeutic agents and radiation affect bone marrow reserves and cause thrombocytopenia. A low platelet count places the client at risk for bleeding, and a transfusion may be indicated.

3. The client with a platelet count less than 20,000 μl is susceptible to spontaneous CNS bleeding.

4. Invasive procedures could cause an injury and trigger prolonged bleeding.

5. The client with a low platelet count needs to take measures to prevent injury. Signs and symptoms of bleeding should be reported to prevent anemia and significant decreases in hemoglobin levels.

6. Testing excretions for blood will identify any occult bleeding. Vitamin C can cause a false-negative result on a stool guaiac test.

OUTCOME CRITERIA
• The client will not have bleeding episodes.
• The client will observe and report any signs and symptoms of bleeding.

Nursing diagnosis: *Impaired skin integrity related to steroid use, radiation, or chemotherapy*

NURSING GOALS: To assess the client's skin for side effects of cancer therapy and to maintain the integrity of the client's skin over irradiated areas

Signs and symptoms
• skin redness, excoriation, and breakdown
• alopecia
• wet or dry desquamation (from radiation therapy)
• phlebitis
• skin photosensitivity (from fluorouracil use)
• striae (from steroid therapy)
• urticaria or pruritus

Interventions

1. Assess the client's skin daily for breakdown, tears, rashes, or abnormal dryness. Pay particular attention to the skin over irradiated areas.

Rationales

1. Radiation therapy impairs the sweat glands, causing skin dryness and susceptibility to fissures and infection. Rashes and skin reactions may indicate an allergic reaction to a chemotherapeutic agent.

2. Teach the client receiving radiation therapy to avoid using soaps, ointments, creams, cosmetics, powder, and deodorants on treated skin, unless prescribed by a physician; to avoid washing off radiation markings; to keep the irradiated area dry; to use a mild soap for bathing while avoiding washing the treated area; and to check irradiated areas for increased erythema, dryness, burning, discomfort, or dry or wet desquamation.

2. Topical preparations may enhance the effects of radiation on the skin and increase the possibility of skin toxicity. External markings identifying the radiation field allow the radiation to be directed to the same region each time. Soap and water on the irradiated area may alter the skin during therapy. Radiation decreases the frequency of epidermal mitosis, which temporarily decreases stem-cell activity in the basal layer of the skin and results in wet desquamation. The elderly client is especially susceptible to radiation damage and is at high risk for infection.

3. Avoid applying heat, such as a hot water bottle, heating pad, or heat lamp, to the treated area during or after radiation.

3. Heat, as well as sunlight and pressure, may exacerbate skin breakdown and toxicity.

4. Teach the client that alopecia may occur with use of radiation therapy. Emphasize that hair loss is temporary and that, although the hair will grow back, it may have a different color or texture.

4. Scalp hair follicles in the area receiving radiation may become damaged, causing alopecia. Hair loss typically begins 2 to 3 weeks after the initiation of therapy and may continue for several months. Hair loss may be permanent, or the regrowth may be retarded, depending upon the dose of radiation.

5. Teach the client to keep his scalp clean by washing with a mild shampoo. Encourage the client with hair loss to wear a wig or scarf.

5. Cleaning the scalp improves circulation in the area. Wigs and scarves camouflage hair loss and help the client adjust to a change in body image.

6. Teach the client to avoid tight-fitting clothing next to the treated area, to wear clothes made of 100% cotton, and to report any skin changes.

6. Constricting garments cause friction and may irritate the treated area. Cotton fabrics absorb skin moisture and allow the skin to breathe. The client needs to observe the skin site for redness, inflammation, and breakdown.

7. Teach the photosensitive client to use a sunscreen and to avoid prolonged exposure to the sun.

7. Some chemotherapeutic agents make the skin more susceptible to the effects of ultraviolet radiation. Sunscreens help block ultraviolet rays.

8. Assess the client who has undergone previous radiation therapy and recent chemotherapy for erythema in the irradiated area.

8. Certain chemotherapeutic agents, such as doxorubicin, may cause a skin reaction in a previously irradiated area (radiation recall).

9. Explain to the client taking steroids that striae, skin fragility, and poor wound healing may occur.

9. Long-term, high-dose steroid therapy can markedly change skin texture and cause weight gain, resulting in striae. Steroid use also causes skin fragility and prevents wound healing.

OUTCOME CRITERIA
- The client's skin over the irradiated area will remain intact throughout therapy.
- The client will practice measures to reduce the possibility of skin breakdown.

Nursing diagnosis: *Potential for vascular, cardiac, and hepatic injury related to chemotherapy infusion*

NURSING GOALS: To prevent tissue sclerosis and to prevent secondary effects of chemotherapeutic agents

Signs and symptoms
- dysrhythmias
- increased cardiac enzyme levels
- congestive heart failure
- phlebitis
- tissue sclerosis
- hepatotoxicity

Interventions

1. Always support the vein when performing venipuncture, and insert the needle less deeply than usual when administering an I.M. injection.

2. To prevent phlebitis and preserve veins, take the following precautions: Flush all chemotherapeutic agents through the vein with an appropriate I.V. solution; alternate I.V. sites every 48 to 72 hours; avoid administering I.V. fluids with a high concentration of potassium; and, if extravasation is suspected, stop the infusion and immediately notify the physician or a nurse skilled in managing extravasation.

3. Monitor the client's blood pressure before, and every 15 minutes during, etoposide infusions. Infuse the medication over 30 minutes to 1 hour. Stop the infusion if the client's blood pressure decreases more than 20 mm Hg, or if his systolic blood pressure falls below 90 mm Hg; restart the infusion at half the original rate when the blood pressure returns to its normal level.

4. Monitor the client for hepatotoxicity by performing an abdominal examination to check for hepatomegaly; monitoring the client's liver function tests; and assessing the client for jaundice and pruritus.

5. Assess the client for signs of cardiac toxicity, such as dysrhythmias, increased cardiac enzyme levels, signs and symptoms of congestive heart failure, and chest pain.

Rationales

1. These measures will help prevent tissue and venous injury. Supporting the arm is necessary because the elderly client has a decreased amount of subcutaneous fat in the arms and hands, which causes veins to roll. Inserting the needle less deeply is necessary because lean muscle mass decreases with aging.

2. Flushing the vein reduces the risk of phlebitis from chemotherapy irritants. If irritants leak into the tissues during administration, permanent, progressive damage will occur. Therefore, meticulous vein selection and accurate catheter placement are essential. Changing I.V. sites frequently prevents the vein from sclerosing and prevents I.V. fluids from leaking into surrounding tissue. Avoiding potassium supplements is necessary because they increase the risk of phlebitis. Sclerosing agents should only be given by skilled phlebotomists via a newly started, free-flowing I.V. Once a site has extravasated, the infusion should be stopped immediately, then restarted by a trained, skilled nurse.

3. Etoposide can cause hypotension if administered rapidly. The elderly client who is dehydrated, anemic, or on antihypertensive medication, may be especially prone to hypotension.

4. Elevated liver function tests are an early sign of hepatotoxicity. An enlarged liver, jaundice, and pruritus are more serious signs that indicate toxicity.

5. Cumulative doses of doxorubicin and daunorubicin, totaling about 550 mg, can irreversibly damage heart muscle. The client with preexisting cardiac disease may develop cardiac toxicity.

OUTCOME CRITERIA
- The client will have no signs of phlebitis related to fluorouracil or etoposide administration.
- The client will have no signs of cardiac toxicity from doxorubicin and daunorubicin.
- The client will remain free of hepatotoxicity.
- The client will not experience hypotension with etoposide administration.

Nursing diagnosis: *Altered nutrition: less than body requirements, related to nausea, vomiting, anorexia, radiation therapy, and chemotherapy*

NURSING GOALS: To prevent or minimize nausea and vomiting associated with cancer or its therapies and to minimize the degree of weight loss while increasing the client's nutritional intake

Signs and symptoms
• lack of appetite
• weight loss
• cachexia
• decreased urinary output
• mucosal dryness and decreased skin turgor
• decreased interest in food
• nausea and vomiting
• confusion

Interventions

1. Monitor the client's fluid intake and output and his weight. Encourage him to drink eight 8-oz glasses (2,000 ml) of fluid a day.

2. Inspect the client's mouth for inadequate dentition, loose teeth, gingivitis, impaired integrity of the oral mucosa, and nutritional deficiencies.

3. Monitor the client's caloric intake for 48 hours, and instruct the client to keep a personal diet history for 1 week.

4. Encourage the client to maintain good oral hygiene and to frequently rinse his mouth with a non-alcohol-based substance, such as baking soda and water.

5. Advise the client with esophagitis to consume thick fluids, such as gelatin and fruit slushes (see "Dysphagia," pages 120 to 127), and to avoid drinking fluids with meals or for 30 minutes afterward.

6. Encourage the client to follow a diet rich in complex carbohydrates, such as whole-grain cereals and fresh fruits and vegetables, and low-fat protein, such as fish, poultry, and skim milk products.

7. Advise the client who typically experiences nausea and vomiting when eating to avoid fried foods, gravies, rich sauces, and lactose-containing foods and to eat pastas, broiled or poached meats, fruits, gelatins, and cold foods.

8. Administer antiemetics and steroids ½ to 1 hour before and after radiation and chemotherapy treatments.

Rationales

1. Normal aging decreases the number of osmoreceptors that conserve water and also decreases the thirst sensation. A client with nausea and vomiting or anorexia secondary to cancer therapy will experience weight loss and decreased fluid intake and output and will be at risk for malnutrition.

2. Cancer therapies lead to tooth loss, fungal infections, and mucosal lesions, which can contribute to difficulties that prevent an adequate nutritional intake.

3. This assessment will reveal the client's nutritional intake and identify deficiencies. Cancer typicallly causes malnutrition and depresses the immune function.

4. These measures help to promote oral health and stimulate salivation, which is necessary for chewing, swallowing, and the initial digestion of food.

5. Esophagitis can result from local radiation therapy to the head, neck, or chest or from chemotherapeutic agents, particularly antimetabolites. Thick fluids are easier to swallow than water or juices. Also, drinking fluids with meals can depress the appetite by causing bloating and feelings of fullness.

6. During radiation therapy, the client typically experiences increased metabolism of both malignant cells and normal cells that compete for available nutrients. Thus, the client requires particular attention to calories and proteins to meet both tumor and body needs.

7. Nausea and vomiting impair oral intake and deplete fluids in the client who is already compromised, as in cancer. Low-fat foods are usually better tolerated during prolonged periods of nausea and vomiting. Cold foods are also tolerated because they produce little odor. Also, the elderly client may be lactose intolerant, and malnutrition, radiation therapy to the abdominal or pelvic area, and chemotherapy exacerbate the problem.

8. Radiation and some chemotherapeutic agents stimulate dopamine uptake in the chemoreceptor trigger zone, causing nausea and vomiting, which contribute to decreased nutritional intake. Antiemetic medications block this action. Chemotherapeutic agents also stimulate prostaglandin production in the brain, also contributing to nausea and vomiting. Steroids inhibit prostaglandin in the brain.

9. Refer the client to a dietitian for help in formulating an individualized meal plan.

9. An individualized meal plan can prevent malnutrition, which is a major contributor to depressed immune function. A depressed immune system increases the client's susceptibility to bacterial, fungal, and viral infections as well as cancer and other autoimmune diseases.

10. Discuss with the physician the need for enteral feedings in the client who is anorectic or has difficulty swallowing, who has received oral radiation, or has an inadequate oral intake.

10. Enteral nutrition provides adequate fluids and nutrition in the client who cannot achieve adequate oral intake on his own.

11. Consult the physician about the client's need for parenteral nutrition, if indicated. Avoid using hypertonic glucose infusions.

11. Parenteral nutrition provides adequate nutrients to the client who is or who may become malnourished. The elderly client has a decreased tolerance to glucose and a decreased ability to clear serum lipids.

OUTCOME CRITERIA
• The client will receive adequate nutrition as evidenced by weight gain and decreased nausea and vomiting.

Nursing diagnosis: *Knowledge deficit related to hospice home care*

NURSING GOAL: To educate the client and his family or caregiver about the client's diagnosis, prognosis, and home care needs.

Signs and symptoms
• lack of understanding regarding the client's disease, prognosis, and treatment
• unawareness of available community resources for caregiving assistance
• underutilization of hospice home care team members

Interventions

1. Arrange for the client and family to meet with the physician and hospice nurse to discuss the client's diagnosis, prognosis, and treatment goals.

2. Inform the client's family or caregiver about community cancer support groups and service organizations.

3. Discuss with the client and caregiver the benefits of the client remaining at home, including physical comfort and privacy, feelings of security, enhanced ties with family and friends, involvement of the family in the client's care, convenience for the client's family and caregiver, and the client's continued autonomy.

Rationales

1. Accurate knowledge should help the client and his family to make short- and long-term medical and financial plans, and to prepare themselves psychologically.

2. These groups can provide information about cancer and the supportive measures available for the client and caregiver.

3. The elderly client may become disoriented in an institutional setting, feel assaulted by blood tests and multiple X-rays, and frequently cannot sleep. Remaining at home helps the client to retain control over his rest and sleep times, privacy, social interactions, and meal selection. Remaining at home also provides a safe refuge and quells fears of abandonment and isolation. Familiar surroundings and people provide the client with a continued sense of identity despite the threat of illness. Also, those who remain at home are better able to enjoy intimacy, sexuality, sharing, and reminiscing and are also able to make last requests. Participation in the client's care allows the family to express their devotion and affection, and assures them, after the client's death, that they enhanced the client's last days. Home care also allows the client's family to avoid limited visiting hours, transportation problems, and a disrupted life-style.

4. Instruct the client's caregivers about appropriate ways to control the side effects of chemotherapy and radiation. Also instruct them on the importance of having the client follow a bowel and bladder management program, preventing pressure sores, and coping with the client's mental status changes.

4. Education decreases the caregiver's fears about routine daily care and emergencies.

5. Explain to the client the specific roles of each hospice team member, including the physician, visiting hospice nurse, home health aide or homemaker, medical social worker, psychologist, chaplain, volunteers, and physical, occupational, and speech therapists. Implement the services specifically needed by the client.

5. Individualized homecare services decrease the client's and family's anxiety and increase their sense of purpose and control.

6. After determining the feasibility of the client remaining at home, provide the family with access to community resources. Outline the costs and caretaking responsibilities involved with hospice home care. If hospice home care is not a viable option, provide them with information regarding alternative living arrangements, and assist them with placing the client.

6. Using community resources enhances the caregiver's physical and psychological resources, decreases caretaker burnout, and increases the caretaker's sense of independence.

OUTCOME CRITERIA
• The client and caregivers will use the resources necessary to maximize home care services.
• The client's family and caregivers will verbalize an understanding of or demonstrate appropriate interventions for helping the client to control adverse effects of the cancer.

Nursing diagnosis: *Ineffective family coping related to the client's terminal illness*

NURSING GOAL: To help the client's family or caregiver to cope with the client's terminal illness

Signs and symptoms
• anger
• depression
• hostility
• tearfulness
• apathy
• anxiety
• silence
• overt references to death and religion

Interventions

1. Assess the client's and family's level of comfort in discussing the issues surrounding death.

2. Use effective communication techniques, especially active listening.

Rationales

1. The nurse needs to assess the client and family to know which level of awareness they are experiencing before interventions can be implemented. The four levels of awareness concerning dying include closed awareness (the client's unawareness that death is imminent), suspected awareness (the client's expectation, but uncertainty, that he will die), mutual pretense (the client's and caregiver's acknowledgment that the client is dying and agreement to act as if this were not so), and open acceptance (the client's and caregiver's free acknowledgment that the client is dying).

2. The client and family often make overt references to death to test the hospice staff's true level of comfort in confronting death and dying issues.

3. Allow the terminally ill client and his family to talk freely about the illness, their suspicions, and their knowledge.

3. The family may doubt their ability to care for a terminally ill client at home and fear that their strength will disappear during an emergency or when the client dies. Encouraging verbalization promotes a trusting environment in which the client and family can share their feelings.

4. Encourage family members to touch and hold the hands of the unresponsive client.

4. Touching conveys feelings and can comfort the client who, because of confusion or a decreased level of consciousness, cannot understand words.

5. Educate the client and the client's family about Kübler-Ross's five phases of grief (denial, anger, bargaining, depression, and acceptance).

5. The client and family need to know that fluctuating among the various stages of grief is normal and that they may be experience conflicting feelings at any given time.

6. Continually assess the family's coping abilities throughout hospice home care to determine whether the client should remain at home or be admitted to a hospice facility (see *Nonhome care options*).

6. The client and family should be aware that, if they cannot effectively cope with their present situation, various health care and home care settings are available to provide adequate hospice care.

7. Reinforce emergency procedures, and teach the signs and symptoms of impending death. Inform the family about the availability of the hospice's 24-hour on-call service.

7. Such instruction helps caregivers feel prepared and lessens their sense of isolation.

8. As a hospice team member, confront your own views on death and religion.

8. Nurses should confront their personal views to prevent any biases and anxieties from inhibiting dialogue.

9. Offer the dying client and his family every opportunity to practice their religious traditions and explore their beliefs.

9. The client and family should be allowed to recognize and appropriately respond to their spiritual concerns at this time.

10. Attempt to discuss spiritual concerns throughout hospice home care.

10. The client sometimes perceives spiritual discussions as one of the last things to do before death, so timing is important.

11. Encourage prayer and rituals.

11. Prayer is a personal form of communication that may express fear, anger, joy, thanksgiving, and requests. Before death, religious rituals associated with reconciliation, forgiveness, and becoming "at one" with the divine become extremely important.

12. Encourage the client's family to use respite care.

12. Respite care supports the family and may reduce the need to permanently institutionalize the client. Respite care allows for the admission of the client to the hospital or a nursing home for a day, a week, a weekend, during family vacations, or during emergencies.

13. Help the client's family to anticipate grieving. Also provide bereavement follow-up after the client's death.

13. Anticipatory grief can reduce the shock of loss and can help the client and his family have a meaningful time together before death. Immediately after the client's death, survivors may need practical help in coping with everyday living or psychological support in coping with their grief. If abnormal grief patterns develop, the family or family member may need the help of a professional therapist.

OUTCOME CRITERIA
• The client will attain psychological and spiritual ease before death.
• The client's family and caretakers will achieve an optimal level of coping with both the physical and psychological aspects of death.

NONHOME CARE OPTIONS

Facility	Client and family participation	Level of care rendered	Financial considerations
After-care programs	*Client:* Active participant in programmed therapy *Family:* Involved with transportation, assisting client in accomplishing goals, easing transition from hospital to home	• Provides hospital services to clients 3 to 5 times weekly for a few hours each visit • Eases transition from hospital to home • Accomplishes specified, therapeutic, short-term tasks	Insurance coverage is variable
Day hospitals	*Client:* Works actively to achieve rehabilitation goals *Family:* Learn how to provide interim personal care	• Provided within a hospital setting • Emphasizes rehabilitation services and instruction for family members and caregivers regarding interim personal care of client; usually offered 5 days a week	Usually expensive; variable insurance coverage
Day-care services	*Client:* Active involvement *Family:* Supportive role; monitors client's level of independent functioning	• Provides ambulatory care and some personal hygiene care • Emphasizes primary prevention services (such as medication and nutrition education, health screening), recreation, and some therapeutic and rehabilitative services (such as speech, physical, and occupational therapies)	Insurance coverage is rare, although some state Medicaid programs pay for daily fees
Intermediate-care facilities	*Client:* Active in rehabilitation and recuperative goals *Family:* Assists client with goal-achievement and return to home setting	• Institutional setting • Emphasizes postconvalescent hospital care; usually rehabilitative on a short-term basis	Variable insurance coverage
Nursing homes and skilled nursing facilities	*Client:* Recipient of skilled care *Family:* Supportive; assist client with adjustment to institutionalization	• Institutional setting • Emphasizes 24-hour medical and skilled nursing care	Insurance coverage depends on holder's policy specifications; state grants are available according to family's level of income
Homes for the aged	*Client:* Healthy, independent *Family:* Supportive	• Homelike setting • Emphasizes 24-hour care, room, board, and recreation	Insurance coverage is rare
Hospices	*Client:* Terminally ill status *Family:* Commitment to client	• Free-standing hospices provide institutionalization 24 hours a day, 7 days a week; emphasizes skilled and supportive care to client and family • Provides control through palliative therapies; offers bereavement services to survivors for a period of at least 1 year.	Insurance coverage depends on policy and private and public donations

MEDICAL COVERAGE FOR THE ELDERLY CLIENT

Program	Eligibility	Characteristics	Coverage
Medicare (Parts A & B)	Automatically at age 65 (application must be made 3 months before birthday); related to the eligibility for Social Security or federal work credits.	Federal program of hospital and medical insurance	Does not cover any type of primary prevention services, such as dental, vision, or hearing care. Does not cover medications. Care in long-term settings and home health care is covered only if skilled nursing care is required. Some examples of skilled nursing include wound care, catheter care, and I.V. administration of fluids and medications. Medicare categorizes any unskilled nursing services as custodial care. Hence, those who require assistance with activities of daily living or ambulation or who have chronic illness without significant physical needs are ineligible to receive reimbursement by Medicare for home care services.
Medicare Part A		Reimburses 4 kinds of care: inpatient hospital care, medically necessary inpatient care in a skilled nursing facility after a hospital stay, home health care, hospice care.	Covers all inpatient hospital costs, skilled nursing facility, home health care, and hospice care. Coverage is for first consecutive 60 days. Skilled nursing care is covered for up to 100 days as long as admission follows a hospital discharge. Clients pay first $520 of hospital bill.
Medicare Part B		Voluntary program, subscribers pay a portion of this cost in the form of monthly premiums. Client pays first $75 of doctor's bills once a year.	Covers 80% of reasonable doctor's services, outpatient hospital care, outpatient physical therapy and speech pathology services, home health care, ambulance service and other health services and supplies not covered by Medicare hospital insurance.
Medicaid	People of all ages in low income categories. Each state determines eligibility and benefits within the constraints of certain federal and state limits. Benefits and eligibility vary from state to state.	Grant-in-aid program in which federal, state, and sometimes local government share the costs of medical care.	Medicaid (also known as Medical Assistance) complements Medicare's Part A by paying all or part of the deductible co-insurance amounts for the low income elderly client who is eligible. It also complements Medicare's Part B program by paying the monthly premiums for Medicaid recipients. Medicaid will cover prescription drugs.
Medigap (supplemental insurance)	Senior citizens, who tend to buy more than one policy	Policyholder must pay annual premiums for policy, which usually averages $200/year.	Offers coverage for services not covered under Medicare. Most supplemental policies follow Medicare guidelines, thereby limiting the coverage provided.
HMOs	All persons	Deductibles and copayments for doctors and hospitals are eliminated.	Covers all hospital and outpatient services.
Long-term care insurance	Clients are excluded who have AIDS, Parkinson's disease, Alzheimer's disease, and epilepsy.	Policies are expensive and premiums are determined by age.	Skilled nursing care is predominant coverage. May also include intermediate nursing care and custodial care.

NURSING ACTIONS IN VARIOUS SETTINGS

Nursing actions for a client with cancer depend on the setting in which care is provided. This section identifies which actions are appropriate in all settings and which pertain to acute care, extended care, or home care situations.

All settings
• Promote screening examinations for common cancers, such as a yearly rectal or breast examination.
• Promote awareness of cancer symptoms.
• Teach elderly clients how to detect the difference between the normal signs of aging and cancer.
• Discuss with the client and his family, while decisions can still be made, the extent of care to be provided during acute and life-threatening events.

Acute care
• Ease the client's transition from hospital to home by explaining and implementing services (such as home care services, physical therapy, occupational therapy, and Meals On Wheels) one at a time.
• Initiate any necessary predischarge teaching, such as for wound care, I.V. therapy, or catheter care.
• Consider the following when determining the feasibility of discharging the client to home care: the level of care needed, financial resources and insurance coverage, client preference, and family and social supports.

Extended care
• Learn the dying client's wishes and needs, and make every attempt to fulfill them.
• Focus nursing care on providing comfort and safety.
• Institute bereavement counseling for clients when a fellow client dies.
• Schedule small group conferences to help clients share their feelings about deceased clients and to provide support to each other.

Home care
• Determine if the state in which the client resides has a program to pay for prescribed medication and medical equipment (see *Medical coverage for the elderly client,* page 294).
• Develop home care services in collaboration with an inpatient facility for backup support.
• Schedule home health aides to provide personal care, light cooking, laundry, and shopping.
• Assess the availability of community volunteers who can donate their time to assist the family with transportation and respite care.

SELECTED REFERENCES

Billings, J.A. *Outpatient Management of Advanced Cancer: Symptom Control Support and Hospice-in-the-Home.* Philadelphia: J.B. Lippincott Co., 1985.

Cancer Facts and Figures. Atlanta: American Cancer Society, 1989.

Caring for the Terminally Ill Patient at Home. Philadelphia: University of Pennsylvania Cancer Center, Hospice and Homecare Program, 1986.

Chernoff, R., and Ropka, M. "The Unique Nutritional Needs of the Elderly Patient with Cancer," *Seminars in Oncology Nursing* 4(3):189-97, August 1988.

Crawford, J., and Cohen, H.J. "Relationship of Cancer and Aging," *Clinics in Geriatric Medicine* 3(3):419-32, 1987.

Cukman, J.M. "Cancer in the Elderly: Systems Overview," *Seminars in Oncology Nursing* 4(3):169-77, August 1988.

Fleck, A.E. "Economic Issues in the Care of the Elderly Cancer Patient," *Seminars in Oncology Nursing* 4(3): 217-23, August 1988.

Hutchins, L.F., and Lipschiltz, D.A. "Cancer: Clinical Pharmacology and Aging," *Clinics in Geriatric Medicine* 3(3):483-503, 1987.

Kübler-Ross, E. *Death: The Final Stage of Growth.* Englewood Cliffs, N.J.: Prentice-Hall, 1975.

Paradis, L.F. *Hospice Handbook: A Guide for Managers of Planners.* Rockville, Md.: Aspen Publications, 1985.

Phillips, L.R., and Rempusheski, V.F. "Caring for the Frail Elderly at Home: Toward a Theoretical Exploration of the Dynamics of Poor Quality Family Caregiving," *Advances in Nursing* 8(4):62-84, July 1986.

Pillemer, K. "Risk Factors in Elder Abuse: Results from a Crosscontrol Study," in *Elder Abuse: Conflict in the Family.* Edited by Pillemer, K., and Wolf, R. Dover, Mass.: Auburn House, 1986.

Quinn, M.J., and Tomita, S. *Elder Abuse and Neglect.* New York: Springer-Verlag Publishers, 1986.

Weinrick, S.P., et al. "Timely Detection of Colorectal Cancer in the Elderly," *Cancer Nursing* 12(3):170-76, March 1989.

Welch-McCaffrey, D., ed. *Nursing Considerations in Geriatric Oncology.* Columbus, Ohio: Adria Laboratories, 1986.

Insomnia and Sleep Apnea

Insomnia and sleep apnea are two common sleep pattern disturbances that affect older adults. Insomnia, a condition characterized by difficulty in falling or remaining asleep, affects as many as 30% of the American population, mostly women. Sleep apnea, a disorder characterized by apneic episodes that last about 10 seconds and may occur as frequently as 300 times a night, affects approximately one-third of all adults over age 65.

Insomnia can be classified according to four major categories: initial insomnia (characterized by the inability to fall asleep because of anxiety, stress, or sleep phobia), maintenance or intermittent insomnia (marked by midcycle interruption of sleep caused by a reaction to internal or external stimuli), terminal insomnia (related to aging or depression and characterized by early morning awakening), and imaginary insomnia (characterized by claims of not sleeping when evidence indicates otherwise). Most elderly clients have terminal insomnia in which they typically awaken early in the morning.

Sleep apnea can be classified according to one of three categories: central sleep apnea (related to central nervous system [CNS] damage), obstructive sleep apnea (resulting from an upper airway obstruction caused by enlarged tonsils or obesity), and mixed sleep apnea (beginning as central apnea but becomes complicated by obstructive apnea). Mixed sleep apnea occurs mainly in men; however, the incidence in women increases after age 80.

Clients suffering from sleep apnea commonly experience the apnea every night. They usually receive no relief from naps and may even feel worse after napping. The most common complaint resulting from sleep apnea is hypersomnolence, or excessive daytime sleepiness, although some clients with sleep apnea deny having this problem. Hypersomnolence typically results from of sleep deprivation or decreased oxygen concentrations during apneic episodes.

ETIOLOGY

Many factors, such as anxiety or anticipation, influence the length and quality of sleep time. Most individuals have conditioned patterns of sleeping, and any interruption in these patterns, such as a change in room temperature or lighting, can affect their ability to sleep. Sleep patterns change with age, commonly affecting the quality of sleep (see *Sleep and aging,* page 301). Also, metabolic activity or the physiologic alterations that occur with certain health problems affect both the length and quality of sleep.

Total sleep time, including both rapid eye movement (REM) and non-REM sleep, remains constant in those between ages 20 and 60. Clients over age 60 have a decreased total sleep time, mainly because of an increased number of awakenings. They must spend more time in bed to achieve restorative sleep, but their sleep tends to be distributed throughout a 24-hour period rather than concentrated in one block of time. These age-related sleep pattern changes may result from CNS changes, especially in the autonomic and hypothalamic centers.

Women appear to have fewer sleep pattern disturbances than men. However, all elderly clients nap more, regardless of sex, working status, living arrangements, health status, exercise, or daily schedule. The frequency of naps increases after age 75; the length, after age 85. Experts believe that naps augment sleep and increase total sleep time, rather than compensate for lost sleep. Morning naps are thought to provide REM, or mentally refreshing sleep, whereas afternoon naps provide Stage IV, or physically restorative, sleep. Therefore, elderly clients involved in an active physical therapy program may require an afternoon nap.

HEALTH HISTORY FINDINGS

In a health history interview, the client may report or the nurse may detect many of these findings:
• use of sedatives or over-the-counter medications
• history of heavy caffeine, alcohol, and tobacco consumption
• history of thyroid disease, chronic renal insufficiency, Alzheimer's disease, duodenal ulcer, hiatal hernia, congestive heart failure, rheumatoid arthritis, chronic obstructive pulmonary disease, or emphysema
• history of depression or schizophrenia

PHYSICAL FINDINGS

In a physical examination, the nurse may detect many of these findings.

Respiratory
• dyspnea
• shortness of breath
• chronic cough

Genitourinary
• enuresis
• nocturia
• impotence

Musculoskeletal
• skeletal muscle weakness
• dysarthria
• lack of coordination

Neurologic
• morning headaches
• sundowner's syndrome (increased agitation and confusion toward late afternoon)
• nocturnal myoclonus (leg twitching occurring every 20 to 40 seconds during sleep)

Psychological
• decreased attention span
• diminished memory
• personality changes (such as irritability, hostility, and violence)

Other
• burning or heaviness of eyelids
• visual distortions, such as auras around light sources or cobwebs on floors

DIAGNOSTIC STUDIES
The following studies may be performed to evaluate the client's health status:
• polysomnographic evaluation (may include an electroencephalogram (EEG), electrooculogram (EOG), or electromyogram (EMG)—to determine abnormalities
• sleep EEG—to identify the stages of sleep, apneic events, arterial oxygen saturation, and dysrhythmias; a face mask with monitoring sensors measures airflow at the mouth and nose and records jaw muscle activity while the client is observed on closed circuit television
• serum blood urea nitrogen (BUN) levels—to identify abnormalities in metabolic function; increased level indicates uremia, which can cause a sleep pattern disturbance

---

Nursing diagnosis: *Sleep pattern disturbance related to environmental stimuli*

NURSING GOAL: To provide a safe, comfortable environment conducive to sleep

Signs and symptoms
• visual disturbances
• apathy
• frequent awakenings during sleep
• frequent napping

Interventions

1. Explain nighttime sights and sounds.

2. Encourage the client to ambulate during the day and to relax after dinner. Advise him to avoid exercising 2 hours before bedtime, to prepare for sleep.

3. Ensure the client's safety during trips to the bathroom by keeping the nurse's call light within the client's reach; using a portable bell system, if necessary; keeping a night light on from early evening through the night, or keeping the bathroom light on with the door almost closed; keeping the path to the bathroom clear at all times; having the client void before bedtime, using a bedside commode, urinal, or bedpan if he has difficulty ambulating more than 6'; and keeping upper side rails raised at all times and lower rails raised if the client is confused or agitated.

4. Keep noise to a minimum.

Rationales

1. Being able to identify nighttime sights and sounds should reduce the client's fear and the number of awakenings, reducing the chance of injury.

2. Ambulation and exercise during the day prepare the body for sleep. Avoiding exercise before bedtime reduces excitement which might interfere with the client's ability to fall asleep.

3. Since the elderly client may awaken frequently during the night to go to the bathroom, ensuring his safety is essential. Call bells or other signal devices allow the client to call the nurse for assistance in getting to the bathroom. Because the elderly client takes longer to accommodate from darkness to light, adequate lighting is necessary to decrease the possibilty of falls. Keeping the path clear also prevents falls. Emptying the bladder before sleep should decrease the number of awakenings; using a bedside commode, urinal, or bedpan will reduce the risk of a fall if nighttime voiding is necessary. Keeping upper side rails raised provides a means of support for the client who can ambulate to the bathroom. Upper and lower siderails should only be used for the confused or agitated client whose movement should be limited.

4. Any unfamiliar sounds may keep the client from falling asleep or may awaken the client during lighter stages of sleep.

5. Keep the room temperature between 70° and 81° F (21° to 27° C).

5. Ths temperature promotes sleep.

OUTCOME CRITERION
• The client will report having adequate sleep within a 48-hour period.

Nursing diagnosis: *Sleep pattern disturbance related to side effects from medications, foods, and chronic disease*

NURSING GOAL: To prevent trauma from repeated nighttime awakening

Signs and symptoms
• fatigue
• sensation of a tight band around the head
• eye burning and heavy eye lids
• muscle tremor and weakness
• lack of coordination
• dysarthria
• diminished facial expression
• decreased atttention span

Interventions

1. Discuss with the physician the possibility of discontinuing over-the-counter sedatives.

2. Warn the client to expect sleep disturbances after a relocation or hospitalization or when hypnotics and sedatives are discontinued.

3. Provide a consistent bedtime and awakening time.

4. Encourage the client to avoid consuming caffeine-containing foods and beverages after 1 p.m.

5. Provide extra pillows, if indicated.

6. Teach the client relaxation techniques, such as progressive relaxation, slow deep breathing, imagery, prayer, and meditation.

Rationales

1. Over-the-counter sedatives may enhance sleep pattern disturbances in the elderly client.

2. Preparing the client for disturbances should make him more receptive to treatments other than medications.

3. A consistent sleep pattern promotes sleep.

4. Caffeine is a stimulant that may disturb sleep.

5. Extra pillows can help the client with a respiratory problem, such as emphysema or sleep apnea, to breathe easier.

6. Relaxation techniques promote sleep.

OUTCOME CRITERIA
• The client will experience no physical injury or worsening of medical problems from lack of sleep.
• The client will obtain restful, adequate sleep without the use of medications.

Nursing diagnosis: *Sleep pattern disturbance related to apneic episodes*

NURSING GOAL: To identify and treat the causes of sleep apnea

Signs and symptoms
- excessive daytime sleepiness
- decreased attention span
- restless sleep
- morning headaches
- loud snoring
- personality changes
- exhaustion
- sleepwalking
- polycythemia
- enuresis
- impotence

Interventions

1. Caution the client to avoid using sedatives, narcotics, hypnotics, or alcohol.

2. Administer low flow rates of oxygen, as ordered; continue to monitor the client's respirations.

3. Support the client's head and torso with two or three pillows during sleep.

4. Apply a soft cervical collar, as ordered.

5. Closely monitor the client for excessively long periods of sleep apnea.

6. Encourage the client to stop smoking.

7. Establish a weight reduction program for the obese client.

Rationales

1. These substances enhance sleep apnea by depressing the arousal response. CNS depressants may be lethal to the client who has impaired breathing for anatomic or autonomic reasons.

2. Low flow rates of oxygen may be necessary in the client who has an inadequate concentration of oxygen. However, oxygen may also depress respirations and therefore requires continual monitoring.

3. Elevation of the head and torso may improve sleep.

4. A soft cervical collar prevents airway obstruction from neck flexion, thereby preventing apnea.

5. Long periods of sleep apnea can result in death.

6. Smoking increases the client's risk for sleep apnea.

7. The upper body fat of the obese client reduces chest wall and total respiratory compliance, causing sleep apnea.

OUTCOME CRITERION
- The client will be free from sleep apnea episodes.

Nursing diagnosis: *Sleep pattern disturbance related to pain*

NURSING GOALS: To prevent pain and to enhance sleep

Signs and symptoms
- chest pain during REM sleep
- musculoskeletal stiffness
- gastric pain between 1 a.m. and 3 a.m.
- migraine headaches during REM sleep
- leg pain immediately before and during sleep

Interventions

1. Determine the cause, location, and frequency of the client's pain, noting how it interferes with the client's sleep.

2. Administer analgesics, such as acetaminophen, ½ hour before the client falls asleep, as ordered.

Rationales

1. Identifying the cause, location, and frequency of the client's pain will help the nurse choose interventions to ease the pain and promote sleep.

2. Analgesics may reduce the pain from bursitis or osteoarthritis.

3. Apply warm or cool compresses to the painful area, as ordered.

4. Provide the client with warm milk at bedtime, if tolerated.

5. If the client has angina, keep nitroglycerin tablets at the bedside.

6. If the client has gastric problems, keep antacids (if ordered) at the bedside.

7. Administer prescribed medications to clients who experience migraine headaches during REM sleep.

8. Help the client who has nocturnal myoclonus (restless leg syndrome) to ambulate before falling asleep.

9. Help the client who has rest pain from decreased arterial pressure to ambulate during the night.

10. For the client who has severe rest pain, explore options for keeping the legs in a dependent position during sleep, such as sleeping in a reclining chair.

3. Warmth or coolness will reduce musculoskeletal pain and helping the client to relax and sleep.

4. Milk contains tryptophan, an amino acid that is linked with serotonin production, which promotes restful sleep. Studies indicate that decreased serotonin is connected to sleep pattern disturbances and that insomniacs may be unable to convert serotonin from foods. Warm milk promotes sleep quicker than cold milk does.

5. Ready access to coronary artery vasodilators will prevent the client who awakens with angina from remaining awake for a long period of time.

6. Using antacids before bedtime or during the night may reduce the number of times the client awakens because of increased gastric secretions.

7. Administering medication before the client goes to sleep may reduce the intensity of his headaches.

8. Nocturnal myoclonus is characterized by leg twitching that occurs every 20 to 40 seconds and is typically noticed by the client's sleeping partner. Such activity commonly results in unsatisfying, nonproductive sleep. Ambulation before sleep reduces the incidence of restless leg syndrome.

9. Ambulation increases arterial pressure and decreases pain.

10. Keeping the client's legs in a dependent position enhances arterial blood flow.

OUTCOME CRITERION
• The client will be free from pain while achieving adequate sleep.

NURSING ACTIONS IN VARIOUS SETTINGS
Nursing actions for a client with insomnia or sleep apnea depend on the setting in which care is provided. This section identifies which actions are appropriate in all settings and which pertain to acute care, extended care, or home care situations.

All settings
• Inform the client and his family about the physiologic patterns of sleep and the typical changes related to aging.
• Discuss the complications of using medications to promote sleep, and teach the client and his family alternative relaxation methods to promote sleep.

Acute care
• Upon admission, explain all the hospital sights and sounds to the client to prepare him for environmental changes.
• Monitor the client's use of sleeping medications to ensure that he does not take them for more than 1 week.
• Prepare the family for the delirium or confusion that may result from environmental changes, disease, or altered sleep patterns.

• Carefully assess the risks and value of performing procedures while the client sleeps.

Extended care
• Promote as much of a homelike environment as possible to promote sleep.
• Discontinue the client's sleeping medications, and teach the client relaxation techniques as an alternative to medications.
• Provide the client with a comfortable mattress or, for the client who must sleep in an upright prosition, a reclining chair.
• Avoid or limit the number of times nursing procedures must be performed during the night.
• Allow sufficient nap time.
• Place clients who have similar sleep patterns in the same room.

Home care
• Instruct the client and his family about the appropriate use of sleep medications.
• Help the client's family to access community support groups, such as meditation groups, yoga classes, or prayer groups, that can enhance the client's sleep.

SLEEP AND AGING

The chart below includes information on common age-related sleep pattern changes that occur during the normal stages of sleep

Normal stages of sleep	Age-related sleep pattern changes
Stage I During Stage I, which is characterized by fleeting thoughts and an unawareness of being sleep, the individual is in a light sleep from which he can be easily awakened. Typically, the pulse rate drops 10 to 30 beats/minute; basal metabolism rate drops 10% to 50%; temperature and respirations begin to deline; blood pressure decreases slightly; knee jerks cease; and muscle tone decreases to a minimum. This stage lasts about 1 to 2 minutes.	Older adults usually take longer to fall asleep and tend to remain in Stage I for a prolonged period before progressing to the deeper stages of sleep. Because older adults also tend to awaken more easily, they frequently need to begin the initial stages of sleep on a recurring basis and commonly spend about 20 minutes of their total sleeping time in Stage I.
Stage II During this transitional stage of sleep, which is characterized by short, fragmented, mundane thoughts and an unawareness of surroundings, the individual can be easily awakened. Typically lasting 5 to 10 minutes, this stage constitutes 50% of the total sleeping time.	Older adults spend more time in this lighter stage of sleep as they age.
Stage III During this stage, which is characterized by a deep sleep from which the individual has difficulty awakening, the pulse rate and temperature drop and the muscles relax. This stage, which constitutes about 10% to 20% of the total sleeping time, typically lasts 10 minutes.	No significant changes noted.
Stage IV During this physically restorative stage of sleep, which is characterized by deep sleep and difficulty awakening, the individual experiences few body movements. The need for this stage increases with the amount of physical activity spent during the day. Typically, the stage lasts 5 to 15 minutes and occurs about 40 minutes after Stage I.	Stage IV sleep declines rapidly with age, commonly decreasing by about 50%. About 25% of those over age 65 skip this stage completely. Because this is considered the physically restorative phase of sleep, many elderly adults feel tired or poorly rested when they fail to experience it.
Rapid eye movement (REM) stage REM sleep, which constitutes about 20% of the total sleep time, is considered the mentally restorative stage of sleep and is especially important for learning, memory, adaptation, and problem solving. During REM sleep, which is characterized by dreaming (particularly in the early morning hours), the individual may experience irregular pulse, respiratory, and heart rates, temperature fluctuations, and blood pressure changes. Because of the potential for such irregularities, vital sign checks are inappropriate during REM sleep. Epileptics must be observed more closely as convulsions are most likely to occur at this time.	Although older adults spend as much time in REM stage sleep as younger adults, older adults seem to experience less dreaming. The loss of REM sleep in the elderly client results in increased agitation, irritability, apathy, or depression.

• Instruct the client and his family to use the bed only for sleep and not for eating, reading, or other activities.
• Discuss the need for consistent sleep and awake times.
• Instruct the client's family to perform massage and back rubs, and teach the client to progressively relax by rhythmically contracting and relaxing the basic muscle groups.
• Provide clients and their families information about sleep diagnostic centers if sleep disturbances continue.

SELECTED REFERENCES

Bahr, R.T., and Gress, L. "The 24-Hour Cycle: Rhythms of Healthy Sleep," *Journal of Gerontological Nursing* 11(4):14, April 1985.

Berry, D.T.R., et al. "Sleep and Cognitive Function in Normal Older Adults," *Journal of Gerontology* 40(3):331, March 1985.

Hayter, J. "To Nap or Not to Nap," *Geriatric Nursing* 6(2):104, March/April 1985.

Hoch, C., and Reynolds, C. "Sleep Disturbances and What to Do About Them," *Geriatric Nursing* 7(1):24, January/February 1986.

Israel, S., et al. "Sleep Apnea and Periodic Movements in an Aging Sample," *Journal of Gerontology* 40(4):419, April 1985.

Johnson, J. "Drug Treatment for Sleep Disturbances: Does It Really Work?" *Journal of Gerontological Nursing* 11(8):9, August 1985.

Oesting, H.H., and Manza, R.J. "Sleep Apnea," *Geriatric Nursing* 4:232-233, July/August 1988.

Steffis, R., and Thralow, J. "Do Uniform Colors Keep Patients Awake?" *Journal of Gerontological Nursing* 40(6):6, July 1985.

GENERAL CARE PLAN
Elder Abuse

Elder abuse, a serious problem affecting about 1 million elderly Americans, refers to the maltreatment of older adults by their caregivers. Although its incidence is slightly less than that of child abuse, only one-sixth of all elder abuse cases are reported to protective service agencies, whereas one-third of all child abuse cases are reported to appropriate agencies.

The term *elder abuse* encompasses both the abuse and neglect of older adults. Regardless of whether the client suffers from actual maltreatment (abuse) or omission of care (neglect), the abused client's health and welfare are at risk.

Abuse can be classified as physical, sexual, psychological or emotional, or material in nature. *Physical* abuse occurs when the client is subjected to trauma, pain, injury, or physical coercion. This type of abuse may include slapping, hitting, cutting, burning, or restraining the client against his will.

Sexual abuse is any form of sexual intimacy involving the client and another person that occurs through force or threatened force or without the client's consent. This includes situations in which the client cannot give adequate consent because of chronic dementia or mental retardation. Unfortunately, because many people, including nurses, are reluctant to acknowledge sexual abuse, it frequently remains an unreported problem in the elderly population.

Psychological or *emotional* abuse is the infliction of mental anguish through yelling, insults, threats, or silence. This type of abuse, which commonly accompanies other types of abuse, is commonly manifested in the elderly client in the form of timidity, fear, depression, or isolation.

Material, or financial, abuse occurs when the caregiver misuses funds or resources intended for the care of the elderly client. For example, the caregiver may refuse to disburse available funds for needed services because he does not want the elderly client's estate depleted, and, instead, uses the elderly client's money to satisfy personal needs.

Neglect, the failure to provide adequate care, can be classified as either passive or active. *Passive* neglect occurs through the caregiver's lack of knowledge about proper care—for example, not knowing that the client needs to ambulate or have his position changed frequently. *Active* neglect occurs when the caregiver knows how to properly care, or obtain proper care, for the elderly client but does not use this knowledge appropriately, such as refusal to obtain medical attention for the client when he is ill.

Although neglect is sometimes viewed as a less serious problem than abuse, it may lead to a life-threatening condition if it continues undetected or untreated.

Inadequate nutrition or medication, oversedation with tranquilizers, inappropriate treatment of pressure sores, untreated urinary tract infections, and fecal impaction, are all examples of neglectful caregiving behaviors that interfere with the elderly client's ability to combat serious illness.

Abuse or neglect may also occur as a result of the elderly client's not providing himself with necessities of life, such as shelter and food, or not seeking medical care for a severe illness. Such behaviors commonly occur in clients who are mentally impaired and in those who abuse alcohol or other substances that impair their ability to make rational decisions concerning their own well-being.

ETIOLOGY
Although no evidence supports one explanation for the cause of elder abuse, several theories have been proposed:
• Impairment of the elderly client: Because of physical or mental impairment, the client may be dependent on others for his care and, therefore, becomes vulnerable to abuse and neglect.
• Abuser pathology: The caregiver cannot make appropriate decisions about caring for the elderly client (constituting neglect) or cares for the older adult in an inappropriate manner (constituting abuse). Examples of abuser psychopathology include personality or character disorders, alcohol or substance abuse, or dementia.
• Transgenerational violence: Dysfunctional families may view violence as a normal or acceptable reaction to stress. Abusers who were victims of child abuse may retaliate with violence against elderly parents.
• Stressed caregiver: A caregiver may be depressed or overfatigued from the work of caregiving. External stresses, such as marital conflict, financial problems, or other caregiving responsibilities, may reduce the caregiver's ability to cope effectively.
• Societal attitudes: Negative attitudes toward elderly, female, and disabled clients may contribute to abuse and neglect. Myths and stereotypes may cause the client to feel that he does not deserve to be treated in a dignified manner.

Clients at risk for abuse include those over age 75, women, those with physical or mental impairment, and those who live with their children. Caregivers at risk of becoming abusers include those who have multiple responsibilities (such as children living at home), those who have undergone a recent life crisis, those with a history of violence, those who are immature, isolated, or living with the client, and those who act as the client's primary or exclusive caregiver.

HEALTH HISTORY FINDINGS
In a health history interview, the client may report or the nurse may detect many of these findings:
• history of frequent urinary tract infections or congestive heart failure
• history of previous injuries
• history of repeated emergency department visits for minor injuries or illnesses
• frequent changes in use of physicians or hospital emergency departments
• accompaniment by someone other than the primary caregiver on medical visits
• history of not obtaining medication refills
• history of mishandling finances or of financial abuse
• confusion
• fear or anxiety
• caregiver uncooperativeness
• fatigue and weakness
• inappropriate clothing
• lack of necessary assistive devices, such as hearing aids or canes
• vaginal discharge or bleeding
• difficulty walking or sitting
• depression
• drastic change in mental status

PHYSICAL FINDINGS
In a physical examination, the nurse may detect many of these findings:

Integumentary
• burns (from immersion in hot water, ropes, cigarettes, or heat)
• bruises or hematomas
• diaper rash or urine burn

Gastrointestinal
• decreased sphincter tone or stool impaction

Genitourinary
• torn, stained, or bloody underclothing
• pain or itching in genital area
• bruises, lesions, bleeding, or discharge involving the genitalia or rectum

Musculoskeletal
• fractures
• whiplash injury
• contractures

Neurologic
• sleep or speech disorders

Psychological
• psychoneurotic reactions (such as obsession, compulsion, or phobias)
• depression
• fear in the caregiver's presence
• habitual or conduct disorder (such as sucking, biting, rocking, antisocial, or destructive behaviors)

Other
• poor hygiene
• patches of missing hair
• eye injury
• septal deviation (possibly from a broken nose)
• missing teeth

DIAGNOSTIC STUDIES
The following studies may be performed to evaluate the client's health history status:
• X-rays—to identify fractures or evidence of physical restraint
• serum electrolyte levels—to identify malnutrition or dehydration
• serum drug levels—to confirm oversedation
• complete blood count (CBC), prothrombin time (PT), and partial thromboplastin time (PTT)—to determine the risk of bleeding and bruising
• computed tomography (CT) scan—to diagnose head trauma or the reason for a change in mental status
• Venereal Disease Research Laboratories (VDRL) test—to diagnose venereal disease if the client has vaginal or penile discharge

POTENTIAL COMPLICATIONS
• ineffective family coping
• post-traumatic response

Nursing diagnosis: *Ineffective family coping related to elder abuse or neglect*

NURSING GOALS: To help the client become aware of resources to prevent or end abuse and neglect and to encourage the abuser to seek help in coping to prevent abuse

Signs and symptoms
• fear in the caregiver's presence
• decreased social interaction
• detachment
• childlike treatment by caregiver
• caregiver's lack of emotional control

Interventions

1. Assess the client for signs and symptoms of abuse or neglect.

2. Assess the family at risk for abuse or neglect, and intervene as necessary before abuse occurs.

3. Develop a trusting relationship with the elderly client and his significant others.

4. Promote a positive therapeutic relationship. Use a nonjudgmental approach with both the client and the suspected abuser, encouraging each to discuss their feelings.

5. Offer guidance in how to care for an ill parent or older adult.

6. Provide information about community resources and alternative living arrangements before an elderly client moves in with an adult child.

7. Encourage the caregiver to seek respite by having other family members help or by using formal respite services, such as adult day care and short-term nursing home placement.

8. Encourage the caregiver to ventilate his feelings about the caregiving experience. Advise him to join a self-help group, such as Children of Aging Parents (CAPS) or a local Alzheimer's disease support group.

9. Teach the elderly client the importance using various support sources to prevent social isolation.

10. Report suspected cases of elder abuse or neglect. Learn all state laws and procedures for reporting suspected or actual abuse.

11. Document suspected abuse accurately by using direct quotes, and give specific descriptions of physical findings. Sketches and photographs of injuries may be extremely helpful.

12. Consult a social worker about referring the client to community agencies or providing alternative living arrangements for the client.

13. Suggest possible alternative living arrangements, such as living with other family members or friends or the possibility of living in a boarding home, retirement community, or nursing home.

Rationales

1. Early identification is essential to break a pattern of abuse or neglect.

2. Prevention through identification of high-risk families can promote the integrity of family relationships. Intervention before the abuse or neglect occurs prevents client injury.

3. A therapeutic environment promotes open discussion about difficult situations.

4. The client and the abuser may not have had previous opportunities to freely discuss the situation and may welcome such discussions at this time.

5. The caregiver may lack information about how to appropriately care for the client and may be coping the only way he knows how.

6. Frequently, knowledge of options and services can reduce stress that can lead to abuse.

7. The caregiver needs to know that it is acceptable to take time for himself.

8. Discussion groups provide education and support. They facilitate the sharing of common feelings and experiences, which helps to relieve the guilt or loneliness experienced by the caregiver.

9. Using other support sources decreases the caregiver's responsibilities and increases the client's sense of independence.

10. Most states have laws mandating the reporting of abuse and neglect. Adult protective service units usually investigate and manage the case initially.

11. Accurate and comprehensive documentation is essential for diagnosis as well as potential intervention by legal or social service agencies.

12. Referrals encourage the client to choose formal support services to maximize their independence and enhance their well-being.

13. The client may need to consider temporary or permanent relocation to prevent abuse and neglect.

14. Refer the abuser for counseling through a geriatric or geropsychiatry program, community mental health center, or private clinician familiar with elder abuse and neglect.

14. Counseling can help the abuser explore alternatives to destructive behavior and choose appropriate coping mechanisms for dealing with the stress of caring for an aging parent. Psychotherapy can also help the abuser with possible overdependence on the parent. The abuser may need more direct therapeutic techniques that emphasize self-control to prevent further violence.

OUTCOME CRITERIA
• The client will not experience abuse or neglect.
• The family and caregiver will develop effective coping mechanisms and support systems.

Nursing diagnosis: *Post-trauma response related to abuse or neglect*

NURSING GOALS: To help the client cope with abuse or neglect and to develop a trusting, caring relationship with the client and caregiver

Signs and symptoms
• chronic anxiety or depression
• self-blame or shame
• fear of repeated abuse or death
• feelings of helplessness and powerlessness
• negative self-concept
• social isolation and withdrawal

Interventions

1. Assess the client's psychological responses to abuse and neglect and his ability to cope with the situation.

2. Inform the client of services available for immediate assistance. Furnish the client with the telephone numbers of hotlines, protective service agencies, and the police, and inform him about legal actions he can pursue.

3. Promote a trusting relationship and long-term follow-up.

4. Encourage the client to make decisions for himself. Maintain a nonjudgmental attitude while supporting the client's values and decisions.

5. Consult a social worker about referring the client to a victim's support group or counseling. Counseling may be provided through a geriatric or geropsychiatry program, a rape counseling program, a domestic violence center, or an elder abuse and neglect program.

6. Advise the client about the availability of appropriate advocacy groups, such as a local bar association's legal services program or a local agency on aging.

Rationales

1. An assessment establishes the elderly client's perceptions of the problem and identifies his expectations of health and social service providers.

2. This knowledge will help the client feel more in control.

3. The nurse should advocate the elderly client's right of self-determination regarding his well-being and care.

4. The client's feelings of hopelessness and powerlessness greatly affects the post-trauma response. The client will learn to trust only if he feels in control and believes that the nurse can help him change the situation. The nurse should always attempt to support the client's decisions.

5. Individual and group counseling can help the abused client feel better about himself and enable him make decisions based on his own best interests.

6. Such information may be necessary to ensure the client's legal rights or to obtain a court order to evict the abuser from the household. Local agencies can also provides continued information and referral services.

OUTCOME CRITERIA
• The client will show signs of coping with abuse or neglect.
• The client will view the nurse as the person to contact when problem situations arise.

NURSING ACTIONS IN VARIOUS SETTINGS

Nursing actions for a client suffering from elder abuse depend on the setting in which care is provided. This section identifies which actions are appropriate in all settings and which pertain to acute care, extended care, or home care situations.

All settings
• Educate the client that he has the right not to be abused or neglected.

Acute care
• Assess all elderly clients for signs and symptoms of abuse or neglect, and consult the physician and social worker about the assessment if abuse or neglect is suspected.
• When planning the client's discharge, assess the need for referral to adult protective services and the need for follow-up through social work and counseling services.

Extended care
• Educate the nursing staff to provide quality nursing care and to prevent the abuse and neglect of all clients.
• Inform clients and their families about the availability of a local ombudsmen program to intervene with complaints about nursing homes. Also inform them that the state department of health may investigate cases of possible abuse.
• Assess the client for signs of abuse by family members or others.

Home care
• Assess the client's home environment for signs of neglect.
• Provide, or refer the client for, home care services to reduce the client's dependency on the caregiver. Also consider community programs or alternative living arrangements.
• Provide, or refer the client for, primary care services to ensure continuity of care.

SELECTED REFERENCES

Breckman, R. *Starting an Elder Abuse Victims' Support Group: A Guide for Facilitators.* New York: Victim Services Agency, 1986.

Council on Scientific Affairs. "Elder Abuse and Neglect," *Journal of the American Medical Association* 257(7):966-71, July 1987.

Fulmer, T., and Ashley, J. "Neglect: What Part of Abuse?" *Pride Institute Journal of Long-Term Home Health Care* 5(4):18-24, April 1986.

Fulmer, T., and O'Malley, T. *Inadequate Care of the Elderly: A Health Care Perspective on Abuse and Neglect.* New York: Springer-Verlag, 1987.

Fulmer, T., and Wetle, T. "Elder Abuse Screening and Intervention," *Nurse Practitioner* 11(5):31-38, May 1986.

Gilbert, D.A. "The Ethics of Mandatory Older Abuse Reporting Statutes," *Advances in Nursing Science* 8(2):51-62, January 1986.

O'Malley, T. "Abuse and Neglect of the Elderly: The Wrong Issue?" *Pride Institute Journal of Long-Term Home Health Care* 5(4):25-28, April 1986.

Phillips, L.R., and Rempusheski, V.F. "Caring for the Frail Elderly at Home: Toward a Theoretical Exploration of the Dynamics of Poor Quality Family Caregiving," *Advances in Nursing* 8(4):62-84, July 1986.

Pillmer, K. "Risk Factors in Elder Abuse: Results From a Cross-Control Study," in *Elder Abuse: Conflicts in the Family.* Edited by Pillemer, K., and Wolf, R. Dover, Mass.: Auburn House, 1986.

Quinn, M.J., and Tomita, S. *Elder Abuse and Neglect.* New York: Springer-Verlag, 1986.

The Beth Israel Hospital Elder Assessment Team. "An Elder Abuse Assessment Team in an Acute Hospital Setting," *Gerontologist* 26(2):115-18, February 1986.

Weiler, K. "Financial Abuse of the Elderly: Recognizing and Acting on It," *Journal of Gerontological Nursing* 15(8):10-15, August 1989.

Wolf, R., et al. "Maltreatment of the Elderly: A Comparative Analysis," *Pride Institute Journal of Long-Term Home Health Care* 5(4):10-18, April 1986.

Surgical Care

Surgery, for many older adults, is a growing concern that increases as a person ages. Nearly 50% of all older adults require surgery at some point in their lifetime, and the need for surgery increases by one-third after age 75. Of all of the elderly clients admitted to acute care facilities, 40% require surgery before discharge. The older the client, the greater the chance for mortality and morbidity, the rates doubling between ages 70 and 90.

In the past, surgery was commonly withheld from elderly clients because of the anticipated risk of complications. However, recent studies have indicated that delay of surgery or a reluctance to perform elective surgery frequently leads to an increased need to perform emergency procedures, which places the elderly client at a much greater risk for death. These studies, coupled with improved surgical procedures, better preoperative and postoperative management, and a greater number of elderly clients, have resulted in a marked shift in attitude concerning surgery and the older adult. Consequently, physicians are now performing more and more elective surgeries on elderly clients.

Despite improvements in surgical equipment and procedures, elderly clients continue to remain at risk for complications associated with anesthesia. Anesthetic agents are known to cause untoward, potentially harmful effects on various body systems regardless of age, and frail elderly clients are at highest risk.

ETIOLOGY

Researchers are unclear on whether aging itself is responsible for increased mortality associated with surgery on the elderly client or whether the increasing incidence of cardiopulmonary, renal, and other diseases accounts for the high risk. They do know, however, that hypertension, heart disease, atherosclerosis, cerebrovascular disease, and renal insufficiency add substantially to the risks of surgery.

The reason for surgery varies, depending on the client. The most common types of surgery performed on elderly clients include orthopedic procedures, cardiovascular surgery, and cataract surgery.

Orthopedic surgery is fast becoming a common procedure for elderly clients. Many clients with osteoarthritis who suffer severe pain and limited motion have undergone successful replacement of damaged joints, in part because of the constant improvement in prosthetic devices. Also, aggressive surgical intervention for elderly clients with hip, knee, or other orthopedic injuries, provides early mobilization, relieves pain, and prevents the development of the complications of immobility. Geriatric clients undergoing total joint replacement do not have a significantly higher morbidity and mortality than do younger clients.

Elderly clients also commonly require cardiovascular surgery. Common procedures include pacemaker insertion, open heart surgery, peripheral vascular reconstruction, and carotid endarterectomy.

Most pacemaker implants are performed on clients between ages 60 and 90, with the average age of placement being 71. Indications for a pacemaker include bradycardia, complete heart block with a slow ventricular response, or asystole. Physicians can insert a pacemaker using regional anesthesia. After insertion, the client's mortality rate declines significantly.

Of the types of open heart surgeries, the two types commonly performed on elderly clients include coronary artery bypass surgery and prosthetic valve replacement. Clients who have severe cardiovascular disease may be poor candidates for coronary bypass surgery, especially because the notion that surgery will prolong life is controversial. Open heart surgery has a 50% success rate in clients over age 65.

Peripheral vascular reconstruction may be performed on an elderly client to help prevent ischemia in the legs, thereby preventing amputation. Carotid endarterectomy, the most common major, noncardiac vascular procedure performed in the United States, can help prevent cerebrovascular accidents (CVAs); however, it is associated with various complications (including CVA, depression, blood pressure deviations, and cranial nerve plexus), and candidacy for this type of surgery is highly controversial.

Cataract surgery, which involves removing the cataract lens after the client's vision has become so impaired that it interferes with activities of daily living, is typically performed in a same-day surgery unit using a local anesthetic. If the client needs bilateral surgery, two separate procedures are usually performed at least 1 month apart. The procedure has a 95% to 98% success rate.

HEALTH HISTORY FINDINGS

In a health history interview, the client may report or the nurse may detect many of these findings:
• history of heart disease, recent myocardial infarction, or recent CVA
• history of active peptic ulcer disease
• history of hepatic insufficiency or pulmonary disease
• use of beta blockers, salicylates, or antidepressants
• history of malnutrition and poor fluid intake
• history of smoking and alcohol consumption
• abnormal breathing pattern
• dementia

PHYSICAL FINDINGS

In a physical examination, the nurse may detect many of these findings:

Integumentary
• dry, flaky skin
• poor skin turgor
• bruises or ulcers
• peripheral edema

Respiratory
• ineffective cough
• shortness of breath
• reduced respiratory muscle strength

Cardiovascular
• systolic murmur
• orthostatic hypotension

Musculoskeletal
• decreased muscle tone and bulk
• impaired motor balance, strength, and range of motion
• use of assistive devices
• curvature of the spine

Other
• recent weight loss
• decreased hearing and visual acuity
• decreased peripheral vision

DIAGNOSTIC STUDIES
The following studies may be performed to evaluate the client's health status:
• complete blood count (CBC), red cell index, and serum albumin studues—to assess the client's nutritional sta-

tus; anemia and a serum albumin level less than 3 g/dl increase the incidence of postoperative complications
• serum electrolyte studies—to identify abnormalities caused by diuretics
• electrocardiogram (ECG)—to provide baseline data and identify any age-related changes or cardiac abnormalities
• arterial blood gas (ABG) studies and spirometry—to evaluate the respiratory status of smokers or those with a history of pulmonary disease
• chest X-ray—to identify an increased anteroposterior chest diameter or cardiomegaly, which increases the risk of postoperative complications
• serum digoxin level—to ensure proper dosage and identify toxicity
• urinalysis—to identify urinary tract infection

POTENTIAL COMPLICATIONS
• CVA
• hypothermia
• atelectasis
• pulmonary emboli
• pneumonia
• shock
• immobility
• pain
• constipation
• urinary incontinence

Nursing diagnosis: *Impaired gas exchange related to chronic tissue hypoxia, postoperative immobility, and pain*

NURSING GOALS: To provide adequate ventilation and to assess the client for excessive central nervous system depression

Signs and symptoms
• agitation and confusion
• increased pulse rate and flushing
• hypotension
• abnormal blood gas levels (decreased PO_2, increased PCO_2)
• use of accessory muscles to breathe
• mouth breathing
• cyanosis
• shallow breathing pattern

Interventions

1. Monitor the client's vital signs hourly during the immediate postoperative period.

Rationales

1. Hypothermia can occur immediately after surgery. Hypotension diminishes the oxygen normally supplied to vital organs and can lead to a cerebral hemorrhage. Tachycardia may indicate abnormal bleeding. Shallow respirations also place the client at risk for hypoxia, atelectasis, and pneumonia.

2. Auscultate the client's heart and lungs.

2. Atelectasis, pneumonia, and congestive heart failure, common among older adults who have undergone surgery, are the most common reasons for respiratory distress in the elderly client.

3. Assess the client's mental status after surgery; compare the findings with those from the preoperative assessment.

3. Confusion, an indication of hypoxia, may be caused by ineffective gas exchange, in which the oxygen demand becomes greater than the reserve.

4. Evaluate the client's laboratory results, including blood gas values.

4. An evaluation will determine any deviation from normal. For example, the client's PCO_2 level may increase from hypoxemia; leukocytosis may result from pneumonia; or decreased hemoglobin and hematocrit levels may signal a hemorrhage.

5. Frequently assess the client's surgical wound.

5. Excessive bleeding depletes the amount of oxygen available necessary for effective gas exchange.

6. Assess the client for signs and symptoms of hypoventilation, including restlessness, hypertension, tachycardia, cardiac dysrhythmias, tachypnea, and dyspnea.

6. Hypoventilation can result from anesthetic use and depress the central respiratory center. This desensitizes the client to the stimulating effects of carbon dioxide and causes insufficient airway clearance.

7. Observe the client for noisy, shallow respirations; changes in skin color or temperature; chest retractions; increased abdominal movement; and the use of accesory muscles for breathing.

7. Anesthetics dull the reflexes, causing airway obstruction from the tongue, saliva, or secretions or from a laryngospasm or bronchospasm.

8. Administer oxygen and call the physician if the client has respiratory difficulty.

8. Supplemental oxygen increases the available oxygen supply and relieves dyspnea.

9. Determine the client's need for postoperative respiratory therapy.

9. Muscle relaxants and anesthetics compromise the respiratory system by decreasing vital capacity, increasing the residual volume, and causing the accumulation of secretions.

10. Encourage the postoperative client to perform coughing and deep-breathing exercises every 2 hours. Provide an incentive spirometer or blow bottles if the client can effectively expectorate secretions.

10. Sustained maximal inspiration and vigorous coughing prevent accumulation of secretions from reduced chest muscle mobility and strength. Coughing and deep breathing improves ventilation, mobilizes secretions, and increases muscle tone.

11. Assess the client's need for a respiratory therapist.

11. Trained personnel can substantially reduce the incidence and severity of atelectasis.

12. Position the client on his side without the aid of a pillow, with his head extended and tilted slightly downward.

12. Proper positioning can promote the drainage of secretions and, if vomiting should occur, vomitus. This position also maintains an open airway by keeping the client's tongue forward.

13. Assist the client to sit in a chair or to ambulate early after surgery.

13. Gas exchange improves when the client is seated upright or moving.

14. Encourage the client to stop smoking.

14. Smoking reduces the oxygen-carrying capacity of hemoglobin and depletes the oxygen supply needed for adequate gas exchange.

OUTCOME CRITERION
• The client will have no signs of impaired gas exchange as evidenced by normal breath sounds, effective coughing, and alertness.

Nursing diagnosis: *Fluid volume deficit related to abnormal fluid loss from surgery*

NURSING GOALS: To replace fluid volume and electrolytes and to maintain a positive fluid balance

Signs and symptoms
- hypotension
- elevated temperature
- oliguria
- muscle weakness
- tachycardia
- poor skin turgor
- dry skin and mucous membranes
- nausea and vomiting
- confusion
- elevated hematocrit level
- excessive wound drainage

Interventions

1. Assess the client's mental status, and notify the physician about any significant changes.

2. Monitor the client's vital signs, and notify the physician about any significant.

3. Monitor the client's oral fluid intake and output and his weight. Increase his fluid intake, if indicated.

4. Obtain hemoglobin and hematocrit levels, and notify the physician of any significant changes.

5. Obtain laboratory results on the client's electrolyte levels, and note any imbalances.

6. Assess the client's incision for bleeding or drainage, and monitor the output from all surgical tubes and catheters.

7. Assess the client's need for I.V. fluids or total parenteral nutrition (TPN).

8. Monitor the client's cardiac status, and administer medication, as ordered, to treat any dysrhythmias.

9. Assess the client's skin turgor to identify interstitial edema in dependent areas.

10. Consider the client's medical history when determining his fluid loss.

Rationales

1. Moderate fluid loss in the elderly client can affect mentation. The physician may order an I.V. infusion to correct any deficits.

2. Fluid loss can cause cardiac problems. The elderly client has a high risk for hypovolemia because of excess antidiuretic hormone and aldosterone caused by the stress of surgery and because the elderly client's cardiovascular system is not as compliant as that of a younger client.

3. Monitoring fluid intake and output and the client's weight is an accurate indication of fluid balance. Urine output helps to determine the degree of hydration. Oliguria almost always indicates hypovolemia in a postoperative client.

4. These values may reveal anemia resulting from intraoperative blood loss or bleeding at the surgical site.

5. Imbalances are most likely to occur when the kidney can no longer easily reabsorb or secrete electrolytes.

6. A moderate blood or fluid loss can create an electrolyte imbalance in an elderly client.

7. TPN can supply complete nutrition for an extended period.

8. Dysrhythmias can cause hypoxia, which can lead to multiorgan system failure.

9. Skin turgor indicates fluid balance; edema signifies an expanded extracellular volume.

10. Chronic medical problems, such as congestive heart failure, affect fluid shifting. The nurse should be aware that water retention and electrolyte imbalances can occur rapidly.

OUTCOME CRITERIA
- The client will maintain an adequate fluid intake.
- The client's electrolyte levels will remain within normal limits.

Nursing diagnosis: *Altered nutrition: less than body requirements, related to preoperative nutritional status and postoperative enteric rest*

NURSING GOAL: To meet the client's nutritional requirements

Signs and symptoms
• weight loss
• poor muscle tone
• pale conjunctiva and mucous membranes
• lack of interest in food
• anorexia

Interventions

1. Auscultate the client's bowel sounds, and palpate his abdomen.

2. Monitor the client's fluid intake and output, and weight. Also determine the client's calorie intake.

3. Modify the client's diet by increasing his protein, carbohydrate, and total calorie intake; offering small meals and snacks; providing nutritional supplements; administering vitamin and iron supplements; offering appetite stimulants, such as wine, if allowed; adding sauces, butter, cream, and oils to food and beverages if the client can tolerate fat.

4. Administer TPN or tube feedings, as ordered.

Rationales

1. These actions identify intestinal distention and help determine whether the client needs decompression and parenteral nutritional support.

2. These measures detect potential imbalances and accurately reflect the client's nutritional needs.

3. Nutritional rehabilitation decreases the incidence of wound infection and dehiscence. It also compensates for the catabolic effects of surgery and postoperative feeding difficulties. Proper healing requires appropriate protein intake.

4. TPN and tube feedings help the client meet his nutritional requirements when he cannot eat.

OUTCOME CRITERION
• The client will receive adequate nutritional intake through oral, enteric, or parenteral methods.

Nursing diagnosis: *Hypothermia related to surgery and fluid and blood loss*

NURSING GOALS: To maintain the client's body temperature during and after surgery and to minimize the risk of hypothermia

Signs and symptoms
• low core body temperature
• oxygen consumption changes (decreased PO_2)
• apathy
• listlessness
• slurred speech
• disorientation

Interventions

1. Increase the temperature to 80° F (26.7° C) in the operating room 30 minutes before bringing the client into the room.

Rationales

1. A low temperature increases the client's risk for hypothermia.

2. Cover the client with warm blankets before surgery.

2. The elderly client is at increased risk for hypothermia because of his decreased metabolism rate and normal low body temperature. Also, preoperative medications and anesthetic agents contribute to the risk.

3. Warm the prep solution before cleaning the surgical site.

3. Evaporation of antiseptic prep solutions can cause heat loss.

4. Cover the client with sterile drapes after cleaning the surgical site. Keep the client's head covered during surgery.

4. Covering the client with drapes helps preserve warmth; about 20% of all body heat loss occurs through the head.

5. Use a warm saline lavage to irrigate wounds, if not contraindicated.

5. A warmed solution prevents body heat loss from evaporation and radiation.

6. Cover the client with warm blankets or use a radiant heat lamp after transferring the client to the postanesthesia unit.

6. Warm blankets and a heat lamp help raise the client's core body temperature.

7. Monitor the client's temperature frequently during surgery and postoperatively.

7. Frequent temperature monitoring is essential because it may be the only indication of hypothermia. Certain anesthetics promote surface blood flow and depress central thermoregulatory structures. Skeletal muscle relaxants prevent shivering, which is normally an obvious sign of hypothermia.

8. Administer warmed I.V. fluids, blood products, and oxygen.

8. Warming these substances decreases the risk of body heat loss.

9. Place warm containers of saline solution near the client's groin or axilla, if necessary.

9. This technique provides additional heat to warm the hypothermic client.

10. Monitor the postoperative client's ECG if the client received a general anesthetic during surgery.

10. Hypothermia can cause cardiac irregularities.

11. Assess the client's need to remain in the postanesthesia unit.

11. The hypothermic client tends to absorb more of the anesthetic because of increased tissue solubility and a delayed emergence from anesthesia and may require more time in the postanesthesia unit.

OUTCOME CRITERION
• The client will be protected from hypothermia before, during, and after surgery.

Nursing diagnosis: *Altered thought processes related to a decreased level of consciousness from general anesthesia*

NURSING GOALS: To help the client return to his preoperative level of mental functioning and prevent self-inflicted injury

Signs and symptoms
• prolonged somnolence
• frequent changes in mental status (such as disorientation, confusion, and irritability)
• incoherence and restlessness
• alternating periods of alertness and disorientation

Interventions

1. Avoid administering long-acting sedatives, such as flurazepam hydrochloride or temazepam, preoperatively. If a sedative is necessary, administer a short-acting agent, such as oxazepam.

2. If the client is semiconscious or unarousable to verbal or external stimuli, continually assess the client's vital signs; properly position the client to promote airway clearance, prevent aspiration, and facilitate circulation; and frequently stimulate the client and encourage him to breathe deeply.

3. If the client is restless, agitated, or incoherent, attempt to calm him and and orient him to person, place, and time; prevent the client from harming himself; and determine the type of anesthetic and preoperative medications the client received.

4. Instruct the family of the client with Alzheimer's disease to have a private duty nurse or a family member remain with the client during the immediate postoperative phase.

5. Provide safety measures for the agitated or confused client.

Rationales

1. Long-acting sedatives contribute to postoperative disorientation and amnesia and hinder the recovery process. Short-acting agents do not potentiate the anesthesia or interfere with the administration of postoperative pain medications.

2. Prolonged somnolence can occur after prolonged use of a highly concentrated anesthetic or a combination of anesthetics. Use of lorazepam and diazepam significantly increases the client's sleep time. Positioning the client and stimulating him to breathe deeply can help prevent postoperative complications, such as pneumonia, infection, and aspiration.

3. The client is probably experiencing emergence delirium, a brief state of postanesthesia excitement in which the client experiences increased motor activity, disorientation, and incoherent vocalization.

4. This person can help orient the client when he awakens in an unfamiliar hospital environment.

5. The confused and disoriented client may injure himself or remove a nasogastric tube or I.V. line.

> **OUTCOME CRITERION**
> • The client will not suffer injury or trauma because of his altered mental status.

Nursing diagnosis: *Sensory-perceptual alteration: visual, related to cataract removal*

NURSING GOALS: To help the client readjust to a normal life-style after cataract surgery and to teach the client how to compensate for changes in visual acuity

Signs and symptoms
• distorted peripheral vision
• pear-shaped pupils
• increased intraocular pressure
• fine, white, half-moon cells in the lower anterior chamber
• clouding of the lens
• reduced vision

Interventions

1. Instruct the client about intracapsular and extracapsular cataract extraction. Explain that, in intracapsular cataract extraction, the physician uses cryoextraction to remove the opaque lens and capsule; this method involves applying a super-cooled metal probe to the lens, causing the cataract to adhere to the moist lens capsule, which allows for easy removal. Also explain that, in extracapsular cataract extraction, the physician uses phacoemulsification (ultrasound) if the lens is soft, or irrigation if the lens is hard, to remove the anterior lens capsule and cloudy lens; the posterior lens capsule remains to provide support for an intraocular lens, if necessary.

Rationales

1. About 70% of all elderly clients have some degree of cataract involvement. Senile cataracts are always bilateral; however, opacity is usually more advanced in one eye. The client should know that surgical removal of the cataract usually results in restored vision.

2. Teach the client to keep his affected eye dressed, patched, and covered with an eye shield for 1 month or longer after surgery.

3. Instruct the client to report any eye bulging or sharp eye pain during the first 5 postoperative days.

4. Instruct the client to avoid activities that increase intraocular pressure, such as vomiting, straining during defecation, or lifting heavy objects.

5. Discuss with the client the need for an intraocular lens, contact lenses, or eyeglasses.

2. An eye shield protects the client's eye from accidental injury or damage from contact with clothing and bed linens.

3. These signs indicate a hemorrhage into the anterior chamber of the eye or a wound rupture.

4. Increased intraocular pressure may rupture the suture line.

5. Because removal of the lens contents or capsule deprives the eye of focusing power, the client may need assistance in focusing. Insertion of an intraocular lens is most desirable because this device resembles a natural lens and provides the client with a full visual field. It is most useful in those over age 70; however, because this type of lens also acts as a foreign body in the eye, it may cause problems in several years. Hard or soft contact lenses help the eye to focus light rays and reestablish visual acuity by magnifying images by 8%. Extended-wear lenses may be preferred for the elderly client because they need to be removed only monthly. Eyeglasses, which magnify images by 30%, are the simplest, safest, and most common means of helping the client to focus. However, because they sit about ¾″ (2 cm) in front of the client's original lens, they typically cause difficulty with depth perception and peripheral vision.

OUTCOME CRITERIA
• The client will be free from complications, such as corneal edema or secondary glaucoma, after implantation of an artificial lens.
• The client will recover as close to normal vision as possible after cataract removal.

Nursing diagnosis: *Altered peripheral tissue perfusion related to vascular reconstruction*

NURSING GOAL: To maintain optimal perfusion to the client's legs

Signs and symptoms
• cold feet
• diminished or absent peripheral pulses
• mottled skin when legs are dependent, pale skin when legs are elevated
• burning pain in feet when warmed
• edema in affected leg
• tropic changes in legs

Interventions

1. Assess the client's legs for increasing edema; ulceration; gangrene; or changes in skin color, temperature, or texture (such as decreased temperature and dryness).

2. Assess the client's peripheral pulses (including the aortic, femoral, popliteal, dorsalis pedis, and posterior tibial), noting the force of each pulse. Also check for capillary refill and dependent changes. Notify the physician of signs of decreased perfusion.

Rationales

1. These signs signal vasoconstriction, impaired venous return, and decreased tissue perfusion.

2. Absent pulses or impaired peripheral circulation may indicate vasoconstriction, thrombus formation, or vessel disruption.

3. Ask the client whether he has pain, numbness, or tingling in his legs.

3. These signs reflect decreased tissue perfusion.

4. Keep the client's room warm while performing all leg assessments.

4. Cool temperatures cause vasoconstriction.

5. Care for the client's affected leg by keeping the leg in a nondependent position; bathing the leg in warm, not hot, water; changing the position of the limb at least every hour; avoiding the use of the bed's knee gatch; instructing the client to avoid crossing his legs at the knee or ankle; removing all constricting items, such as stockings; and instructing the client to avoid sitting for prolonged periods.

5. Keeping the client's legs in a nondependent position reduces pain and prevents further tissue damage. Bathing in warm water prevents the risk of injury from the inability to sense hot temperatures. Changing position hourly promotes venous return by decreasing vasoconstriction and augmenting tissue perfusion. Avoiding the use of a knee gatch or crossing the legs prevents a decreased blood supply to the client's legs. Avoiding tight clothing or leg garters prevents impeded blood flow. Avoiding prolonged sitting prevents venous stasis and interstitial edema, which would further compress the arteries.

6. Refer the client to a podiatrist for treatment of thickened nails or skin calluses.

6. Treatment will help prevent ulceration, infection, and trauma.

7. Encourage the client to stop smoking.

7. Smoking results in vasoconstriction of already compromised arteries.

OUTCOME CRITERIA
- The client will be free of leg pain, tissue damage, and infection.
- The client will maintain the highest level of physical function possible.

Nursing diagnosis: *Impaired tissue integrity related to leg amputation*

NURSING GOALS: To teach the client postoperative stump care and to help him initiate necessary lifestyle changes and adapt to the treatment regimen

Signs and symptoms
- above or below-the-knee amputation
- apprehension
- phantom limb pain

Interventions

1. In the evening, clean the client's stump with mild soap and warm water.

2. Teach the client who has edema in the stump to perform upward and downward motions; wrap the stump with an elastic bandage when not wearing the prosthesis; and elevate the stump (if a below-the-knee stump) when sitting.

3. Instruct the client with a below-the-knee amputation to keep the affected leg straight when sleeping. Instruct the client with an above-the-knee amputation to avoid prolonged sitting or hip bending while in bed and to sleep on his abdomen whenever possible.

4. Teach the client with phantom limb pain to apply pressure to the end of the stump, to try to wiggle the painful "toes," and to stretch both legs.

Rationales

1. Washing will remove the dirt and perspiration built up during the day.

2. Upward and downward exercises pump fluids back up the leg. Wrapping the stump acts as an external pump to control edema, promote wound healing, and maintain the proper shape of the stump. Elevating the stump prevents further edema.

3. These measures inhibit the development of hip or knee contractures.

4. Phantom limb sensation or pain, feelings in the part of the leg that has been amputated, frequently occurs after an amputation. Applying pressure and exercising the limb may alter phantom limb sensations.

5. Instruct the client to wear a cotton sock on his stump whenever he wears his prosthesis.

5. Stump socks provide extra padding and help prevent trauma to the affected leg.

6. Promote and encourage early ambulation, as soon as possible after the amputation.

6. Early ambulation prevents flexion contractures and disuse atrophy. The client with a below-the-knee amputations can walk and bear weight early. Weight bearing before the stump has healed can weaken and rupture the suture line.

7. Recommend the use of a walker or cane if the limb loss causes the client to experience difficulties with perception and balance. Advise the client to install a raised toilet seat, grab bars, and a shower stool at home.

7. These measures promote ambulation and prevent falls that can lead to skin lacerations and tears.

OUTCOME CRITERIA
• The client with an above-the-knee amputation will not develop a hip contracture.
• The client with a below-the-knee amputation will not develop a knee contracture.
• The client will have no evidence of stump edema.

Nursing diagnosis: *Impaired physical mobility related to joint replacement, postoperative activity intolerance, and pain*

NURSING GOALS: To prevent falls or other trauma, to maintain the client's optimal function and mobility, and to encourage ambulation with limited assistance

Signs and symptoms
• impaired coordination
• limited range of motion
• decreased endurance
• improper body alignment
• verbalization of pain and fatigue
• decreased activity
• exertional dyspnea or discomfort

Interventions

1. Assess and maintain the client's skin integrity.

2. Maintain the client's body in proper alignment postoperatively.

3. Encourage the client to perform active and passive range-of-motion exercises.

4. Progressively increase the client's activities, allowing for rest periods.

5. Administer pain medications, as needed. Encourage the client to ask for medication when he attempts to increase activity.

6. Encourage the client to start ambulating by the second or third postoperative day, if possible.

Rationales

1. Immobility can impair the elderly client's skin integrity by causing pressure sores and skin breakdown.

2. Proper alignment prevents deformities and injuries that can cause immobility.

3. Muscle wasting accelerates with prolonged bed rest.

4. Increased activity promotes ambulation, thus preventing immobility. Rest periods help conserve the client's energy and reduce fatigue.

5. Pain medication helps to ease the discomfort associated with postoperative activity. Administering medication when the client tries to increase activities enables him to tolerate movement better.

6. Early ambulation stimulates deep breathing and increases the client's lung capacity by 15% to 20%. It also helps prevent pressure sores, venous thrombi, and pulmonary complications associated with immobility.

OUTCOME CRITERIA
• The client will ambulate with limited assistance.
• The client will not fall or suffer other trauma.
• The client will practice measures to conserve energy and decrease fatigue.

Nursing diagnosis: *Altered patterns of urinary elimination related to postoperative immobility*

NURSING GOALS: To eliminate unnecessary episodes of urinary incontinence, to restore bladder function, and to decrease dependency on caregivers

Signs and symptoms
• urinary frequency and urgency
• urinary incontinence
• frequent falls
• use of an indwelling urinary catheter

Interventions

1. Review the client's preoperative voiding pattern, and assess for postoperative changes.

2. Place a bedpan, urinal, and nursing call bell within the client's reach.

3. If the client cannot ambulate, keep the bed side rails lowered; place a commode next to the client's bed at night; install a night light, or leave the bathroom light on; and avoid using sedatives and restraints.

4. Remove the client's catheter as soon as possible, and institue a bladder retraining program (see "Urinary Incontinence," pages 128 to 137).

5. Avoid leaving the catheter in until the day of discharge.

Rationales

1. An assessment enables the nurse to initiate an appropriate bladder retraining program.

2. Placing a bedpan and urinal near the client's bedside allows the client to urinate independently. Keeping a call bell within easy reach enables the client to ask for assistance to the bathroom and prevents falls.

3. Instituting these measures should help the client function independently. Restraints and diminished lighting increase the client's risk for falling.

4. The elderly client requires bladder retraining after catheterization because of lost tonicity and bladder capacity. Instituting a program promptly usually is less traumatic to the client.

5. Removing a catheter on the day of discharge does not allow the time needed to identify a voiding dysfunction or to institute a bladder retraining program.

OUTCOME CRITERIA
• The client will return to a preoperative voiding pattern.
• The client will be discharged from the hospital without an indwelling catheter.

Nursing diagnosis: *Anxiety related to the incision and results of surgery*

NURSING GOAL: To help the client overcome his anxiety and recognize his limitations and capabilities

Signs and symptoms
• missing body part
• ignoring affected body part
• preoccupation with loss
• fear of rejection
• negative self-image
• focusing on past strengths, function, and appearance
• feelings of helplessness, hopelessness, or powerlessness

Interventions

1. Encourage the client to express his concerns and anxieties about surgery and about his postoperative condition.

2. Provide the client with opportunities to interact with others.

3. Avoid administering medications, such as narcotics, anticholinergics, or barbiturates, for preoperative anxiety.

4. When changing the client's dressing, inform the client of the wound's appearance of the wound and allow him to look at it.

5. Refer the client to appropriate support groups, as indicated.

Rationales

1. Verbalization decreases the client's anxieties and fears and provides the nurse with the opportunity to correct any misconceptions.

2. Social interaction helps the client to remain oriented to person, time, and place and helps the client meet his socialization needs.

3. The elderly client is sensitive to the central nervous system and opthalmic effects of these drugs, which can cause postoperative complications, such as pneumonia, delirium, and vision loss.

4. This allows the client perceive himself accurately.

5. Support groups allow the client to socialize with others who have similar conditions.

OUTCOME CRITERIA
• The client will verbalize his concerns about the planned surgery.
• The client will accept postoperative changes.

Nursing diagnosis: *Knowledge deficit related to planned surgery*

NURSING GOALS: To educate the client and the client's family about the planned surgery and to alleviate the client's anxiety

Signs and symptoms
• request for information about the surgery
• inappropriate or exaggerated behaviors (such as hostility and aggression)
• insomnia
• facial tension

Interventions

1. Assess the client's mental status and ability to provide informed consent.

2. Assess the client for hearing and vision changes, slowed reaction time, slowed learning, decreased short-term memory, and the impact of illness on his life.

3. Assess the client's and family's understanding of the disease and impending surgery.

Rationales

1. An assessment provides information about the client's ability to understand, interpret, and retain information. Regardless of age, no one is authorized to give consent for an elderly client unless the client has been declared incompetent and has been appointed a legal guardian.

2. Normal aging can alter the client's understanding of teaching regarding the consent form and impending surgery.

3. Such assessment establishes a basis on which the nurse can begin teaching. Determining the client's and family's understanding of the postoperative phase helps to determine their anticipated need for support systems and rehabilitative services.

4. Identify the expected results from the planned surgery. Inform the client that recovery usually occurs within 4 to 6 months.

4. Anxiety over the impending surgery may decrease the client's perception of how long recovery should take.

5. Allow the client to express his feelings, attitudes, and beliefs about life.

5. Verbalization allows the client to recognize and begin to resolve his fears. The client who wishes to die or who sees little purpose in life is a poor surgical risk.

6. Explain the procedure to the client and family, using visual aids, if available.

6. Accurate information relieves the client's and family's anxieties and fears about the surgical procedure.

7. Review the expected postoperative course with the client, such as coughing and deep breathing and the need for pain relief.

7. Informing the client of expected events beforehand helps with compliance during the postoperative period.

OUTCOME CRITERION
• The client and family will understand the surgery and the expected postoperative course.

NURSING ACTIONS IN VARIOUS SETTINGS
Nursing actions for a client undergoing surgery depend on the setting in which care is provided. This section identifies which actions are appropriate in all settings and which pertain to acute care, extended care, or home care situations.

All settings
• Reinforce postoperative teaching with the client and his family or caregiver.
• Determine the client's need for assistance. Remember that elderly clients may not be receptive to major life changes and may not ask for help because of the fear of threatened independence.
• Prepare the client for the temporary need for nursing care at home.

Acute care
• Refer the client to a social worker before discharge to determine the programs and resources available to the client.
• Assess the client's need for physical therapy or medical follow-up.
• Evaluate the client for placement in an extended care or rehabilitation facility after discharge.
• Arrange for a home health nurse to visit the client regularly until the client's condition stabilizes.

Extended care
• Assess the client's level of rehabilitation, and determine whether he needs continued physical or occupational therapy.
• Help the client learn as much as possible to allow him to achieve an optimal level of self-care and independence.
• Manage the client's pain, as necessary, to facilitate cooperation with therapy and rehabilitation.
• Help the client to incorporate disease management into his activities of daily living.

Home care
• Assess the client's home for the location of stairs and accessibility of the kitchen and bathroom. Determine whether the client's home can be easily adapted to accommodate his mobility problems.
• Determine the client's ability to live alone and care for himself.
• Determine the availability of family members or neighbors to help.
• Assess the client's need for such services as physical therapy, occupational therapy, homemakers, or Meals On Wheels.

SELECTED REFERENCES
Burden, N. "Regional Anesthesia: What Patients and Nurses Need to Know," *RN* 51(5):56-62, May 1988.

Burkle, N.L. "Inadvertent Hypothermia," Journal of *Gerontological Nursing* 14(6):26-30, 1988.

Dean, A. "The Aging Surgical Patient: Historical Overview, Implications and Nursing Care," *Perioperative Nursing Quarterly* 3(1):1-7, March 1987.

Fraulini, K.E. "Guide to Solving Post-Anesthesia Problems," *Nursing88* 18(5):66,69-76,78,81-86, May 1988.

Galazka, S.S. "Pre-operative Evaluation of the Elderly Surgical Patient," *Journal of Family Practice* 27(6):622-32, June 1988.

Jackson, M. "High Risk Surgical Patients," *Today's O.R. Nurse* 10(2):26-33, February 1988.

Kupferer, S., et al. "Geriatric Ambulatory Surgery Patients: Assessing Cognitive Function," *AORN Journal* 47(3):752-64, August 1987.

Latz, P.A., and Wyble, S.J. "Elderly Patients, Perioperative Nursing Implications," *AORN Journal* 46(2):238-53, August 1987.

Lubin, M.F. *Medical Management of the Surgical Patient.* Boston: Butterworths, 1988.

Miller, R.A., and Evans, W.E. "Nurse and Patient: Allies Preventing Amputation," *RN* 51(7):38-42, July 1988.

Omerod, B. "Perioperative Nursing Care of the Elderly Outpatient," *Perioperative Nursing Quarterly* 3(2):22-26, June 1987.

Waugaman, W.R. "Surgery and the Patient with Alzheimer's Disease," *Geriatric Nursing* 4:227-29, July/August 1988.

Hypothermia

Hypothermia refers to the state in which an individual's core body temperature drops below the normal range, typically below 96.8° F (36° C) rectally. Normal body temperatures usually range from 98.6° to 100.4° F (36° to 38° C), depending on the individual's age, sex, activity level, state of health, and basal metabolic rate as well as on the environment and time of day.

Because elderly clients cannot easily adjust to extremes in environmental temperature, they are at high risk for hypothermia. The types of hypothermia include acute, or accidental, hypothermia (which occurs from exposure to cold); senile hypothermia, or relative poikilothermia (which occurs from impaired hypothalamic and autonomic functioning); and functional hypothermia (which occurs from an inability to compensate for heat loss).

Hypothermia can be classified according to the degree of core body temperature. For example, mild hypothermia refers to a core body temperature of 89.6° to 95° F (32° to 35° C); moderate hypothermia, a core body temperature of 86° to 89.5° F (30° to 32° C); and severe hypothermia, a core body temperature below 86° F (30° C).

Clients with severe hypothermia have a mortality rate of greater than 50%, the rate increasing with age or underlying disease.

ETIOLOGY

Certain physiologic changes associated with aging predispose the elderly client to hypothermia. These include a diminished amount of active tissue mass per unit of body surface area; decreased capacity for activity; thinned skin and decreased subcutaneous fat, which reduces the insulating power of the integumentary system; atrophied sweat glands, which reduce the body's ability to sweat; and decreased skin circulation, especially in the arms and legs, which occurs as a compensatory response to reduced cardiac output.

Physiologic factors that contribute to the elderly client's inability to maintain normal body heat include a reduced basal metabolic rate, an impaired shiver response, an impaired ability to discern temperature fluctuations quickly, and a diminished sensation of cold.

Hypothermia in the elderly client can also be precipitated by cold exposure, illness or trauma, malnutrition, inappropriate dress for cold weather, consumption of alcohol or medications that cause vasodilation, evaporation of water from the skin in a cool environment, and inactivity. It occurs most commonly in those of lower economic standing.

HEALTH HISTORY FINDINGS

In a health history interview, the client may report or the nurse may detect many of these findings:
- chronic cough
- decreased muscle bulk and strength
- immobility
- chest pain or palpitations
- vertigo
- weakness or fatigue
- complaints of feeling cold
- history of recurrent upper respiratory infections or septicemia
- recent acute illness
- history of hypothermia
- history of bronchopneumonia or pulmonary embolism
- history of congestive heart failure, myocardial infarction, or peripheral vascular disease
- history of myxedema, hypoglycemia, or diabetic ketoacidosis
- recent general surgery
- use of phenothiazines, barbiturates, diazepam, or thioridazine hydrochloride
- history of malnutrition and vitamin deficiencies
- consumption of alcohol, caffeine, and tobacco
- lack of environmental heat

PHYSICAL FINDINGS

In a physical examination, the nurse may detect many of these findings:

Integumentary
- shivering (early sign)
- pale, ashen, or waxy appearance
- cool skin in exposed and unexposed areas
- cyanosis (late sign)

Respiratory
- dyspnea
- hypoventilation
- increased respirations with apneustic episodes

Cardiovascular
- dysrhythmias
- chest pain
- hypotension
- bradycardia (late sign)

Gastrointestinal
- decreased bowel sounds
- cold, marblelike skin over the abdomen

Genitourinary
• polyuria or oliguria (late sign)

Musculoskeletal
• slowed gait (early sign)
• muscle rigidity (late sign)

Neurologic
• slurred speech (early sign)
• confusion (early sign)
• cranial nerve deficits
• involuntary flapping tremors in the arms and legs
• decreased pupillary responses (late sign)
• coma (late sign)

Psychological
• disorientation
• hallucinations

Other
• fatigue and weakness (early sign)
• rectal temperature below 95° F (35° C)
• facial puffiness resembling myxedema

DIAGNOSTIC STUDIES
The following studies may be performed to evaluate the client's health status:

• blood studies (including serum glucose levels; thiamine levels; hepatic function studies; serum blood urea nitrogen (BUN), creatinine, and electrolyte levels; thyroid function studies; basal metabolic rate; complete blood count (CBC) and platelet count; and serum calcium levels)—to determine the metabolic causes of hypothermia; all reveal abnormal levels
• urinalysis—to indicate urine specific gravity; value is abnormal in hypothermia
• blood cultures—to identify bacteria and possibly septicemia; results may be positive
• electrocardiogram (ECG)—to identify bradycardia, atrial or ventricular fibrillation, premature ventricular contractions, or a prolonged PR interval and QT segment and a widened QRS complex
• chest X-ray—to reveal pneumonia
• magnetic resonance imaging (MRI) or computed tomography (CT) scans—to rule out diseases that may be causing the hypothermia

POTENTIAL COMPLICATIONS
• bronchopneumonia
• cardiac arrest
• acute renal failure
• pulmonary edema
• coma

Nursing diagnosis: *Ineffective thermoregulation related to lowered body temperature*

NURSING GOALS: To increase the client's core body temperature and to prevent further complications of hypothermia

Signs and symptoms
• rectal temperature lower than 95° F (35° C)
• decreased pulse rate, respiratory rate, and blood pressure
• sluggish pupillary responses
• dysarthria
• hyperreflexia
• ataxia
• inability to shiver
• clouded consciousness
• slurred speech
• muscle rigidity
• facial puffiness
• cool abdominal skin
• mottled skin

Interventions

1. Warm the client slowly using heat generated by his own body. Methods include placing the client in a room warmed to 80° F (26.7° C); covering the client with blankets or warm, nonconstricting clothing; giving the client warm beverages, foods, or I.V. fluids; and performing passive range-of-motion exercises.

2. Check the client's rectal temperature hourly.

Rationales

1. Rewarming slowly reduces the risk of a sudden loss of high vasomotor tone, which could result in vasomotor collapse, decreased blood pressure, and a further drop in core body temperature.

2. The client's body should warm gradually at a rate of 1° F (0.5° C) per hour.

3. Avoid using techniques that cause rapid external rewarming, such as electric blankets, hot water bottles, or immersion in hot water.

3. Rapid external rewarming produces rapid cutaneous vasodilation.

4. Avoid using cardioversion or drug therapy to correct any cardiac dysrhythmias.

4. Hypothermia reduces the client's metabolic rate, which makes the body resistant to cardioversion and drug therapy.

5. Transfer the client to an intensive care unit; obtain arterial blood gas measurements if his temperature falls below 86° F (30° C).

5. Intensive care provides immediate support; blood gas measurements help to evaluate the client's respiratory function.

OUTCOME CRITERION
• The client's rectal temperature will increase to 96.8° F (36° C) within 12 to 24 hours.

Nursing diagnosis: *Knowledge deficit related hypothermic condition*

NURSING GOAL: To educate the client and the client's family or caregiver about the causes and prevention of hypothermia

Signs and symptoms
• cold, drafty living environment
• inadequate knowledge about hypothermia
• sedentary life-style
• inappropriate dress for cold weather
• evidence of poor nutrition
• lack of mobility

Interventions

1. Teach the client and caregiver about the dangers, causes, symptoms, treatment, and prevention of hypothermia.

2. Advise the client to avoid smoking tobacco and drinking caffeine-containing beverages.

3. Advise the client to avoid consuming alcoholic beverages during hypothermic periods.

4. Instruct the client to retain body heat by wearing appropriate clothing that covers the head and fits snugly around the neck, wrists, and ankles; wearing several layers of lightweight clothing; using several layers of bedding rather than one heavy layer; immediately changing any damp or wet clothing; winterizing the client's home; performing some type of physical activity, such as isometric exercises; and eating a diet high in protein, minerals, and vitamins.

Rationales

1. Knowledge about hypothermia should help prevent its occurrence or recurrence.

2. These behaviors reduce the flow of warm blood to the hands and feet, which can cause a drop in skin temperature of 7° to 8° F (3.5° to 4° C).

3. Alcohol causes gastric and peripheral dilation, which increases heat loss.

4. The elderly client requires more clothing, especially around the extremities, because of his reduced skin circulation. Dry clothing provides needed warmth, especially in cold weather. Adequate insulation keeps cold air out of the home. Exercise increases peripheral blood circulation. Adequate nutrition maintains body metabolism and prevents a drop in core body temperature.

OUTCOME CRITERIA
• The client will wear appropriate clothing to prevent hypothermia.
• The client will identify environmental factors that can contribute to hypothermia.

NURSING ACTIONS IN VARIOUS SETTINGS

Nursing actions for a client with hypothermia depend on the setting in which care is provided. This section identifies which actions are appropriate in all settings and which pertain to acute care, extended care, or home care situations.

All settings
• Teach the client and caregiver the signs and symptoms of hypothermia.

Acute care
• Monitor the client's rectal temperature hourly.
• Initiate measures to prevent heat loss during the client's admission assessment.
• Upon admission, determine the precipitating factors of the hypothermia.
• Upon discharge, assess the client's living environment for possible causes of hypothermia.

Extended care
• Check the client's rectal temperature monthly.
• Maintain environmental temperatures at 78° F (25.6° C).
• Identify clients at risk for hypothermia.
• Alert the physician when signs of hypothermia occur.
• Provide adequate nutrition and fluids.
• Monitor the client's medication use for possible causes of hypothermia.

Home care
• Evaluate the client's bed coverings and clothes. If the client needs additional clothes or blankets, contact local thrift shops and such organizations as Goodwill and the Salvation Army.
• Contact social services for supplemental assistance for food, clothing, and utilities. Fuel-assistance programs can provide funds for fuel.
• Assess the client's home for air leaks, and plug them with newspapers or cover them with plastic.
• Arrange for the client's family or friends to check in on the client daily during cold weather.
• Instruct the client to check his room temperature daily using a thermometer separate from the thermostat.

SELECTED REFERENCES

Avery, C., and Pestle, R. "Hypothermia and the Elderly: Perceptions and Behaviors," *The Gerontologist* 27(4):523-26, April 1987.

Burkle, N.L. "Inadvertent Hypothermia," *Journal of Gerontological Nursing* 14(6):26-30, June 1988.

Calkins, E., et al. *The Practice of Geriatrics.* Philadelphia: W.B. Saunders Co., 1986.

Christ, M.A., and Hohloch, F. *Gerontological Nursing.* Springhouse, Pa.: Springhouse Corp., 1988.

Matteson, M.A., and McConnell, E.S. *Gerontological Nursing.* Philadelphia: W.B. Saunders Co., 1988.

Rossman, I. *Clinical Geriatrics,* 3rd ed. Philadelphia: J.B. Lippincott Co., 1986.

Slotman, G.J., et al. "Adverse Effects of Hypothermia in Postoperative Patients," *American Journal of Surgery* 149:495-501, April 1985.

APPENDIX AND INDEX

NANDA Taxonomy of Nursing Diagnoses

A taxonomy for discussing nursing diagnoses has evolved over several years. The following list contains the approved diagnostic labels of the North American Nursing Diagnosis Association (NANDA), as of summer 1988.

A
Activity intolerance
Activity intolerance, potential
Adjustment, impaired
Airway clearance, ineffective
Anxiety
Aspiration, potential for

B
Body image disturbance
Body temperature, potential altered
Breast-feeding, ineffective
Breathing pattern, ineffective

C
Cardiac output, decreased
Communication, impaired verbal
Constipation
Constipation, colonic
Constipation, perceived
Coping, defensive
Coping, family: potential for growth
Coping, ineffective family: compromised
Coping, ineffective family: disabling
Coping, ineffective individual

DE
Decisional conflict (specify)
Denial, ineffective
Diarrhea
Disuse syndrome, potential for
Diversional activity deficit
Dysreflexia

F
Family processes, altered
Fatigue
Fear
Fluid volume deficit (1)
Fluid volume deficit (2)
Fluid volume deficit, potential
Fluid volume excess

G
Gas exchange, impaired
Grieving, anticipatory
Grieving, dysfunctional
Growth and development, altered

H
Health maintenance, altered
Health seeking behaviors (specify)
Home maintenance management, impaired
Hopelessness
Hyperthermia
Hypothermia

IJ
Incontinence, bowel
Incontinence, functional
Incontinence, reflex
Incontinence, stress
Incontinence, total
Incontinence, urge
Infection, potential for
Injury, potential for

KLM
Knowledge deficit (specify)

N
Noncompliance (specify)
Nutrition, altered: less than body requirements
Nutrition, altered: more than body requirements
Nutrition, altered: potential for more than body requirements

O
Oral mucous membrane, altered

PQ
Pain
Pain, chronic
Parental role conflict
Parenting, altered
Parenting, potential altered
Personal identity disturbance
Physical mobility, impaired
Poisoning, potential for
Post-trauma response
Powerlessness

R
Rape-trauma syndrome
Rape-trauma syndrome: compound reaction
Rape-trauma syndrome: silent reaction
Role performance, altered

S
Self-care deficit, bathing/hygiene
Self-care deficit, dressing/grooming
Self-care deficit, feeding
Self-care deficit, toileting
Self-esteem, chronic low
Self-esteem disturbance
Self-esteem, situational low
Sensory/perceptual alterations (specify: visual, auditory, kinesthetic, gustatory, tactile, olfactory)
Sexual dysfunction
Sexuality patterns, altered
Skin integrity, impaired
Skin integrity, potential impaired
Sleep pattern disturbance

(continued)

NANDA Taxonomy of Nursing Diagnoses *(continued)*

Social interaction, impaired
Social isolation
Spiritual distress (distress of the human spirit)
Suffocation, potential for
Swallowing, impaired

T

Thermoregulation, ineffective
Thought processes, altered
Tissue integrity, impaired
Tissue perfusion, altered (specify type: renal, cerebral,
  cardiopulmonary, gastrointestinal, peripheral)
Trauma, potential for

U

Unilateral neglect
Urinary elimination, altered patterns of
Urinary retention

VWXYZ

Violence, potential for: self-directed or directed at others

Index

Notes

Notes

Notes

Notes

Notes

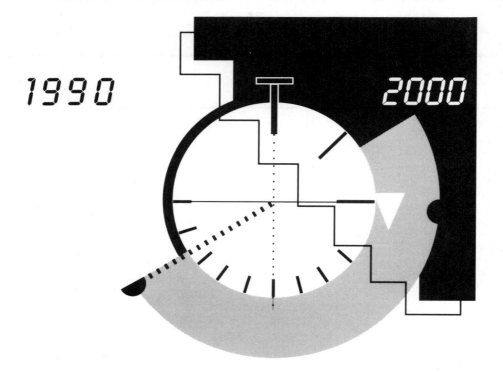